Handbook of Dermatology

Handbook of Dermatology
A Practical Manual

SECOND EDITION

Margaret W. Mann, MD

Associate Professor and Director of Aesthetic Dermatology
University Hospitals, Case Western School of Medicine
Cleveland, OH, USA

Co-Founder
Innova Dermatology
Hendersonville, TN, USA

Daniel L. Popkin, MD PhD

Assistant Chief of Dermatology, Louis Stokes VA Medical Center
Assistant Professor of Dermatology
University Hospitals, Case Western School of Medicine
Cleveland, OH, USA

Co-Founder
Innova Dermatology
Hendersonville, TN, USA

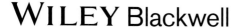

WILEY Blackwell

Dedication

This second edition is dedicated to our son Samuel. Without you, completing this second edition would have been so much faster and less fun.

Contents

Part 3 Drugs and Therapies, 293

Color plate section can be found facing page 206

Preface

Welcome to the second edition of *The Handbook of Dermatology: A Practical Manual*, a pocket guide designed for practicing dermatologists, dermatology residents, medical students, nurses, health care providers, and physicians in other fields who may be interested in dermatology.

New to second edition: We appreciate thoughtful feedback from our readers resulting in extensive revisions including the following: Part 1 sections were reorganized so that information could be found more quickly and intuitively; many sections were added including Workup Quick Reference Table, Melasma Workup and Management Algorithm, Propranolol, Contact Dermatitis, and Dermatologic Signs and Dermoscopy; all sections were updated to reflect new gene discoveries and other interval advancements. Part 2 includes updated fillers and toxins, UV and sunscreen updates, peeling agents, and a venous disease section. In Part 3, Drugs and Therapies was extensively updated.

Our first edition was created and edited by graduating residents at Washington University School of Medicine, Division of Dermatology. Our handbook started as an in-house resident handbook. Our goal was to compile and consolidate need-to-know dermatologic information for daily use in both patient care and resident and fellow education. As such, it represents the indispensable pocket-sized quick reference which we had wanted during our training and which we now use in our practices.

Currently, there are multiple in-depth dermatology textbooks and atlases, most of which are too bulky to be carried around in the clinic. Our manual concisely presents data in outline, bullet-point, and table formats such that information is manageable and easily retrievable. The compact design is lightweight, allowing information to be accessible in seconds during clinics, facilitating patient care. We have tried to balance space limitations with the need to cover a subject in sufficient detail.

Our manual has three main sections – medical dermatology, surgical dermatology, and pharmacology/treatment. Each section is designed to give the reader concise information for patient care. The content is up-to-date, comprehensive yet succinct. In addition to core material, we sought to consolidate the information which we found ourselves most often looking up, which our attendings most often quizzed us on, and which were most emphasized on the dermatology board exam. The manual consolidates the essential algorithms, protocols, guidelines, staging, and scoring systems of dermatology. Each section is designed for easy reference, with tabular and graphic information throughout. The diseases covered are those which we most often encountered in clinic, on call, during morning conferences, and on board exams.

We hope you will find this manual helpful to you in providing care to your patients. We welcome your input as this manual continues to evolve.

Acknowledgments

We thank Michael McBride for his assistance in updating Part 1 General Dermatology sections and Part 3 Drugs and Therapies.

Special thanks to Drs. David Berk and Susan Bayliss, who helped make the first edition possible; without you, this book would never have happened. Finally, we wish to thank the many people who have inspired us to write this book and supported us in our careers–our mentors, our colleagues and especially the residents and students we have had the pleasure of working with–for this book is written for you.

Part 1
General Dermatology

Handbook of Dermatology: A Practical Manual, Second Edition.
Margaret W. Mann and Daniel L. Popkin.
© 2020 John Wiley & Sons Ltd. Published 2020 by John Wiley & Sons Ltd.

COMMON WORK-UPS, SIGNS, AND MANAGEMENT

Dermatologic Differential Algorithm

Courtesy of Dr. Neel Patel

1. Is it a rash or growth?
2. If it is a rash, is it mainly epidermal, dermal, subcutaneous, or a combination?
3. If the rash is epidermal or a combination, try to define the characteristics of the rash. Is it mainly papulosquamous? Papulopustular? Blistering?
   After defining the characteristics, then think about causes of that type of rash: CITES MVA PITA:
   Congenital, **I**nfections, **T**umor, **E**ndocrinologic, **S**olar related, **M**etabolic, **V**ascular, **A**llergic, **P**sychiatric, **I**atrogenic, **T**rauma, **A**utoimmune. When generating the differential, take the history and location of the rash into account.
4. If the rash is dermal or subcutaneous, then think of cells and substances that infiltrate and associated diseases (histiocytes, lymphocytes, mast cells, neutrophils, metastatic tumors, mucin, amyloid, immunoglobulin, etc.).
5. If the lesion is a growth, is it benign or malignant in appearance? Think of cells in the skin and their associated diseases (keratinocytes, fibroblasts, neurons, adipocytes, melanocytes, histiocytes, pericytes, endothelial cells, smooth muscle cells, follicular cells, sebocytes, eccrine cells, apocrine cells, etc.).

Direct Immunofluorescence (Dif)

Diseases	Where to biopsy
LE, MCTD, PCT, LP, vasculitis	Erythematous border of active lesion/involved skin (avoid old lesions, facial lesions, and ulcers)
Pemphigus group, pemphigoid group, linear IgA	Erythematous perilesional skin (avoid bullae, ulcers, and erosions)
DH	Normal-looking perilesional skin (0.5–1 cm away)
Lupus band	Uninvolved, non-photoexposed skin (buttock)

Source: http://www.mayoclinic.org/dermatology-rst/immunofaqs.html

False positive/negative DIFs:
False negative in BP: (i) low yield of biopsy on distal extremity (esp. legs) (controversial) and (ii) predominantly IgG4 subclass of auto-antibody (poorly recognized on DIF)

False positive in LE: chronically sun-exposed skin of young adults

To increase DIF yield: transport in saline (reduces dermal background) – cannot do DIF on formalin-fixed specimen

Workup Quick Reference Orders (guided by clinical presentation)

Acanthosis nigricans	CBC/CMP, lipid panel, HgA1C, TSH, CEA, LH/FSH
Alopecia (see "Alopecia Workup, p. 6–9 for further details)	CBC/CMP, Fe/TIBC/Ferritin, TSH, free and total testosterone, 17-OH progesterone, VDRL,FSH, LH, DHEA-S, ANA, ESR, prolactin, Vitamin D
Anetoderma	CBC, ANA, anti-dsDNA, anti-SSA/B, TSH, RPR, Lyme titer, HIV, fasting AM cortisol, C3/C4/CH50, protein C/S, anti-thrombin III, anti-cardiolipin abs, lupus anticoagulant, B2-glycoprotein
Angioedema	CBC, C1 est inhib, C1,C2,C4
	Hereditary: C1-nl; C2,C4,C1 est inhib- ↓ (C1-INH levels may be nl but nonfunctional)
	Acquired: C1-↓; C2,C4,C1 est inhib- ↓
CTCL	CBC with peripheral smear (Sezary Prep), AST/ALT, LDH, CXR, HIV, HTLV-1, CD4/8 flow cytometry (CD5, CD7, CD45RO, CD26: CTCL protocol)
Dermatitis herpetiformis	anti TTG-IgG, IgA > endomysial ab, anti-Gliadin ab (IgG and IgA), total IgA, CBC, CMP, Vitamin D
Dermatomyositis	*Antisynthetase panel:* (Anti-Jo-1 PL-7, EJ, OJ PL-12), anti-Mi-2, CK, aldolase, LDH, CRP, anti-SRP PFTs, anti-aminoacyl-tRNA synthetases (interstitial lung disease (ILD) association), anti P-155 (cancer association), anti-CADM (ILD association), anti-MDA5 (RA-like associations)
Flushing	24-hour urine 5-HIAA and metanephrines, norepinephrine, VMA, prostaglandin D2, dopamine, tryptase, histamine, plasma VIP, UA, serotonin, calcitonin (if thyroid nodule)
Hypercoagulability and thrombogenic vasculopathy	ANA, protein C/S, lupus anticoagulant, anti-phospholipid ab, β2 glycoprotein ab, anti-cardiolipin, hepatitis B/C, SPEP/UPEP, Factor V Leiden, prothrombin gene mutation, homocysteine level, MTHFR gene mutation
Hyperhidrosis (diffuse/sudden)	CBC, HbA1c, cortisol, TSH, GH, serotonin, urine 5-HIAA, urine 24-hour catecholamines
LCV	ROS neg: CBC, CMP, UA, ANA, HBV/HCV, Skin Bx +/- DIF
	ROS pos: add ANCA, Cryo, ASO, HBV, ESR, RF, Complement, age-appropriate cancer screening
MCTD	Anti-U1RNP, anti-Ku, ANA, RF, CRP
PCOS	Total and free testosterone, DHEA-S, LH/FSH, sex hormone-binding globulin, β-HCG

PCT/ pseudoporphyria	HCV, Fe, 24-hour urine porphyrins *(Uro:copro> 8:1)*, CBC, LFT, lead levels, quantitative plasma porphyrins, stool porphyrins
Photosensitivity	ANA, ENA (SSa/b)
Pruritus	CBC/CMP, LFTs, TSH, bilirubin, CXR, UA, hepatitis B/C, peripheral blood smear, Fe, β-HCG, ESR, HIV
	SPEP/UPEP, stool ova and parasite, age-appropriate cancer screening
Purpura	CBC w/ peripheral smear, CMP, TSH, ANA, PT/PTT, bleeding time, c-ANCA, p-ANCA, SPEP/UPEP, cryoglobulins, vitamin K level, D-dimer
Pyoderma gangrenosum	CBC/CMP, UA, peripheral smear, ANA, RF, SPEP/UPEP, ANCA, antiphospholipid ab, RF, colonoscopy, Hep B/C
Recurrent furunculosis/ carbunculosis	Skin culture w/ gram stain, CMP, blood glucose, HIV, hepatitis B/C, CH50, peripheral smear, SPEP, IgG/IgM/IgE, nitroblue tetrazolium (if concern for CGD)
Sarcoidosis	CBC, CMP, Ca+, Serum ACE level, 1,25 Vit D, PTH, Alk Phos, ESR, ANA, CXR, QuantiFERON Gold
Scleroderma/CREST syndrome	Anti-Scl-70, ANA, anti-Jo-1, anti-centromere, RNA, polymerase I/III, RF, esophageal motility, PFTs, BUN/creatinine
Sjogren's syndrome	ANA, anti-Ro/La, CRP, RF, anti-alpha-fodrin ab
Syphilis	RPR/VDRL – primary; FTA-ABS – secondary
SLE	CBC/CMP, ANA, anti-smith, dsDNA, UA, BUN/ creatinine, ESR, ENA panel, C3/C4/CH50
TEN	Check for IgA deficiency if Tx = IVIG as GammaGard needed (IgA depleted):
	IVIG 2–4 g/kg (total dose, divided over 2–5 d, see TEN protocol pg. 227
Urticaria	CBC, IgE, anti-FcεRI (CUI), sinus X-ray, hepatitis B/C, TSH, anti-TPO, anti-thyroglobulin, *H. pylori*, cryoglobulins
	In children often due to strep: Check ASO, Rapid Strep
Urticarial vasculitis	ESR, C4/CH50, anti-FcεRI (CUI), anti-C1q, ASO, RF, ANA, UA, SPEP, Hep B/C, CRP, C3/C4/CH50
Vitiligo	CBC, TSH/Free T4, anti-thyroid peroxidase (TPO), fasting blood glucose, 25-OH Vitamin D, B_{12}/folic acid, anti-parietal gastric cell antibody (APGC)

Source: Adapted from Comprehensive Laboratory Disease Workups. Graham PM, Wilchowski S and Fivenson D. Directions in Residency. Spring 2016, pp.1–4.

Management of acne

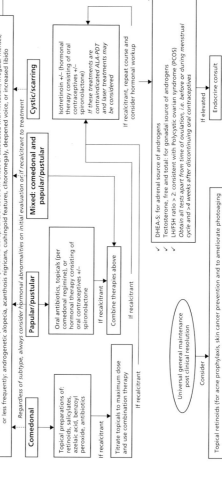

In all cases, consider hormonal workup if acne in a female patient is abrupt and/or severe in onset or associated with hirsutism, irregular menses, or less frequently: androgenetic alopecia, acanthosis nigricans, cushingoid features, clitoromegaly, deepened voice, or increased libido

Regardless of subtype, always consider hormonal abnormalities on initial evaluation or if recalcitrant to treatment

Comedonal

Topical preparations of: retinoids, salicylates, azelaic acid, benzoyl peroxide, antibiotics

If recalcitrant

Titrate topicals to maximum dose and use combination therapy

If recalcitrant

Papular/pustular

Oral antibiotics, topicals (per comedonal regimine), or hormonal therapy consisting of oral contraceptives +/− spironolactone

If recalcitrant

Combine therapies above

If recalcitrant

Mixed: comedonal and papular/pustular

Cystic/scarring

Isotretinoin +/− (hormonal therapy consisting of oral contraceptives +/− spironolactone)

If these treatments are contraindicated ALA-PDT and laser treatments may be considered

If recalcitrant, repeat course and consider hormonal workup

› DHEA-S: for adrenal source of androgens
› Testosterone, free and total: for gonadal source of androgens
› LH/FSH ratio > 2: consistent with Polycystic ovarian syndrome (PCOS)
› *Obtain all tests apart from time of ovulation, i.e. before or during menstrual cycle and >4 weeks after discontinuing oral contraceptives*

If elevated

Endocrine consult

Universal general maintenance post clinical resolution

Consider

Topical retinoids (for acne prophylaxis, skin cancer prevention and to ameliorate photoaging)

Thiboutot D. Acne: hormonal concepts and therapy. *Clin Dermatol* 2004 22(5);419–28

Alopecia Workup

Hair	Duration	% of hair	Microscopic/hair pull
Anagen	2–6 yr	85–90	Sheaths attached to roots
Catagen	2–3 wk	<1	Intermediate appearance (transitional)
Telogen	3 mo	10–15	Tiny bulbs without sheaths, "club" root
Exogen	Active shedding of hair shaft		
Kenogen	Rest period after shedding telogen; empty follicle		

A. Associations

1. Medications? Telogen effluvium associated medications: anticonvulsants, anticoagulants, chemotherapy, psychiatric medications, antigout, antibiotics, and beta-blockers
2. Hormones (pregnancy, menstruation, and OCPs)?
3. Hair care/products?
4. Diet (iron or protein deficiency)?
5. Systemic illness/stress?

B. Cicatricial or non-cicatricial?

1. **Non-cicatricial**: Is hair breaking off or coming out at the roots? Is hair loss focal or diffuse?

Breakage	Coming out at roots
Hair shaft defects, trichorrhexis nodosa, hair care (products, traction, and friction), tinea capitis, trichotillomania, anagen arrest/chemotherapy	Telogen effluvium, alopecia areata, androgenetic, syphilis, loose anagen, OCPs

Focal loss	Diffuse loss
Hair care (traction), tinea capitis, trichotillomania, alopecia areata, syphilis, hair shaft defects	Telogen effluvium, anagen effluvium, androgenetic alopecia, hair shaft defects

2. **Cicatricial**: Is biopsy predominately lymphocytic, neutrophic, or mixed?

Classification of cicatricial alopecia

Lymphocytic	Neutrophilic	Mixed
• Lichen planopilaris/LPP (including classic, frontal fibrosing, Graham-Little)	• Folliculitis decalvans	• Folliculitis/acne keloidalis
• Central centrifugal cicatricial alopecia (CCCA)	• Dissecting cellulitis/ folliculitis	• Folliculitis/acne necrotica
• Alopecia mucinosa		• Erosive pustular dermatosis
• Keratosis follicularis spinulosa decalvans		
• Chronic cutaneous LE		
• Pseudopelade (Brocq)		

Source: Adapted from Olsen EA, *et al.* North American Hair Research Society Summary of Sponsored Workshop on Cicatricial Alopecia. *J Am Acad Dermatol.* 2003;48:103–110.

C. Associated hair fragility?

Structural hair abnormalities by hair fragility

Increased fragility	No increased fragility
Trichorrhexis invaginata (bamboo)	Loose anagen
Monilethrix	Pili annulati
Trichorrhexis nodosa	Uncombable hair (spun-glass)
Trichothiodystrophy	Woolly hair
Pili torti	Pili bifurcati
	Pili multigemini
	Acquired progressive kinking

Source: Adapted from Hordinsky MK. Alopecias. In: Bolognia JL, Jorizzo JL, Rapini RP. Dermatology Vol. 1, Mosby; London. 2003, p. 1042.

D. Pull test and hair mount
1. **Pull test** – Telogen hairs in telogen effluvium, Anagen hairs in loose anagen syndrome. Helpful in identifying active areas in cicatricial alopecia or alopecia areata.
2. **Hair mount**

Disorder	Hair mount findings
Monilethrix	Beaded, pearl necklace, knots
Trichorrhexis nodosa	Fractures, paint brushes
Trichorrhexis invaginata	Bamboo/golf tee hair
Trichothiodystrophy	Trichoschisis, tiger-tail on polarization
Loose anagen	Anagen hairs with ruffled cuticles and curled ends and lacking root sheaths
Pili torti	Flattened, 180° irregularly spaced twists

Disorder	Hair mount findings
Uncombable hair	Pili canaliculi et trianguli, triangular in cross-section
Pili annulati	Abnormal dark bands on polarization, air bubbles in cortex
Elejalde	Pigment inclusions
Griscelli	Pigment clumping
Menkes	Multiple – pili torti, trichorrhexis nodosa, trichoptilosis

E. **Hair count** – helpful in quantifying hair loss
  1. Daily hair count: collect all hairs before shampooing (Normal <100)
  2. 60-second hair count: comb for 60 seconds (Normal 10–15 hairs)
F. **Biopsy** – helpful in persistent alopecia, may help determine if cicatricial alopecia
  1. 4 mm punch biopsy for horizontal sectioning
     a. Hair count: Caucasians should have ~40 total hairs (20–35 terminal, 5–10 vellus) while African-Americans should have fewer (18 terminal, 3 vellus)* – assess catagen vs. telogen at the isthmus level and terminal vs. vellus at the infundibular level
     b. Look at terminal to vellus** hair ratio:
        Normal >4 (~7–10T: 1V)
        Androgenic <2–4T: 1V
     c. Look for characteristic findings:
        Alopecia areata: lymphocytes around anagen bulbs
        Trichotillomania: pigment casts, trichomalacia, catagen hairs, dermal hemorrhage
        Androgenetic alopecia: miniaturized follicles
G. **Labs** – TSH, CBC, iron, TIBC, ferritin; consider RPR, ANA
   Check hormones (testosterone, DHEAS, and prolactin) – if irregular menses, infertility, hirsutism, severe acne, galactorrhea, or virilization
   Consider checking "nutrition labs" – Vitamin D, thiamine, zinc, total protein

Ethnic differences in hair

	Hair shaft structure	Hair shaft cross-section	Others
African-American	Coiled, curved	Elliptical, flattened	Lowest water content, slower growth, fewer cuticular layers at minor axes (only 1–2 not 6–8), longer major axis, less dense, large follicles

continued p.10

	Hair shaft structure	Hair shaft cross-section	Others
Asian	Straight	Circular	Largest follicular diameter; fewer eyelashes with lower lift-up/curl-up angles and greater diameter
Caucasian	In between	In between, oval	More dermal elastic fibers anchoring hair

*Vellus hairs – true vellus hairs (small and lack melanin) and miniaturized terminal hairs – histologically identical.

Telogen effluvium – workup and treatment

1. History: Medical/surgical; Stressors (stress scale 1–10), drugs, pregnancy, diet, weight loss/gain, metabolic/nutritional deficiency, endocrine dysfunction
    a. Drugs: majority of drugs implicated, important to determine change in dose, and history of adverse reaction
2. Etiology:
    a. Normal hair cycle is asynchronous – each follicle is independent
    b. TE – altered follicular growth cycle shedding:
        a) Telogen shed > 35% loss – common
        b) Anagen shed > 80% loss – rare
    c. Immediate release – seen in fever, drugs, and stress
    d. Delayed release – prolongation of anagen phase, then synchronized telogen phase in postpartum female
3. Labs: CBC, CMP, TSH, DHEAS, free and total Testosterone, Ferritin, Zinc, Vitamin D, Vit A, ANA, microsomal AB
4. Physical exam/Bx:
    a. Look at scalp, eyebrow, eyelash, and body hair
    b. Hair pull test: pull 40–60 hairs at 3 areas, <6–10 pull is positive
    c. Look for nail changes
    d. Bx: >7–35% telogen hairs
5. Treatments:
    a. Treat seb derm (healthy skin, healthy hair) – ketoconazole shampoo
    b. Treat deficiency: Biotin forte 3 with zinc, Vit D, iron supplement
    c. High DHEAs – use spironolactone
    d. Find and remove triggers
    e. Minoxidil 5% liquid or foam

Androgenic alopecia – workup and treatment

1. Autosomal dominant – 23–28% prevalence
2. Androgen influence on hair follicle and sebaceous glands
    a. Alopecia: scalp – change from terminal to vellus hair

   b. Hirsutism: increase sexual terminal hairs
   c. Acne: increase sebaceous gland
3. Risk of androgen excess – PCOS, infertility, hyperlipid, metabolic syndrome, insulin resistance, and diabetes
4. Labs: DHEA-s, testosterone (total and free), androstenedione, and prolactin
5. Treatment
   a. Minoxidil – 5% more effective in both men and women but may cause facial hair growth in women
   b. Finasteride (Propecia) 1 mg PO QD.
      a) Effective in men
      b) Effective in young women with SAHA (seborrhea, acne, hirsutisum, and alopecia), Finesteride 0.5 mg/d. Must use with OCP
      c) Avoid in pregnant females (causes ambiguous genitalia in male fetus)
      d) Not effective in postmenopausal women
   c. Spironolactone may be helpful in women with hyperandrogenism – dose 50–300 mg/d (Preg category D)
   d. OCP – suppress gonadotrophins, reduce testosterone
   e. Cyproterone acetate – Progestin, high anti-andorgen activity. Usually combined with estrogen (Preg category D). Increase risk of venous thromboembolism
   f. Metformin – 500–1000 mg/d in combination with spironolactone
   g. Weight loss – decrease insulin and testosterone
   h. Healthy scalp/healthy hair – consider ketoconazole/zinc pyrithione, green tea

Alopecia areata – workup and treatment

Associated with nail pitting, exclamation point hair, and yellow dots on dermoscopy

No approved FDA treatment. Guided by age of pt, location of loss, disease extent, disease activity, other medical issues, and pt choice

Patchy AA	Extensive AA
Topical or IL corticosteroid	Topical, IL, Oral corticosteroids
Steroid in shampoo	Anthralin
Minoxidil	Minoxidil
Anthralin	Immunotherapy
Topical immunotherapy	Phototherapy/Excimer laser
	Immunosuppressive-MTX, CSA
	Biologics

1. Watchful waiting
2. Intralesional kenalog 2.5–10 mg/cc (preferred 5 mg/ml, max 3 ml). Use 0.1 ml per injection site about 1 cm apart; every four to six weeks. Response 71%; relapse rate 29% in focal AA, 72% in totalis.
3. Topical steroid. Class I–II BID × three weeks, week off, then QD alternate week on and week off for two months. Response rate 75%; relapse 37–63%.
4. Oral steroid – reserve for rapid onset/acute progression, high relapse
5. Monoxidil 5% solution – use in conjunction with above treatments
6. Anthralin ointment or cream (0.5–1%) to affected area daily, start with 5–15 minutes, then wash off with soap or remove with mineral oil on cotton ball. Increase time by five minutes per night to two hours max as tolerated. Stop application if irritated until skin returns to normal. Need to produce mild irritation to be effective.
7. Immunotherapy with squaric acid dibutylester (SADBE) or diphenylcyclopropenone (DPCP)
   a. Initial sensitization to 2% (2 × 2 cm area to scalp)
   b. Apply lowest concentration 0.001% to scalp every one to three weeks to produce a mild eczematous rxn.
   c. If no rxn, increase to 0.01%, then 0.1, 0.5, 1, and 2%.
   d. If no regrowth after 6–12 months, treatment is discontinued.
8. Methotrexate – 15–25 mg weekly dose, takes three months to see regrowth. Response 57% along, 63% if used with low-dose oral steroid. Relapse 57%.
9. Cyclosporin – Response 25–76%, relapse rate up to 100%
10. JAK inhibitors (oral tofacitinib) – off-label use. Response rate 50–65%. Consider topical JAK inhibitor: Tofacitinib 2% in Versabase.
11. Simvastatin/ezetimibe 40 mg/10 mg (Vytorin) – off-label use. Anti-inflammatory effect, modulate JAK pathway. Variable response rate.
12. Fexofenadine (Allegra) 60 mg BID – H1 receptor antagonist decrease IFN-g and ICAM-1. Variable response rate.

Other alopecia treatments

A. Central centrifugal cicatricial alopecia (CCCA)/Folliculitis decalvans
1. Noninflammatory: potent topical steroid + Tetracycline
2. Inflammatory: Rifampin 300–600 BID and Clindamycin 150–300 BID × 10–12 weeks

B. Discoid lupus
1. Sun avoidance/physical sunblock such as zinc oxide
2. High-potency topical steroid and IL kenalog 10 mg/ml q4–6 weeks
3. Hydroxychloroquine 200 mg BID
4. Acitretin/isotretinoin for recalcitrant and/or hyperkeratotic disease

C. Dissecting cellulits of the scalp
  1. Tetracycline + IL kenalog
  2. Isotretinoin – 0.5–1.5 mg/kg/d – variable response
  3. Rifampin 300–600 BID and Clindamycin 150–300 BID
  4. Surgical – incision and drainage, CO_2 laser

D. Erosive pustular dermatosis
  1. Topical steroid and topical psoriatic medications
  2. Avoid traumatic manipulation and phototherapy – may aggravate condition

E. Lichen planopilaris
  1. Corticosteroid – intralesional kenalog 3–10 mg/ml; oral prednisone
  2. Tetracycline
  3. Hydroxychloroquine 200 BID
  4. Mycophenolate mofetil 500 BID × 4 weeks, then 1 g BID
  5. Compounded tacrolimus 0.1% solution

Aphthosis Workup and Treatment

Adapted from Letsinger *et al. J Am Acad Dermatol.* 2005 Mar;52(3 Pt 1):500–508.

Morphologic classification
- **Minor aphthae**: single to few, shallow ulcers (<1 cm) which spontaneously heal in ~ one to two weeks
- **Major aphthae** (Sutton's, periadenitis mucosa necrotica recurrens): single to few, deep ulcers (>1 cm) which heal over weeks – months and scar
- **Herpetiform aphthae**: 10–100, clustered, small (≤3 mm) ulcers which heal in days–weeks, may scar (not associated with HSV)

Classification by cause
- **Simple aphthae**: recurrent minor, major, or herpetiform aphthae, often in healthy, young patients
- **Complex aphthae**: >3, nearly constant, oral aphthae OR recurrent genital and oral aphthae AND exclusion of Behcet and MAGIC syndrome
  - Primary: idiopathic (stress, trauma, hormonal changes, acidic foods, EBV, and CMV potential cause)

- Secondary: IBD, HIV, cyclic neutropenia, FAPA (fever, aphthous stomatitis, pharyngitis, and adenitis), gluten sensitivity, ulcus vulvae acutum, vitamin deficiencies (B_1, B_2, B_6, and B_{12}, folate), iron, and zinc deficiencies, and drugs (NSAIDS, alendronate, beta-blockers, and nicorandil)

Workup for complex apthae

- HSV PCR/Cx
- CBC
- Iron, folate, vitamin B_{12}, and zinc
- UA
- Consider HIV, HLA-B27, and antigliadin/antiendomysial Ab
- Consider biopsy
- Consider GI, Rheum, Ophtho, and Neuro consults
- If considering dapsone, check G6PD

Local factors promoting aphthae: chemical/mechanical injury, sodium lauryl sulfate-containing dental products, inadequate saliva, and cessation of tobacco

Treatment

1. Avoid trauma (soft foods, atraumatic brushing, and avoid acidic foods)
2. Topical:
   - Corticosteroids (hydrocortisone hemisuccinate pellets 2.5 mg; triamcinolone dental paste, betamethasone sodium phosphate 0.5 mg tablet dissolved in 15 cc water for mouth rinse)
   - Anesthetics for pain
   - Tacrolimus
   - Tetracycline rinses (doxycycline 100 mg or tetracycline 500 mg dissolved in 10 cc of water) QID may reduce severity of ulcers
   - Other mouth rinses (chlorhexidine, betadine, salt water, and hydrogen peroxide)
   - B complex vitamins
3. Systemic: colchicine, dapsone, and thalidomide (HIV)

Dermatologic Signs

Sign	Disease association	Site
Albright's dimpling	Albright's hereditary osteodystrophy	Dimpling over knuckles, enhanced by fist clenching
Albright's	Nevoid BCC syndrome/Gorlin's	Short fourth metacarpal digits
Asboe–Hansen	+: in pemphigus and other blistering dx (BP, DH, EBA, CP, DEB, bullous drug, SJS/TEN) −: usually for Hailey–Hailey and Staph scalded Skin	Existing blister, extension to adjacent unblistered skin with mechanical pressure on top of bulla
Auspitz	Plaque psoriasis, but also Darier's disease and actinic keratosis	Red, glossy surface with pinpoint bleeding on removal of the scale by scraping or scratching
Battle's	Basal skull fracture	Discoloration at mastoid process
Blue dot	Torsion of testicular epididymis and appendices	Blue or black nodule visible under the skin on the superior aspect of the testis or epididymis and area will be tender
Butterfly	Lupus erythematosus on face; atopic dermatitis on upper back	Erythema over the malar eminence and nasal bridge; butterfly-shaped area of sparing observed over the upper central back, corresponding to the zone that is difficult to reach by hands
Buttonhole	Cutaneous neurofibroamas, but also syphilitic chancre and old pigmented nevi	Invaginate the tumor into the underlying dermal defect with digital pressure
Cluster of jewels	Early stage of chronic bullous disease of childhood	New lesions at margin of older ones, aka "string of pearls," "rosettes sign"
Corn-flake	Kyrle's and Flegel's diseases	Polygonal irregular configuration of lesions that tend to occur over the lower extremities
Crowe's	Type II neurofibromatosis	Axillary freckling, may occur in perineum, typically appears later than café au lait macules
Darier's	Condns with increased mast cells in the dermis (urticaria pigmentosa, systemic mastocytosis, insect bite reactions, neurofibroma, juvenile xanthogranuloma, acute neonatal lymphoblastic leukemia)	Whealing, circumferential erythema, and localized pruritis elicited by scratching or rubbing of a lesion

COMMON WORK-UPS, SIGNS, AND MANAGEMENT

continued p.16

Sign	Disease association	Site
Deck chair	Cutaneous Waldenstrom's macroglobulinemia	Widespread eruption of erythematous papules that coalesce into rectangular plaques. Sparing of the natural skin folds, resembling the slats of a deck chair
Dimple	Dermatofibromas	Lateral compression with the thumb and index finger leads to depression of the lesion. This dimpling is secondary to the lesion being attached to the subcutaneous fat
Dirty neck	Chronic atopic dermatitis	Reticulate pigmentation of the neck with the anterolateral aspects of the neck typically affected secondary to melanin incontinence
Doughnut	Scleromyxedema	Central depression surrounded by an elevated rim of skin on the extended proximal interphalageal joint
Dubois'	Dermatitis artefacta	Produced by corrosive liquids. Patterned burned areas correspond to the areas of dripping of the liquid when applied by the patient
Ear lobe	Contact dermatitis	Substance applied with the hand to the face and neck leads to sparing of the diagonal crease of the ear lobe on the ipsilateral side, whereas the contralateral side is affected. Secondary to hand-sweeping movement made during application of the substance
Enamel paint	Kwashiorkor	Sharply demarcated hyperpigmented desquamating patches and plaques resembling enamel paint occur on the skin, predominantly in areas of pressure and irritation
Exclamation mark hair	Alopecia areata	Proximal tapering of hair where the dot represents the remains of the bulb

Sign	Disease association	Site
Flag	Nutritional deficiencies (kwashiorkor) intermittent high dosage of methotrexate or following chemotherapy and ulcerative colitits	Horizontal alternating bands of discoloration in the hair shafts corresponding to periods of normal and abnormal hair growth. Discoloration may be reddish, blonde, gray, or white depending on the original hair color
Forchheimer's	Rubella	Enanthem of red macules or petechiae confined to the soft palate
Frank's	Coronary disease and coronary artery disease or retinopathy in DM type II	Diagonal groove across the ear lobe in adults
Gorlin's	Ehlers–Danlos syndrome	Ability to touch the tip of the nose with the extended tongue
Gottron's	Dermatomyositis, but also systemic lupus	Symmetric confluent macular violaceous erythema occurring over the knuckles, hips, knees, and medial ankles
Grey Turner's	Acute hemorrhagic pancreatitis and other causes of retroperitoneal hemorrhage	Induration and bruising seen on the skin over the costovertebral angle secondary to the spread of blood from anterior pararenal space
Groove	Lymphogranuloma venereum in heterosexual males	Inflammatory mass of femoral and inguinal nodes separated by a depression or groove made by Poupart's (inguinal) ligament
Hair collar	Neural tube closure defects on the scalp (such as aplasia cutis, encephalocele, meningocele, or hetertropic brain tissue)	Ring of dark coarse hair surrounding a malformation. Defect is typically midline and the occipital or parietal scalp is typically affected
Hanging curtain	Pityriasis rosea	When the skin is stretched across the long axis of the herald patch, the scale is noted to be finer, lighter, and attached at one end, which tends to fold across the line of the stretch
Heliotrope	Dermatomyositis	Violaceous erythema involving the periorbital skin

continued p.18

Sign	Disease association	Site
Hertoghe's	Atopic dermatitis, trichotillomania, ectodermal dysplasia, alopecia areata, alopecia mucinosa, leprosy, syphilis, ulerythema ophryogenes, systemic sclerosis and hypothyroidism	Lack of hair at the outer 1/3 of the eyebrows
Hoagland's	Infectious mononucleosis	Early and transient bilateral upper lid edema
Holster	Dermatomyositis	Pruritic, macular, violaceous erythema affecting the lateral aspects of the hips and thighs
Hutchinson's nail	Subungual melanoma	Periungual extension of brown-black pigmentation onto the proximal and/or lateral nail folds
Hutchinson's nose	Herpes zoster	Presence of vesicles occurring on the tip of the nose
Jellinek's	Hyperthyroidism	Hyperpigmentation of the eyelid
Leser–Trelat	Internal malignancy (typically adenocarcinomas, lung cancer, melanoma, and mycosis fungoides)	Sudden eruption of multiple seborrheic keratoses, which are often pruitic
Muehrcke's	Nephritic syndrome, GN, liver disease, and malnutrition	Paired, transverse, narrowed white bands that run parallel to the lunula of the nails and are seen in patients with hypoalbuminemia or those receiving chemotherapy agents
Neck	Scleroderma	Ridging and tightening of the neck forming a visible and palpable tight band that lies over the platysma in the hyperextended neck
Necklace of casal	Pellagra	Hyperpigmentation on the neck extending as a broad collar-like band around the entire circumference of the neck
Nikolsky's	Pemphigous foliaceus	Pulling the ruptured wall of the blister it is possible to take off the horny layer for a long distance on a seemingly healthy skin and rubbing off of the epidermis between the bullae by slight friction without breaking the surface of the skin and leaving moist surface of the granular layer

Sign	Disease association	Site
Nose	Airbone contact dermatitis, severe atopic dermatitis, and exfoliative dermatitis	Sparing of the nose in the eruption distribution
Oil drop	Psoriasis	Translucent, yellow-red discoloration and circular areas of onycholysis in the nail bed that fail to reach the free border and look like oil drops underneath the nail
Panda	Laser therapy complication	Nevus of Ota in the periorbital location
Pastia	Preeruptive stage of scarlet fever	Pink or red transverse lines found in the antecubital fossae and axillary folds
Pathergy	Pyoderma gangrenosum or Behcet's syndrome	Elicitation of new lesions or worsening of existing lesions by superficial trauma
Racoon	Basilar skull fracture	Periorbital ecchymosis from subconjunctival hemorrhage
Romana's	Chagas' disease	First clinical sign of sensitization response to the bite of the Trypansoma cruzi insect presenting as severe unilateral conjunctivitis and palpable, painless lid edema
Rope	Interstitial granulomatous dermatitis with arthritis	Inflammatory indurations appearing like cords that extend from the lateral trunk to the axillae
Round fingerpad	Scleroderma	Disappearance of the peaked contour on the fingerpads and progression to a hemisphere-like finger contour
Russell's	Bulimia nervosa	Lacerations, abrasions, and callosities that are found on the dorsum of the hand overlying the metacarpophalangeal and interphalangeal joints due to repeated contact of the incisor teeth with the skin during self-induced vomiting
School chair	Contact dermatitis to nickel	Rash occurring over the posterior thighs, corresponding to contact with a school chair

continued p.20

Sign	Disease association	Site
Shawl	Dermatomyositis	Vonfluent, symmetric, macular violaceous erythema on the posterior shoulders and neck, giving a distinctive shawl-like appearance
Slapped cheek	Children with fifth disease	Confluent, erythematous, edematous plaques on the cheeks
Sternberg's thumb	Arachnodactyly and Marfan syndrome	Completely opposed thumb in the clenched hand projects beyond the ulnar border
Tent	Benign appendageal tumor pilomatricoma	Solitary, asymptomatic, firm nodule. When the overlying skin is stretched, the lesion appears to be multifaceted and angulated, giving a "tent" appearance. The tent sign is due to calcification occurring in the lesion
Thumbprint	Disseminated strongyloidosis	Periumbilical purpura resembling multiple thumbprints
Tin-tack	Discoid lupus erythematosus	Hyperkeratotic scale extending into the follicular infundibulum creates keratotic spikes when viewed from the scale's undersurface, resembling a carpet tack
Tripe palms	Internal malignancy (carcinoma of the stomach and lung)	Rugose thickening of the palmar surface of the hands, with accentuation of the normal dermatoglyphic ridges, thus resembling the ridging of the interior surface of a bovine foregut
Trousseau's	Visceral malignancy (predominantly pancreatic cancer)	Development of successive crops of tender nodules in affected blood vessels secondary to intravascular low-grade hypercoagulation usually affecting upper extremities or trunk
Ugly duckling	Melanoma	A nevus that does not resemble a patient's other nevi

Sign	Disease association	Site
V	Dermatomyositis	Erythema secondary to photosensitivity seen in the V area of the upper chest
Walzel	Acute and chronic pancreatitis	Livedo reticularis
Winterbottom's	Gambian form of African trypanosomiasis	Occasionally visible enlargement of lymph nodes in the posterior cervical group

Source: Adapted from Freiman et al. *J Cutaneous Med Surg* 2006; 10(4).

Folliculitis

Type	Clinical presentation	Treatment
Staph	Multiple follicular-based erythematous papules/pusules	Mupirocin cream to nares Chlorhexidine wash Dicloxacillin or cephalexin for MSSA Trimethoprim/ sulfamethoxazole, clindamycin, or doxycycline for MRSA
Gram-negative	Multiple small pustules in the perinasal region, chin, and cheeks. Classic scenario: acne patient treated with long-term antibiotics	Isotretinoin Ampicillin, trimethoprim/ sulfamethoxazole, and ciprofloxacin
Pseudomonas	Exposure to contaminated water in pools/hot tub	Usually resolve without treatment in 7–10 d Ciprofloxacin for severe cases
Demodex	Rosacea-like papules and pustules with periorificial accentuation on a background of erythema. Facial perifollicular scaling.	Permetherin 5% cream Metronidazole Ivermectin
Pityrosporum	Very pruritic small monomorphous papules and pustules on upper trunk. Commonly found in hot and humid environment or with immunocompromised patient or those on long-term antibiotics	Ketoconazole cream/ shampoo Selenium sulfide shampoo May need systemic antifungals

continued p.22

Type	Clinical presentation	Treatment
Eosinophilic folliculitis	1. Ofuji – in Asian descent, discrete papules and pustules that coalesce to form circinate plaques with central clearing on the face, back, and arms 2. HIV positive/immunocompromised – persistent papules and pustules favoring face, scalp, and upper trunk. 3. Infantile – male, self-limiting. Cyclic course. Scalp and eyebrows	Tacrolimus 0.1% ointment Cyclosporin Indomethacin 25–75 mg qd for 1–8 wk Isotretinoin Metronidazole Phototherapy
EGFR induced	Four stages of eruption – dysesthesia, erythema, edema; erythematous papules and pustules; purulent crusting; telangiectasia. Lesions can be painful and pruritic.	Doxycycline 200 QD prescribed with EGFR inhibitor to prevent folliculitis

Melasma

(From Sheth VM and Pandya AG. *JAAD* 2011;65: 689–697)

A. Etiology/pathogenesis
1. **Skin type** – Melasma is more common in Fitz III and IV.
2. **Genetics** – highly reported incidence in family members
3. **UV exposure** – induces melanocyte proliferation, migration, and melanogensis. Increase production of IL-1, endothelin-1, a-MSH, and ACTH which upregulates melanocyte proliferation and melanogensis.
4. **Hormones** – no definitive association of serum hormone levels to melasma. Definite association of melasma with OCP and pregnancy. If pt notes onset/worsen with OCP, should stop OCP when possible.
5. **Vascular component** – bx of melasma skin show greater vascular endothelial growth factor expression

B. Differential diagnosis
1. PIH
2. Solar lentigines
3. Ephelides
4. Drug-induced pigmentation (i.e. MCN pigmentation)
5. Actinic lichen planus
6. Acathosis nigracans
7. Frictional melanosis
8. Acquired nevus of Ota (Hori's nevus)
9. Nevus of Ota

C. **Assessment tools**
   1. **Melasma Area and Severity Index (MASI)**
      MASI $= 0.3A\,(D+H) + 0.3A\,(D+H) + 0.3A\,(D+H) + 0.1A\,(D+H)$
         [Forehead]   [L malar]   [R malar]   [chin]
      Score range 0–48
      a. Divide face into four areas – forehead (30%), L malar area (30%), R malar area (30%), and chin (10%).
      b. Area of involvement (A) from 1 (<10%) to 6 (90–100%)
      c. Darkness of pigment (D)
      d. Homogeneity of pigment (H)
   2. **Quality of life assessment – MelasQoL**

Principles of melasma therapy

1. Set realistic expectations
   - Melasma is a chronic skin disease
   - Recurrence is common
   - Requires daily commitment
   - Rotational regimen based on flare and remission

2. Avoid triggers
   - **Broad-spectrum sunscreen –** UVA and UVB protection SPF 30 + physical blocker – improves melasma and enhances efficacy of HQ.
   - **Wear protective hats and clothing**
   - **Iron oxide** sunscreen and makeup (tinted) – protect from high-energy visible (HEV) light, esp. important for Fitz IV–VI.
     - Avene, Femme Couture and Get Corrected, Elta MD.
     - Visible light may play a role – visible light (400–700 nm) and UVA1 (340–400 nm) induce hyperpigmentation in Type V skin (Mahmoud JID 2010).
     - Iron oxide improves MASI in conjunction with HQ4% (Bissonnette Derm Surg 2008; Castanedo-Cazares PPP 2014).
   - **Camouflage makeup –** Dermablend, Covermark, and CoverFx
   - **OCP –** If onset associated with OCP and no family history, consider stopping OCP.

3. Topicals
   - Triple combination cream – first line for eight weeks (more effective than HQ alone)
     - Kligman: HQ 5%, tretinoin 0.1%, and dexamethasone 0.1%
     - Triluma: HQ 4%, tretinoin 0.05%, and fluocinolone 0.01%
   - For resistant melasma *(adapted from Dr. Alison Tam)*
     - Start with compounded cream (i.e. HQ8%/Kojic acid 6%, vitC, HC 2.5%) BID dosing
     - Take photos prior to initiation of therapy, followup in six to eight weeks

- o If no improvement, titrate HQ by 2–4%
- o If improved, decrease usage frequency from BID → QD → QOD → TIW. Give drug holiday.

4. Resistant cases
   - Tranexamic acid – synthetic lysine analog (available in 650 mg in the United States)
     - o 250 mg BID or 650 mg break in half BID × three months
     - o FDA approved for menorrhagia, off-label for melasma
     - o Blocks plasminogen activator/plasmin pathway
     - o SE: nausea, diarrhea, GI upset, and oligomenorrhea
     - o Must assess risk of thromboembolism in patient: ask about personal and family history of DVT/PE, stroke, miscarriages, complications of pregnancy
   - Chemical peels
   - Lasers
     - o Vascular component of melasma, consider PDL
     - o IPL, Fraxel, and Q-swithced Nd:YAG have been used for melasma

5. Maintenance therapy
   - Decrease HQ concentration to 2% or off HQ to avoid risk of exogenous ochronosis
   - Azelaic acid 20% (off-labeled), similar efficacy as HQ 2%
     - o Direct cytotoxic effect on hyperactive melanocytes
     - o Can be used during pregnancy/breastfeeding
     - o Does not cause depigmentation in normal skin
   - Kojic acid combination with lower strength HQ
     - o More irritating than HQ, use with steroid
   - Lignin peroxidase/Melanozyme (Elure)
   - Other agents: Soy, Arbutin, Green tea, Ascorbic acid, and Niacinamide
   - Polypodium leucotomos – Heliocare, may be photoprotective

IMMUNOLOGY AND IMMUNOLOGIC DISEASE

Lupus Erythematosus

Systemic lupus erythematosus criteria (4 of 11)

Adapted from the American College of Rheumatology 1982 revised criteria

Mucocutaneous
1. Malar rash (tends to spare nasolabial folds)
2. Discoid lesions
3. Photosensitivity
4. Oral ulcers (must be observed by physician)

Systemic
5. Arthritis – nonerosive arthritis of 2+ joints
6. Serositis – pleuritis, pericarditis
7. Renal disorder – proteinuria > 0.5 g/d or 3+ on dipstick
8. Neurologic – seizures or psychosis
9. Hematologic
   a. hemolytic anemia with reticulocytosis
   b. leukopenia (<4 K) on 2 occasions
   c. lymphopenia (<1.5 K) on 2 occasions
   d. thrombocytopenia (<100 K)
10. Immunologic – anti-dsDNA, anti-Sm, false positive RPR
11. ANA+

Acute cutaneous lupus erythematosus
Clinical findings: transient butterfly malar rash, generalized photosensitive eruption, and/or bullous lesions on the face, neck, and upper trunk.
Associated with HLA-DR2, HLA-DR3
DIF: granular IgG/IgM (rare IgA) + complement at DEJ

Subacute cutaneous lupus erythematosus
Clinical findings: psoriasiform or annular non-scarring plaques in a photodistribution.
Associated with:
- HLA-B8, HLA-DR3, HLA-DRw52, HLA-DQ1
- SLE, Sjögren, RA, C2 deficiency
- Medications: HCTZ, Ca+ channel blocker, ACE inhibitors, griseofulvin, terbinafine, anti-TNF, penicillamine, glyburide, spironolactone, piroxicam
DIF: granular pattern of IgG/IgM in the epidermis only (variable)

Chronic cutaneous lupus erythematosus
Discoid lupus
Clinical findings: erythematous plaques which progress to atrophic patches with follicular plugging, scarring, and alopecia on sun-exposed skin.
Progression to SLE: 5% if above the neck; 20% if above and below the neck
DIF: granular IgG/IgM (rare IgA) + complement at DEJ, more likely positive in actively inflamed lesion present × 6–8 weeks

Lupus panniculitis
Clinical findings: deep painful erythematous plaques, nodules, and ulcers involving proximal extremities and trunk. Overlying skin may have DLE changes.
Progression to SLE: 50%
DIF: rare granular deposits at the DEJ. May have deposits around dermal vessels.

Tumid lupus

Clinical findings: erythematous indurations of fat with no scale or follicular plugs.

DIF: nonspecific

Lupus band: strong continuous antibody deposits at the DEJ on nonlesional skin; found in >75% of SLE patients on sun-exposed skin and 50% SLE patients on non-sun-exposed skin

Autoantibody

Autoantibody sensitivities and specificities

Condition	Autoantibody	Sensitivity (%)	Specificity (%)
SLE	ANA	93–99	57
	Histone	60–80	50
	dsDNA*	50–70	97
	U1-RNP	30–50	99
	Ribosomal-P	15–35	99
	Sm	10–40	>95
	SS-A	10–50	>85
	SS-B	10–15	
SCLE	ANA	67	
	SS-A	60–80	
	SS-B	25–50	
DLE	ANA	5–25	
	SS-A	≪10	
Drug-induced LE	ANA	>95	
	Histone	>95	
	dsDNA		1–5
	Sm	1	
Neonatal lupus	SS-A**	95	
	SS-B	60–80	
MCTD	ANA	100	
	U1-RNP	>95	
Scleroderma	ANA	85–95	55
	Scl-70	15–70	100
	U3-RNP	12	96
	Centromere	<10	
CREST	Centromere	>80	
	Scl-70	15	

Condition	Autoantibody	Sensitivity (%)	Specificity (%)
Progessive systemic sclerosis	Scl-70	50	
	Centromere	<5	
Sjögren	ANA	50–75	50
	SS-A	50–90	>85
	SS-B	40	>90
	RF	50	
Polymyositis (PM)	ANA	85	60 (DM/PM)
	Jo-1	25–37	
Dermatomyositis (DM)	ANA	40–80	60 (DM/PM)
Rheumatoid arthritis	CCP	65–70	90–98
	RF	50–90	>80
	ANA	20–50	55
	Histone	15–20	
Secondary Raynaud	ANA	65	40

Sensitivity and specificity for different antibiodies varies depending on the assay used. The % reported here are estimated averages from the referenced text below.

*Correlates with SLE activity and renal disease.

**Risk of neonatal lupus among babies of SS-A+ mothers: 2–6%.

ANA titers of 1:80, 1:160, and 1:320 are found in 13, 5, and 3%, respectively, of healthy individuals. Among healthy elderly patients, ANA titers of 1:160 may be seen in 15%.

Sheldon J. Laboratory testing in autoimmune rheumatic disease. *Best Pract Res Clin Rheumatol.* 2004 Jun;18(3): 249–269.

Lyons et al. Effective use of autoantibody tests in the diagnosis of systemic autoimmune disease. *Ann N Y Acad Sci.* 2005 Jun;1050:217–228.

Kurien BT, Scofield RH. Autoantibody determination in the diagnosis of systemic lupus erythematosus. *Scand J Immunol.* 2006 Sep;64(3):227–235.

Habash-Bseiso et al. Serologic testing in connective tissue diseases. *Clin Med Res.* 2005 Aug;3(3):190–193.

Autoantibodies in connective tissue diseases

Autoantibody or target	Activity	Clinical association
LAC, β2-glycoprotein I, Prothrombin, Cardiolipin, Protein S, and Annexin AV	Phospholipids	Antiphospholipid antibody syndrome*
Rheumatoid factor	Fc portion of IgG	Low level nonspecific (SLE, SSc, MCTD, neoplasm, chronic disease)
		High level – associated with erosive RA
Ku	DNA end-binding repair protein complex	Overlap DM/PM, SSc, LE
U2-RNP		Overlap DM/PM, SSc
Alpha-fodrin	Actin-binding protein	Specific for Sjögren
Jo-1/PL-1	Histidyl-tRNA synthetase	DM/PM** (20–40% sensitive) – increased risk of ILD, but no increased rate of malignancy
Mi-2	Nuclear helicase	DM with malignancy, better prognosis than anti-synthetase
PDGF		SSc, cGVHD
SRP	Signal recognition protein	Anti-SRP syndrome (rapidly progressive necrotizing myopathy); association with cardiac disease not confirmed
155 K-EB antigen	Transcriptional intermediary factor-1	DM (20% sensitive in adult-onset classical form), may be associated with internal malignancy

Source: Adapted from Jacobe H et al. Autoantibodies encountered in patients with autoimmune connective diseases. In: Bolognia J, et al. *Dermatology*. Philadephia: Elsevier; 2003. pp. 589–599.

*__Antiphospholipid antibody (APA) syndrome__ – Primary (50%), SLE (35%); Skin: livedo reticularis, ulcers, gangrene, and splinter hemorrhages.

Diagnosis requires at least one clinical criterion:

- Clinical episode of vascular thrombosis
- Pregnancy complication: unexplained abortion after week 10, premature birth at or before week 34, or ≥3 unexplained, consecutive SAB before week 10

And at least one lab criterion: anticardiolipin, lupus anticoagulant, or anti-β2-glycoprotein I Abs on 2 occasions six weeks apart.

**__Polymyositis/Dermatomyositis__ – ≥0% ANA+, 90% auto-Ab. Anti-synthetase syndrome (tRNA): ILD, fever, arthritis, Raynaud disease, and machinist hands.

Anti-nuclear antibodies
(Sn: sensitive Sp: specific)

Pattern	Antibody target	Disease	Notes
Homogenous	Histone	**Drug-induced LE*** (>90% Sn), SLE (>60% Sn), Chronic Dz	
	dsDNA	**SLE** (60% Sp), **Lupus nephritis**	IC in glomeruli = nephritis, follows disease activity, test performed on *Crithidia luciliae*
Peripheral nuclear (Rim)	Nuclear lamins	**SLE**, Linear Morphea	
	Nuclear pore	**PM**	
Centromere/ true speckled	Centromere	**CREST** (50–90% Sn), SSc, Primary billiary cirrhosis (50% Sn), Idiopathic Raynaud, PSS	
Speckled/ particulate nuclear (ENA)	U1RNP	**Mixed connective tissue disease** (near 100% Sn)	Titer > 1:1600 in 95–100% MCTD
		SLE (30% Sn), DM/PM, SSc, Sjögren, RA	
	Smith (snRNP)	**SLE** (99% Sp but only 20% Sn)	
	Ro/SS-A (E3 ubiquitin ligase, TROVE2)	**SCLE** (75–90% Sn), **Sjögren**, Neonatal LE, Congenital Heart Block, C2/C4 deficient LE	Photosensitivity workup
	La/SS-B (binds RNA newly transcribed by RNA Pol III)	**Sjögren, SCLE**	
Nucleolar	SCL-70 (Topoisomerase I)	**SSc** (diffuse)	Poor prognosis
	Fibrillarin (U3-RNP)	SSc (localized > diffuse)	
	PM-SCL	PM/SSc overlap syndromes	Machinists hands, arthritis, Raynaud, and calcinosis cutis
	RNA Pol I	SSc	Poor prognosis, renal crisis

*Drug-induced ("Dusting Pattern"): Allopurinol, aldomet, ACE-I, chloromazine, clonidine, danazol, dilantin, ethosuximide, griseofulvin, hydralazine, isoniazid, lithium, lovastatin, mephenytoin, mesalazine, methyldopa, MCN, OCP, *para*-amino salicylic acid, penicillamine, PCN, phenothiazine, pheylbutazone, piroxicam, practolol, procainamide, propylthiouracil, quinidine, streptomycin, sulfasalazine, sulfonamides, tegretol, and TCN.

ANCA (Anti-neutrophil cytoplasmic antibodies)

	Granulomatosis with polyangiitis (formerly Wegener's)	Microscopic polyangiitis	Churg–Strauss syndrome
ANCA (% sensitivity)	C-ANCA (85%) > P-ANCA (10%)	P-ANCA (45–70%) > C-ANCA (45%)	P-ANCA (60%) > C-ANCA (10%)
Classic features	Upper respiratory (sinusitis, oral ulcers, rhinorrhea), glomerulonephritis (GN), saddle-nose, strawberry gingiva, ocular	Necrotizing GN (segmental and crescentic), pulmonary hemorrhage (esp. lower), neuropathy	Asthma, allergies, nasal polyps, eosinophilia, PNA, gastroenteritis, CHF, mononeuritis multiplex
Skin	Palpable purpura, SQ nodules, pyoderma gangrenosum-like lesions	Palpable purpura	Palpable purpura, SQ nodules
Pathology	Perivascular necrotizing granulomas, LCV	No granulomas, LCV with few/no immune deposits	Eosinophils, extravascular granulomas, LCV
Respiratory	Upper and lower respiratory, fixed nodular densities	Lower respiratory, alveolar hemorrhage	Patchy, transient interstitial infiltrates
Treatment	High-dose corticosteroids; Cytotoxic agents if severe (no controlled trial demonstrating benefits)	High-dose corticosteroids; Cytotoxic agents if severe (no controlled trial demonstrating benefits)	High-dose corticosteroids combined with cytotoxic agent (cyclophosphamide) with proven benefit in survival

C-ANCA = cytoplasmic (IIF) = proteinase 3.
P-ANCA = perinuclear (IIF) = myeloperoxidase.
Other conditions which may be ANCA positive: SLE, RA, chronic infection (TB, HIV), digestive disorders (inflammatory bowel disease, sclerosing cholangitis, primary biliary cirrhosis, autoimmune hepatitis), drugs (propylthiouracil, hydralazine, methimazole, minocycline, carbimazole, penicillamine), silica/occupational solvents
Titers might indicate disease activity, relapse.

Treatment of ANCA-associated vasculitis

- Induction: Cyclophosphamide 2 mg/kg/d, Prednisolone 1 mg/kg/d tapered to 0.25 mg/kg/d by 12 weeks
- Maintenance: Azathioprine 2 mg/kg/d, Prednisolone 7.5–10 mg/d

Frequent life-severe adverse events with cyclophosphamide (Cytoxan), nitrogen mustard, and alkylating agent:

1. Hemorrhagic cystitis (10%) and risk of bladder cancer (5% at 10 years, 16% at 15 years): minimize by using copious fluids, mesna, acetylcysteine and not using h.s. dosing.
2. Bone marrow suppression: Onset 7 days, nadir 14 days, recovery 21 days.
3. Infection
4. Infertility

Vasculitis

Initial workup: Detailed history, physical exam, ROS, skin biopsy ± DIF, CBC, ESR, BMP, UA, consider drug-induced vasculitis.
Further studies guided by ROS and type of vasculitis suspected:
CRP, SPEP, UPEP, cryo, LFT, HBV, HCV, RF, C3, C4, CH50, ANA, ANCA, ASO, CXR, guaiac, cancer screening, HIV, ENA, echo, electromyogram, nerve conduction, biopsy (nerve, respiratory tract, kidney)

Small vessel vasculitis

Disease	Symptoms	Etiology Associations	Treatment
Cutaneous small vessel vasculitis	Palpable purpura, lower legs/ankles/ dependent areas, +/− livedo reticularis, urticaria, edema, ulcers, +/− pruritic, painful/burning, fever, arthralgias	Drugs, infections, connective tissue diseases, and neoplasms	Usually self-limited, rest, elevation, compression, NSAIDs, anti-histamines, corticosteroids, colchicine, dapsone, and immunosupressants
Henoch–Schönlein purpura	Palpable purpura on extensors and buttocks, pts 4–7 yrs old polyarthralgia (75%), GI bleeding, fever, hematuria, edema, renal dysfunction, pulmonary hemorrhage, and headache	1–2 weeks after respiratory infection, allergens/food, drugs; usually unknown	Primarily supportive. corticosteroids, other immunosuppressants, dapsone, factor XII
Acute hemorrhagic edema of infancy	Large, annular, purpuric plaques and edema on face, ears, extremities, usually in patients <2 yo	Infections (especially respiratory), drugs, vaccines; usually unknown	Self-resolving

continued p.32

Disease	Symptoms	Etiology Associations	Treatment
Urticarial vasculitis	Painful >pruritic, lasts >24 h, post-inflammatory hyperpigmentation, +/− bullae, systemic dz in hypocomplementemic version (anti-C1q precipitin, F>M, ocular, angioedema, COPD), F>M	Autoimmune/ CTD (30% of Sjogren, 20% of SLE pts), drugs (serum sickness), infections (HBV, HCV, EBV), neoplasms, Schnitzler syndrome	Oral corticosteroids, antimalarials, dapsone, colchicine, anti-histamines, and NSAIDs
Hyperimmuno-globulinemia D syndrome	Periodic fever, arthralgia, GI sxs, LAN, erythematous macules/papules/ nodules/urticaria on extremities, onset <10 yo, ↑ IgD and IgA levels	AR; Mevalonate kinase deficiency	NSAIDs, anti-IL-1 Ab, and corticosteroids
Familial mediterranean fever	Periodic fever, arthritis, serositis, erysipelas-like rash on legs, myalgias, AA amyloidosis, renal failure, PID sxs; unlike Hyper-IgD, no LAN and nl IgD level	AR; Pyrin deficiency	Colchicine, anti-IL-1
Erythema elevatum Diutinum	Yellow/brown/red papules, plaques, and nodules over joints	Various associations: hematologic diseases, HIV, IBD, CTD, and streptococcal infections	Dapsone, niacinamide, and topical/ intralesional corticosteroids
Granuloma faciale	Brown/red plaques on face Middle-aged, M>F, Caucasian	Unknown	Treatment-resistent, intralesional steroids, dapsone, and surgery
Serum sickness	Fever, lymphadenopathy, arthralgias, urticaria, maculopapular, scarlatiniform, purpura, and myalgias	Type III hypersensitivity, commonly following streptokinase, IVIG, Abx (cefaclor, PCN, MCN, rifampin, and cefprozil)	Avoidance, anti-histamines, anti-pyretics, and corticosteroids

Medium (± small) vessel vasculitis

Polyarteritis nodosa (systemic)	SQ nodules on legs, livedo reticularis, "punched-out" ulcers, digital gangrene, p-ANCA positive, universal multisystemic involvement: myocardial/GI/renal infarction, polyneuritis, CNS, arthralgias, weight loss, HTN, (renal) microaneurysms, orchitis (esp. with HBV)	Various infections/inflammatory conditions: streptococcus, HBV, HCV, CMV, HIV, SLE, IBD, and hairy cell leukemia	Corticosteroids, cyclophosphamide
Polyarteritis nodosa (cutaneous)	SQ nodules, starburst pattern of livedo reticularis, mild fever, nerve and muscle involvement	As above (cPAN represents 10% but is most common form in children, more often strep)	Topical/intralesional steroids, PCN
Microscopic polyangiitis	Palpable purpura, ulcers, splinter hemorrhages, crescentic necrotizing segmental GN, fever, weight loss, myalgias, neuropathy, HTN, p-ANCA (60%); c-ANCA (40%)		Corticosteroids, cyclophosphamide
Granulomatosis with polyangiitis (formerly Wegener's)	Respiratory, renal, sinus, ocular, otologic, CNS, cardiac, joints, nasal nodules/ulcers/saddle nose, pulmonary infiltrates/nodules, SQ nodules, and c-ANCA (85%)	Unknown – distinguish from lymphomatoid granulomatosis – severe EBV+ angioinvasive B-cell lymphoma of skin and lungs	Corticosteroids, cyclophosphamide (treat staph infection and nasal carriage to minimize relapse)
Churg–Strauss syndrome (Allergic granulomatosis)	Asthma, sinusitis, allergic rhinitis, eosinophilia, arthritis, myositis, CHF, renal/HTN, mononeuritis multiplex, palpable purpura, infiltrated nodules, p-ANCA (60%)	Vaccination, leukotriene inhibitors, desensitization therapy, rapid steroid taper	Corticosteroids, cyclophosphamide

Large vessel vasculitis

Giant cell arteritis (temporal)	Tender, temporal artery, polymyalgia rheumatica, unilateral HA, jaw claudication, blindness, F > M, Northern European	Unknown	Corticosteroids
Takayasu arteritis	Constitutional sxs, pulselessness, signs/sxs of ischemia, EN-like nodules, and pyoderma gangrenosum-like lesions	Associations: RA, other CTD	Corticosteroids, cyclophosphamide, surgical revascularization

Other causes of vasculitis: Infections (bacterial – meningococcemia, gonnococcemia, strep, mycobacterial; viral – HSV; fungal), Rheumatoid vasculitis, drug-induced, Lupus, Paraneoplastic, Buerger, and Mondor.

Lymphocytic vasculitis: Pityriasis lichenoides, Pigmented purpuras, Gyrate erythemas, Collagen vascular dz, Degos, Perniosis, Rickettsial, TRAPS

Neutrophilic dermatoses: Sweet, Marshall (+ acquired cutis laxa), Behcet, Rheumatoid, Bowel-associated dermatosis–arthritis syndrome.

Vasculo-occlusive/Microangiopathies: Cryos, Anti-phospholip syndrome, Atrophic blanche/Livedoid, DIC, Purpura fulminans, Coumadin necrosis, TTP, Sneddon (livedo reticularis + cerebrovascular ischemia), Cholesterol emboli, CADASIL, Calciphylaxis, and Amyloid.

Cryoglobulinemia

Cryoglobulinemia type	Monoclonal or polyclonal	Immunoglobulins	Diseases
1 ("Simple/Single")	Single monoclonal	IgM > IgG > IgA or light chain	**Associations:** Lymphoproliferative disorders: lymphoma, CLL, myeloma, and Waldenstrom macroglobulinemia **Manifestations:** Retiform necrotic lesions, acrocyanosis, Raynaud phenomenon, cold urticaria, livedo reticularis, retinal hemorrhage, and arterial thrombosis

Cryoglobulinemia type	Monoclonal or polyclonal	Immunoglobulins	Diseases
2 ("Mixed")	Monoclonal and polyclonal	Monoclonal IgM (RF) complexed to polyclonal IgG	**Associations**: HCV > other autoimmune (Sjögren, SLE, and RA), infections (CMV, EBV, HIV, HBV, and HAV), and lymphoproliferative disorders
			Manifestations: LCV with palpable purpura, arthralgias/arthritis involving PIPs, MCPs, knees and ankles, diffuse GN
3 ("Mixed")	Polyclonal	IgG and/or IgM	**Associations**: HCV, other autoimmune (Sjögren, SLE, and RA), infections (CMV, EBV, HIV, HBV, and HAV), and lymphoproliferative disorders
			Manifestations: LCV with palpable purpura, arthralgias/arthritis PIP, MCP, knees and ankles, and diffuse GN

Rheumatoid factor = Antibody against Fc portion of IgG = Cryoglobulinemia Types 2 (monoclonal RF) and 3 (polyclonal RF)

Meltzer Triad = Purpura, arthralgia, and weakness

Workup: Serum specimen must be obtained in WARM tubes. Immunoglobulins precipitate at cold temperature. Type 1 precipitates in 24 hours, Type 3 may require 7 days.

Cryoglobulinemia: Immunoglobulins which reversibly precipitate on cold exposure
Cryofibrinogen: Fibrinogen, fibrin, and fibronectin which precipitate in the cold
Cold agglutinins: IgM antibodies which promote agglutination of RBCs on exposure to cold, triggering complement activation and lysis of RBCs.
All three groups cause occlusive syndromes in the skin triggered by cold exposure.

Bullous Disorders

Intracorneal/subcorneal

- *Impetigo* – PMNs + bacteria
- *SSSS* – Epidermolytic/exfoliative toxins cleave Dsg 1 (160 kd) (ETA – chromosomal, ETB – plasmid-derived), strain type 71 of phage group II, organisms not usually present on bx, kids <six years or immunosuppressed/renally insufficient adults
- *Staphylococcal toxic shock* – superantigens activate T-cell receptor through Vβ
- *Streptococcal toxic shock* – grp A including (strep pyogenes), 60% have + blood cx (unlike Staphylococcal toxic shock)
- *P. foliaceous* – Dsg 1 (160 kd) (upper epidermis), may have "grains"-like dyskeratotic cells in granular layer of older lesions
  - Endemic – fogo selvagem
  - DIF – intercellular IgG/C3
- *P. erythematosus* (Senear–Usher) – Features of lupus + PF
  - DIF – intercellular IgG/C3 + lupus band
- *Subconeal pustular dermatosis (SPD)* (Sneddon–Wilkinson)
  - Distinguish Sneddon–Wilkinson from pustular psoriasis and IgA pemphigus – IgA Pemphigus has two variants: SPD variant (Ab's to desmocollin 1) and intraepidermal neutrophilic (IEN) variant (AB's to Dsg 1 or 3), 20% IgA monoclonal gammopathy, intercellular IgA (upper epidermis in SPD type but less restricted in IEN type)
- *Infantile acropustulosis*
- *Erythema toxicum neonatorum* – eosinophils, may be intraepidermal
- *Eosinophilic pustular folliculitis*
- *Transient neonatal pustular melanosis* – neutrophils
- *AGEP* – β-lactams, cephalosporins, macrolides, and mercury
- *Miliaria crystalline*

Intraepidermal

- *Palmoplantar pustulosis*
- *Viral blistering diseases*
- *Friction blister* – Acral, just beneath SG
- *EBS* – May be suprabasilar
- *Amicrobial pustulosis associated with autoimmune disease (APAD)*
- *Coma blisters* – May be subepidermal, sweat gland necrosis (EM-like)

Suprabasilar

Acantholysis – *P. vulgaris, P. vegetans*, Hailey–Hailey, and acantholytic AK

Acantholysis + dyskeratosis – Darier, Grover, paraneoplastic pemphigus, and warty dyskeratoma

Other blistering diseases with acantholysis – SSSS, *P. foliaceous*

- *P. vulgaris* – Dsg 3 (130 kd), ~50% also have Ab to Dsg 1 (160 kd), "tombstoning" with adnexal involvement unlike Hailey–Hailey, DIF: intercellular IgG/C3, IIF: 80–90% positivity, fishnet on monkey esophagus (more sensitive than Guinea pig)
- *P. vegetans* – Dsg 3 (130 kd), Dsg 1 (160 kd), Histo: eos > pms (esp. in early pustular lesions), DIF = P. vulgaris,
  Two types of P. vegetans:
  - Neumann type – more common, starts erosive and vesicular, then becomes vegetating
  - Hallopeau type – starts pustular, more benign course
  Should distinguish P. vegetans from pyodermatitis–pyostomatitis vegetans – associated with IBD, DIF-
- *Hailey–Hailey* (Benign familial pemphigus) – Dilapidated brick wall, DIF–
- *Darier* – Acantholytic (more than PV) dyskeratosis (less than H–H)
- *Grover* – Four histo patterns: Darier-like, H–H-like, PV-like, and spongiotic
- *EBS*
- *Pemphigus-like blisters + PPK* – Case report with Ab to Desmocollin 3, BPAg1, LAD

Subepidermal with little inflammation

- *EB*
  - EBS – fragmented basal layer at base of blister, floor: BP Ag, Col IV, laminin, and PAS+ BM
  - JEB – subepidermal, cell-poor, roof: BP Ag; floor: Col IV, laminin, PAS+ BM
  - DEB – subepidermal, cell-poor, roof: BP Ag, Col IV, laminin, PAS+ BM
  - EB types may also demonstrate supepidermal blisters with eos
- *EBA* – Ab to Col VII (290 kd), DIF: linear IgG/C3 at BMZ, EBA variant may also demonstrate supepidermal blisters with PMNs
- *PCT/pseudo-PCT*
- *Burns and cryotherapy*
- *PUVA-induced*
- *TEN*
- *Suction blisters*
- *Bullous amyloidosis*

- *Kindler*
- *Vesiculobullae over scars*
- *Bullous drug*

Subepidermal with lymphocytes

- *EM*
- *Paraneoplastic pemphigus* – Can demonstrate suprabasaliar acantholysis or subepidermal clefting, dyskeratosis, basal vacuolar change, band-like dermal infiltrate, DIF: intercellular IgG/C3 + IgG/C3 at BMZ (~P. erythematosus), IIF: intercellular staining on rat bladder
- *LS&A*
- *LP pemphigoides*
- *Fixed drug*
- *PMLE*
- *Bullous tinea*

Subepidermal with eosinophils

- *BP* – DI: linear BMZ + IgG/C3, Abs to BPAg1 (230 kd, 80% of patients) and/or BPAg2 (180 kd, contains Col 17 and NC16A domain, 30% of patients)
- *Pemphigoid gestationis* (herpes gestationis) – DIF similar to BP, BPAg2 – placental matrix antigen
- *Arthropod bite* – esp. with chronic lymphocytic leukemia

Subepidermal with neutrophils

- *DH* – IgA endomysial ab, DIF: IgA at the dermal papillae (perilesional and uninvolved skin)
- *Linear IgA* – Various antigens including 97 kd (ladinin) or 120 kd (LAD-1) = BPAg2 degradation products (in lamina lucida form), DIF: linear IgA at BMZ (non-lesional skin)
- *CP* (benign mucosal pemphigoid)
- Brunsting–Perry = localized form, head/neck, w/o mucosa
- *Deep lamina lucida (anti-P105) pemphigoid*
- *Anti-P200 pemphigoid*
- *Bullous LE* – Clinically, may be similar to DH or have large hemorrhagic bullae, Ab to Col VII (like EBA), Histo: like DH and often lacks vacuolar change of other forms of LE
- *Sweet*
- *Orf* – May have eos, DIF: C3/IgG at DEJ, IIF: anti-BMZ IgG (binding dermal side of SSS)

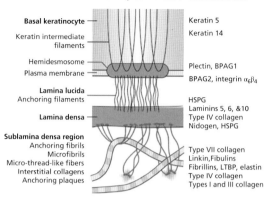

'Laminated' model of the epidermal basement membrane

Basal keratinocyte	Keratin 5
	Keratin 14
Keratin intermediate filaments	
Hemidesmosome	Plectin, BPAG1
Plasma membrane	BPAG2, integrin $\alpha_6\beta_4$
Lamina lucida	
Anchoring filaments	HSPG
	Laminins 5, 6, &10
Lamina densa	Type IV collagen
	Nidogen, HSPG
Sublamina densa region	
Anchoring fibrils	Type VII collagen
Microfibrils	Linkin, Fibulins
Micro-thread-like fibers	Fibrillins, LTBP, elastin
Interstitial collagens	Type IV collagen
Anchoring plaques	Types I and III collagen

Subepidermal with mast cells
• *Bullous mastocytosis*

From JL Bolognia, JL Jorizzo, RP Rapini [Editors], Dermatology. Elselvier, 1st Edition, 2003. p. 436, Figure 30.2, with permission.

Epidermolysis bullosa
Simplex ("epidermolytic EB") – split basal layer tonofilament clumping in basal layer on EM, 40% of EB patients, sxs worse in summer/heat, typically no scarring and not severe (except Dowling–Meara and AR forms)

>   **Mutations:** KRT5 or 14, plectin, mainly AD (99%)
>   **IF**: Col IV, laminin, BPAg on floor of blister

Localized forms:
1. *Weber–Cockayne* (AD) – most common, hyperhidrosis, palms/soles, usually due to KRT5 or 14 mutations, rarely may be due to ITGB4 (integrin β4) mutations
2. *Kallin* (AR) – anodontia/hypodontia, hair/nail anomalies
3. *Autosomal recessive EBS* (AR) – KRT14

Generalized forms:
1. *Koebner* (AD) – mild, (–) Nikolsky, mucous membrane and nails are nl
2. *Dowling–Meara* (AD) – herpetiform pattern, hemorrhagic bullae, milia, oral involvement, dystrophic/absent nails, alopetic areas, confluent PPK,

improves at ~10 years-old and in adulthood (becomes more restricted to acral/pressure sites)
3. *Ogna* (AD) – hemorrhagic blister and bruising, *plectin* defect but no MD, closely linked to glutamic pyruvic transaminase
4. *Mottled pigmentation* (AD) – reticulated hyperpigmentation
5. *Muscular dystrophy* (AR) – *plectin* defect, blisters at birth with scarring, neuromuscular dz
6. *Pyloric atresia* (AD, AR) – *plectin* defect, may be lethal, single family reported (*J Invest Dermatol.* 2005 Jan;124(1):111–115)

Junctional – split lamina lucida, defect in hemidesmosome, <10% of EB patients, oral lesions, absent/dystrophic nails, dysplastic teeth, usually no scarring/milia
   Mutations: laminin 5, α6β4 (ITGA6, ITGB4), BPAg2, all AR except Traupe–Belter–Kolde–Voss
   IF: Col IV, laminin on floor; BPAg on roof

1. *Herlitz* (EB letalis or gravis) – defect: laminin 5, very severe generalized dz – may be fatal (often during infancy or childhood), manifest at birth, stereotypical stridor/cry, nonhealing erosions (often large and zygomatic), GI, gallbladder, corneal, vaginal, laryngeal (>esophageal), and bronchial lesions, dystrophic/absent nails, exuberant granulation tissue and bleeding
2. *Non-Herlitz* (non-lethal) – defect: laminin 5, moderately severe generalized dz worse pretibially, bullae smaller and healing, dystrophic nails, risk of SCC, large acquired melanocytic nevi (seen in JEB > DEB or EBS; asymmetric, irregular)
3. *JEB with pyloric atresia* – defect: α6β4, severe mucocutaneous fragility and gastric outlet obstruction, manifest at birth, polyhydramnios during pregnancy
4. *Generalized atrophic benign EB* – defect: COL XVIIA1 (BPAg2), moderately severe generalized dz + enamel defects/oral lesions and atrophic alopecia (~ male-pattern), survive to adulthood, dystrophic nails, "Localized Atrophic" variant also due to COL XVII mutations
5. *JEB letalis with congenital muscular dystrophy* – *Eur Neurol* 1993;33(6):454–460.
6. *Laryngo–Onycho–Cutaneous/Laryngeal and Ocular Granulation tissue in Children from the Indian subcontinent (LOGIC)/Shabbir* – hoarse cry as newborn, erosions and bleeding at tramatic sites, onychodystrophy, conjunctival and laryngeal chronic granulation tissue, symblepharon, blindness, dental enamel hypoplasia, and anemia
7. Others: *Acral, Inversa, Cicatricial, Late-Onset/Progressiva.*

Dystrophic ("dermolytic EB") – split sublamina densa (papillary dermis), >50% of EB patients, defective anchoring fibers, scars and milia.

Mutation: Col VII*

IF: Col IV, laminin, BPAg on roof

Dominant dystrophic EB: manifest at birth, bullae on extensor surfaces, (+) Nikolsky, (onion) scars and atrophy, milia on ears, hands, arms, and legs, mucous membrane/esophagus involved, nail dystrophy, scarring tip of tongue, improve w/ time.

1. *Albopapuloid* (Pasini, Pretibial with lichenoid features) – white papules on trunk not preceded by bullae, more severe, present in adolescence
2. *Cockayne–Touraine* – hypertrophic scars, more limited
3. *Bart* – aplasia cutis (legs), blisters, and nail deformities, rarely with JEB
4. *Dominant transient bullous dermolysis of the newborn* – vesiculobullae at birth, recover by four months, no scars
5. *Pruriginosa* - pruritis, prurigo-like lesions, nail dystrophy, and may have albopapuloid lesions, may be AR
6. *EBD with subcorneal cleavage* = EBS-superficialis

Recessive dystrophic EB

1. *Generalized – mitis (non-Hallopeau–Siemens)* – severe blisters, generalized, esophageal strictures, ±digital cicatricial pseudosyndactyly
2. *Generalized – gravis (Hallopeau–Siemens)* – very severe, generalized, skin and mucous membrane bullae as newborn, high risk of SCC (primary cause of death), mitten deformity, esophageal stricture, anemia, cardiomyopathy, and fatal amyloidosis (AA type)
3. Others: *Inversa* (axilla, groin), *Centripetal, Recessive Transient Bullous Dermolysis of the Newborn*

*Tumorigenesis in RDEB is increased with production/retention of Col VII containing the NC1 domain (in laminin five-dependent process).
Non-EB genodermatoses with infantile bullae: Kindler, Ichthyosis Bullosa of Siemens, BCIE, Gunther

Major bullous diseases – clinicopathologic findings

Disease	Manifestation	Antigen(s)	Size (kD)	Path	DIF	Rx
Pemphigus foliaceus	Crusted, scaly erosions, seborrheic distribution, positive Nikolsky, non-mucosal	Dsg 1 Plakoglobin	160 85	Acantholysis in upper epidermis, split in SG or right below SC	Intercellular IgG/C3, often superficial, may be throughout epidermis	Topical steroids if mild, systemics similar to PV if generalized
Pemphigus vegetans	Flaccid bullae, erosions, fungoid vegetations, intertriginous, head, mucous membrane, two subtypes: Neumann – severe, Hallopeau – mild	Dsg 3 Dsg 1 Plakoglobin	130 160 85	Like PF	Like PF	Like PF
Pemphigus vulgaris Drug-induced (usually PF-like): penicillamine, IL-2, PCN, thiopurine, rifampin, ACE-I	Flaccid bullae, mucous membrane, + Nikolsky, + Asboe–Hansen	Dsg 3–100% Dsg 1–~50% Plakoglobin	130 160 85	Suprabasilar acantholysis can follow hair, + tombstones	Intercellular IgG (also C3, IgM, and IgA) throughout epidermis. Follow progression with IIF (Dsg 3) (monkey esophagus)	Prednisone, azathioprine, cyclophosphamide, mycophenolate mofetil, and CSA
IgA pemphigus	Flaccid vesicles, superficial pustules in annular/serpentine patterns, trunk (axilla, groin), proximal extremities	SPD variant – Desmocollin 1; IEN variant – Dsg 1/3	105, 115	Pustules: subcorneal or suprabasilar, no acantholysis, PMNs	IgA in upper epidermis (intercellular), no IgG	Dapsone, sulfapyridine, etretinate, UV, and steroids

Disease	Clinical features	Antigen	MW (kDa)	Histology	Immunofluorescence	Treatment/Notes
Pemphigus erythematosus (Senear–Usher)	Erythematous, crusted, erosions, often malar, originally PE = PV + LE	Dsg 1 Plakoglobin	160 85	Like PF	Intercellular and DEJ IgG/C3+ lupus band sometimes	Prednisone
Paraneoplastic pemphigus Associations: NHL, CLL, Castleman, sarcoma, and thymoma	Bullae, erosions, EM-like, lichenoid, SJ-like in mucous membranes	Plectin Desmoplakin 1 BPAg1 Envoplakin Desmoplakin 2 Periplakin Dsg 1,3	500 250 230 210 210 190 170 160, 130	Suprabasilar acantholysis, dyskeratotic keratinocytes, sometimes basal layer degeneration/band-like infiltrate	Intercellular IgG/C3 in epidermis and at BMZ IIF: IgG rat bladder	Treat-associated neoplasm May die from bronchiolitis obliterans
Epidermolysis bullosa acquisita Associations: myeloma, colitis, DM2, leukemia, lymphoma, amyloid, and cancer	Fragile skin, blisters with trauma, atrophic scars, milia, and nail dystrophy	Col VII (also an antigen in bullous LE)	290/145	Noninflammatory subepidermal bullae, PMN >Eos	IgG/C3 linear BMZ IIF anti-BMZ Salt split skin: immunoreactants on dermal side, type IV collagen on roof	Immunosuppression, wound care

continued p.44

Disease	Manifestation	Antigen(s)	Size (kD)	Path	DIF	Rx
Bullous pemphigoid Drug-induced: lasix, PCN, ACE-I, sulfasalzine, and nalidixic acid	Large, tense bullae on trunk and extremities	BPAg1 BPAg2 BPAg2 worse prognosis.	230 180	Subepidermal bullae, eosinophils in superficial dermis (more likely acral in infants)	Linear IgG/C3 at BMZ Salt split skin: immunoreactants on epidermal side, type IV collagen on base	Topical steroids, prednisone, MTX, mycophenolate mofetil, azathioprine, nicotinamide, TCN, sulfapyridine, dapsone
Herpes gestationis/ gestational pemphigoid Associations: HLA-DR 3,4, B8	Pruritic, urticarial plaques on trunk, starts near umbilicus, flares with delivery/OCP, increased risk of prematurity/ SGA, 10% of newborns with skin lesions	BPAg1 BPAg2	230 180	Subepidermal bullae, eosinophils, perivascular infiltrate	Linear C3 ± IgG at BMZ IIF: anti-BMZ IgG by complement-added IIF.	Topical/oral steroids
Dermatitis herpetiformis	Grouped, pruritic papules and vesicles on extensors, HLA+B8, DR3, and DQ2	Endomysial Ag (tissue transglutaminase) Anti-gliadin	—	Subepidermal bullae, PMNs in dermal papillae	Granular IgA ± C3 (tips of papillae)	Gluten-free diet, dapsone, sulfapyridine, TCN, nicotinamide, and colchicine

		Antigen	kDa	Histology	Immunofluorescence	Treatment
Linear IgA Drug-induced: vancomycin, lithium, amiodarone, ACE-I, PCN, PUVA, lasix, IL-2, oxaprozin, IFN-γ, dilantin, diclofenac, and glibenclamide	DH-like vesicles (crown of jewels), BP-like bullae, 50% mucous membrane involvement, children: self-limited	Ladinin LAD-1 BPAg1 BPAg2 Col VII	97 120 230 180 290/145	Subepidermal bullae, PMNs in dermal papillae ± Eos	Linear IgA at BMZ, maybe IgG, no C3	Dapsone, steroids, TCN, nicotinamide, IVIg, and colchicine
Cicatricial pemphigoid (benign mucosal pemphigoid) Drug-induced: penicillamine, clonidine	Primarily mucous membrane, vesicles, erosions, ulcers, scars, erosive gingivitis, and chronic	BPAg1 BPAg2 Laminin-6 Epiligrin (Lam-5) Integrin $\beta4$	230 180 165, 220, 200 165, 140, 105 200	Like BP plus scarring in upper dermis	C3/IgG at BMZ in 80%; IIF+ in 20%, usually IgG	Topical steroids, dapsone, cyclophosphamide, oral steroids, and surgery.

Complement

Complement type	Action
C1q	Binds antibody, activates C1r
C1r	Activates C1s
C1s	Cleaves C2 and C4
C2	Cleaves C5 and C3
C3a	Basophil and mast cell activation
C3b	Opsonin, component at which classical and alternative pathways converge
C4a	Basophil and mast cell activation
C4b	Opsonin
C5a	Basophil and mast cell activation
C5b, 6, 7, 8, 9	Membrane attack complex
C5, 6, 7	PMN chemotaxis
C5b	Basophil chemotaxis

Classical pathway: C1qrs, C1 INH, C4, C2, C3
   Activated by: antibody–antigen complex
      IgM > IgG (except IgG4 does not bind C1q)
Alternative pathway: C3, Properdin, factor B, D
   Activated by: pathogen surfaces
Lectin pathway: Mannan-binding lectin and ficolins serve as opsonins, analogous to C1qrs. Leads to activation of the classical pathway without antibody.
   Activated by: pathogen surfaces
Membrane attack complex: C5–9
C3NeF: Autoantibody that stabilizes bound C3 convertase (C3Bb). IgG isotype against Factor H, inhibits its activity to also drive complement activation. Associated with mesangiocapillary GN and/or partial lipodystrophy.

Angioedema and complement levels

	C1	C1 INH	C2	C3	C4
HAE − 1	Nl	↓	↓	Nl	↓
HAE − 2	Nl	Nl/↑ (but nonfunctional)	↓	Nl	↓
HAE − 3*	Nl	Nl	Nl	Nl	Nl
AAE − 1**	↓	↓	↓	Nl/↓	↓
AAE − 2***	↓	↓	↓	Nl/↓	↓
ACEI-induced	Nl	Nl	Nl	Nl	Nl

*HAE-3 = estrogren-dependent form
**AAE-1 = associated w/ B-cell lymphoproliferation
***AAE-2 = autoimmune form, Ab against C1-INH

Treatments:

- Acute: C1-INH concentrate, FFP, epinephrine, and terbutaline
- Severe Rxn: steroids, antihistamines (H1 and H2 blocker)
- Hereditary angioedema: androgens for acute attacks (stanozolol or danazol), antifibrinolytics (epsilon-aminocaproic acid or tranexamic acid)

Complement deficiencies

Most are AR, except hereditary angioneurotic edema (HAE) which is AD

Complement deficiency	Disease
Early classical pathway (C1, C4, C2)	SLE without ANA, increased infections (encapsulated organisms)
C1 esterase	HAE
Decreased C1q	SCID
C2	Most common complement deficiency, SLE (sometimes HSP, JRA)
C3	Infections, SLE, partial lipodystrophy, Leiner disease
C4	SLE with PPK
C3, C4, or C5	Leiner disease (diarrhea, wasting, and seborrheic dermatitis)
C5–9	Recurrent Neisseria infections

GVHD (Graft vs. Host Disease)

Biopsy for GVHD vs. lymphocyte recovery vs. drug eruption

- In general, path is indistinguishable between GVHD, lymphocyte recovery, and drug eruption except high-grade GVHD.
- Lymphocyte recovery occurs in the first two weeks after transplant.
- Acute GVHD occurs between 3 weeks and 100 days (or longer in persistent, recurrent, or late-onset forms).
- Chronic GVHD classically was considered to occur after 40 days but has no time limit.
- Eosinophils may be found in both drug eruption and acute GVHD.

Marra, DE, et al. Tissue eosinophils and the perils of using skin biopsy specimens to distinguish between drug hypersensitivity and cutaneous graft-versus-host disease. JAAD 2004, 51(4): 543–545.

Zhou, Y et al. Clinica significance of skin biopsies in the diagnosis and management of graft vs host disease in early postallogeneic bone marrow transplantation. Arch Derm 2000, 136(6): 717–721.

HLA associations

Disease	Associated HLA(s)
Abacavir-induced hypersensitivity syndrome	B*5701
Actinic prurigo	DR4 (DRB1*0401), DRB1*0407
Acute generalized erythematous pustulosis	B5, DR11 and DQ3
Allopurinol-induced SJS/TEN	
– Han Chinese	B*5801
Alopecia areata	
– all types	– HLA-DQB1*0301 (DQ7), HLA-DQB1*03 (DQ3), and HLA-DRB1*1104 (DR11)
– severe alopecia totalis/universalis	– DRB1*0401 (DR4) and HLA-DQB1*0301 (DQ7)
Behçet's disease	B51
Bullous pemphigoid	
– Caucasians	– DQB1*0301
– Japanese	– DRB1*04, DRB1*1101, and DQB1*0302
Carbamazepine-induced SJS/TEN	
– Asians and East Indians	– B*1502
– Europeans	– A*3101
Chronic urticarial	DR4, DQ8
Dermatitis herpetiformis	DQ2, B8
Dermatomyositis	
– Juvenile	– DR3, B8
– with anti-JO antibodies	– DR52
– with anti-Mi-2 antibodies	– DR7, DRw53
– adults with dermatomyositis overlap	– B14, B40
– Japanese with juvenile dermatomyositis	– DRB1*15021
Epidermolysis bullosa aquisita	
– Caucasians and African Americans	– DRB1*1501, DR5
– Koreans	– DRB1*13
Erythema dyschromium perstans	
Mexican patients	DR4
Erythema multiforme	DQw3, DRw53, and Aw33
Generalized granuloma annulare	Bw35
Granulomatosis with polyangiitis (formerly Wegener's)	DPB1*0401
Henoch–Schonlein purpura	
With renal disease	B35

Disease	Associated HLA(s)
Juvenile idiopathic arthritis	
– Type II oligo/pauciarticular arthritis	– B27
– Enthesitis-related arthritis	– B27
Leprosy	
– Lepromatous form	– DQ1
– Tuberculoid form	– DR2, DR3
Lichen planus	
– Oral and cutaneous	– DR1
– Oral	
– English patients	– B27, B51, and Bw57
– Japanese and Chinese patients	– DR9
– HCV patients	– DR6
Mixed connective tissue disease	DR4, DR1, and DR2
Mucous membrane pemphigoid	DQw7
Pemphigoid gestationis	DR3, DR4
Pemphigus vulgaris	
– Caucasians	– DRB1*0402, DRB1*1401 and DQB1*0302
– Japanese	– DRB1*14 and DQB1*0503
Psoriasis	
– Early onset	Cw6 (also in late-onset), DRB1*0701/2
Relapsing polychondritis	DR4
– Negatively associated w/ organ involvement	DR6
Rheumatoid arthritis	DR1, DR4, and DRB1
Sacroiliitis	
– Psoriasis	
– Crohns	
– UC	
– SAPHO	
– Reactive arthritis	B27
Sarcoidosis	1, B8, DR3, DRB1, and DQB1
Stevens–Johnson syndrome	
With ocular complications	DQB1*0601
Still's disease, Adult-onset	B14, B17, B18, B35, Bw35, Cw4, DR2, DR7, DR4, and Dw6
Subacute cutaneous lupus erythematosus	B8, DR3
Systemic lupus erythematosus	A1, B8, and DR3

Adapted from *Bolognia JL, Jorizzo JL, Schaffer JV. Dermatology. 3rd Edition. Elsevier; 2012.*

Th profiles

Th profile	Cytokines	Associated diseases
Th1	IL-2, IFN-γ, IL-12	Tuberculoid leprosy, Cutaneous leishmaniasis, Erythema nodosum, Sarcoidosis, Behcet, and MF
Th2	IL-4, IL-5, IL-6, IL-10, IL-9, IL-13	Atopic dermatitis, Lepromatous leprosy, Disseminated leishmaniasis, and Sezary
Th17*	IL-6, IL-15, IL-17, IL-21, IL-22, IL-23, TGFβ	Psoriasis, ACD, and Hyper-IgE
T regulatory	IL-10 or TGFβ (also CD25+ and FOXP3+)	IPEX

*Th17 and Treg differentiation are both TGFβ-dependent, but retinoic acid inhibits Th17 and promotes Treg differentiation.

SPECIAL SITES: GLANDS, NAIL, BONE, MUCOSA

Glands

Glands	Apocrine	Eccrine	Sebaceous
Derivation	Ectodermal (~weeks 16–24)	Ectodermal (~week 14)	Ectodermal (~week 14)
Secretion	Decapitation	Merocrine	Holocrine
Innervation	Sympathetic adrenergic	Sympathetic cholinergic and cholinergic	Androgenic hormones (not innervated)
Purpose	Pheromones	Temperature regulation	Lubricate, waterproof
Locations	Axillary, breast (mammary), external ear (ceruminous), anogenital, eyelid (Moll)	Widespread (especially soles) excluding vermilion border, labia minora, glans, nail beds, and inner prepuce	Everywhere except palms and soles
	Nevus sebaceous		Associated with hair follicles except on mucosa
			Montgomery tubercles – nipples, areola
			Meibomian – deep eyelid; granuloma
			Glands of Zeis – superficial eyelid
			Tyson – foreskin, labia minora
			Fordyce spots – vermilion, buccal
Secretion contents	Fatty acids, cholesterol, triglycerides, squalene, androgens, ammonia, iron, carbohydrates, antimicrobial peptides	NaCl, potassium, bicarbonate, calcium, glucose, lactate, urea, pyruvate, glucose, ammonia, enzymes, cytokins, and Ig's	Ceramides, triglycerides, free fatty acids, squalene, sterol and wax esters, free sterols
Stains*	GCDFP, EMA, CEA, keratins	CEA, S100, EMA, keratins (CAM 5.2, AE1)	EMA, CK15, lipid stains

continued p.52

Glands	Apocrine	Eccrine	Sebaceous
Nonneoplastic conditions	• Fox Fordyce (apocrine miliaria) • Apocrine chromhidrosis – ochronosis, stained undershirts • Axillary bromhidrosis – (E)-3-methyl-2-hexanoic acid, Micrococcus or Corynebacterium, M>F, postpuberty, more common than eccrine bromhidrosis except during childhood	• Neutrophilic eccrine hidradenities: chemo, palmoplantar (pediatric), pseudomonas • Syringolymphoid hyperplasia with alopecia • Miliaria • Lafora – PAS+ granules • Bromhidrosis – drugs (bromides, PCN), food, metabolic, or bacterial degradation of softened keratin • Uremia – small eccrine glands • PAS+ granules in hypothyroidism • Degeneration in lymphoma, heat stroke, coma blister • Ebola particles	• Acne • Vernix caseosa • Juxtaclavicular beaded lines • Chalazion – granuloma involving Meibomian glands • Internal hordeolum (stye) – infection/inflammation of Meibomian glands • External hordeolum (stye) – infection/inflammation of Zeiss or Moll (apocrine)

*Specificity of apocrine vs. eccrine stains is controversial.

52

Nail terminology

Sign	Definition/due to	Associated conditions
Nail plate/nail shape abnormalities		
Anonychia	Absence of nail plate or nail unit	—
Angel wing deformity	Central portion of nail is raised and lateral portions are depressed. Due to nail plate thinning	Lichen planus
Beau line	Transverse (horizontal) ridges affecting all nail plates due to intermittent injury to the nail matrix	Acute systemic illness
Brachyonychia	Short, wide nails (racquet nails)	Rubinstein–Taybi
Clubbing	Bulbous fusiform enlargement of the distal portion of the digit with exaggerated curvature of the nail and flattening of the angle between the proximal nail fold and nail plate	Idiopathic (pahcydermoperiostosis, familial clubbing, hypertrophic osteoarthropathy); Secondary (systemic disease)
Koilonychia	Concave, spoon-shaped nails	Normal variant, iron deficiency anemia (Plummer–Vinson associated with esophageal webbing), diabetes, protein deficiency, connective tissue disease, and acitretin
Habit tic deformity	Longitudinal furrow with multiple transverse parallel lines in the center	Habitual picking of the proximal nail fold, most common the thumb
Longitudinal groove	Central longitudinal groove/ median canaliform dystrophy	Growth at the nail matrix such as myxoid cyst or wart
Longitudinal splitting	Extension of ridging	Lichen planus, psoriasis, darier, and fungal infection
Median nail (canaliform) dystrophy	Central longitudinal ridge with feathering, like branches of a Christmas tree	Unknown, trauma may play a role
Onychocryptosis	Ingrown nail with granuloma	Aggravated by oral retinoids
Onychorrhexis	Longitudinal ridging	Lichen planus, psoriasis, darier, and fungal infection
Onychogryphosis	Thick curved nail plate (ram's horn)	Aging, psoriasis, trauma, and ill-fitting shoes

continued p.54

Sign	Definition/due to	Associated conditions
Onychomadesis	Transverse full thickness break in the nail from temporary growth arrest of the nail plate (unlike Beau line – partial thickness)	Viral infection such as hand–foot–mouth disease
Onychauxis	Thick nail plate	Psoriasis, trauma, and fungal nail infection
Onychoschizia	Splitting/brittle nail	Water damage
Pincer nail	Transverse over-curvature of the nail plate, sometimes causing pain at the lateral nail plates curving into the nail bed/fold	Psoriasis, SLE, Kawasaki disease, cancer, and paronychia congenita
Pitting	Inflammatory condition affecting the nail matrix or bed	Alopecia areata, eczema, and psoriasis
Trachyonychia	Rough opaque nails	Lichen planus, Twenty nail dystrophy (if all nails affected), alopecia areata, atopical dermatitis, and psoriasis
Transverse ridging	—	Eczema, paronychia, and psoriasis
Nail discoloration		
Blue nail	—	Wilson disease (blue lunula), argyria, oral medications (minocycline, AZT, HIV, antimalarials, and busulfan)
Green nail	Striking blue-green color to 1 or 2 nails	Pseudomonas or candida infection
Yellow nail syndrome	Yellow, hard, hypercurved (classic hump), thickened nail	Due to lymphatic obstruction associated with lymphedema, pleural effusion, and ascites. Biotin 10 mg qd and fluconazole may be helpful
Yellow nail	Yellow discoloration	Funal nail infection, yellow nail syndrome, and quinacrine (fluorescent on black light)
Oil drop sign	Salmon colored "oil" spots in the nail bed. Caused by exudation of a serum glycoprotein in psoriasis	Psorasis
Orange streak	Orangish/yellow patch	Dermatophytoma (dermatophyte abscess)

Sign	Definition/due to	Associated conditions
Brown nail	—	Staining (nicotine, potassium permanganate, nail varnish, and podophyllin); chemotherapy, hyddroxyurea
Leukonychia (white nail)	White spots or white discoloration (see also Mee lines and Muehrcke lines)	Trauma (especially to the cuticle that does not follow contour of the matrix), superficial onychomycosis (*T. mentagrophytes* in immunocompetent; *T. rubrum* in HIV and kids)
Transverse leukonychia	Multiple parallel white lines	Manicuring, associated with beau lines
Mee lines	Partial leukonychia. Transverse white bands on several nails (follows the contour of lunula because of matrix growth) These grow out	Arsenic, thallium, or other heavy metal poisoning, systemic disease, chemotherapy, thallium and antimony intoxication, and etretinate therapy
Muehrcke lines	Apparent leukoychia – Double band. Disappears with digital pressure	Hypoalbuminemia, correlates with serum albumin below 2.2 g/100 ml
Half and half nail (Lindsay nail)	Apparent leukonychia: white proximal nail, brown or pink distal nail	Renal failure
Terry nail	White proximal nail (about 2/3), reddened distal nail	Liver cirrhosis
Onycholysis	Lifting of the distal nail plate. Appears white or yellow.	Idiopathic, trauma, contact dermatitis, photoonycholysis (tetracycline, psoralens) and drug reaction (5FU, doxorubicin, captopril, etretinate, isotretinoin, indomethacin, isoniazid, and griseofulvin). Partial onycholysis can occur in psoriasis, thyrotoxicosis, and candida infection.

continued p.56

Sign	Definition/due to	Associated conditions
Melanonychia striata/ Longitudinal melanonychia	Longitudinal hyperpigmented band(s) extending from the proximal nail plate to the distal end of the nail plate	Normal physiologic variant, trauma, pregnancy, Addison disease, post inflammatory hyperpigmentation, Laugier–Hunziker, and Peutz–Jeghers. Can be associated with doxorubicin, 5FU, AZT, and psoralen. Can occur in benign melanocytic nevi and malignant melanoma (Hutchinson sign – extension of the hyperpigmentation through the lunula to the proximal nail fold and cuticle) Candida can sometimes cause candida black melanocyhia at the lateral edge. Exposure to hydroquinone and vitamin C can cause multiple melanonychia that scrapes off
Erythronychia (Red nail)	Longitudinal thin red/brown line beneath the nail plate	• Single nail: Most common – onychopapilloma (V nicking, longitudinal streak, and spincter hemorrhoage), glomus tumor, wart, Bowen's disease, BCC, and melanoma • Multiple nails = inflammation/systemic disease such as subacute bacterial endocarditis (SLE), rheumatoid arthritis, antiphospholipoid syndorome, malignancy, OCP use, pregnancy, psoriasis, and trauma
Splinter hemorrhage (Red nail)	Multiple longitudinal thin red/ brown lines beneath the nail plate	Multiple nails = inflammation/ systemic disease; SLE, rheumatoid arthritis, antiphospholipoid syndorome, malignancy, OCP use, pregnancy, psoriasis, and trauma

Sign	Definition/due to	Associated conditions
Abnormalities of the cuticle, lunula, and nail fold		
Pterygium	V formation scarring from the proximal nail outward	Due to scarring in the nail matrix. Seen in lichen planus, Stevens–Johnson, after trauma.
Ragged cuticle	—	Connective tissue disease, parakeratosis pustulosa
Blue lunula	—	Wilson disease (dark blue); Diabetes (pale blue)
Red lunula	—	Cardiovascular disease, collagen vascular disease, and hematologic malignancy
Absent lunula	—	Anemia or malnutrition
Nail fold telangiectasia	Dilated capillaries at the ponychium (just proximal to the cuticle)	Connective tissue disease (SLE, rheumatoid arthritis, dermatomyositis, and scleroderma)

Disorders or drugs associated with nail, bone, or ocular findings

	Ocular	Skeletal/oral	Nail
5-FU, AZT, Phenophthalein, antimalarials, Hydroxyurea, MCN	—	—	Blue lunulae (also argyria, Wilson, Hgb M dz)
Acitretin	—	—	Koilonychia, onychocryptosis (ingrown/unguis incarnatus, granuloma)
Acne fulminans	—	Osteolytic lesions (clavicle, sternum, long bones, ilium)	—
Albright hereditary osteodystrophy	—	Short stature, brachydactyly, subcutaneous ossifications	—
Alkaptonuria	Osler sign (blue/gray slerae)	Arthritis, blue/gray ear cartilage, calcified cartilage	—

continued p.58

	Ocular	Skeletal/oral	Nail
Alezzandrini	Unilateral retinitis pigmentosa, retinal detachment	—	—
Alopecia areata	Asx punctate lens opacities	—	Pitting, trachyonychia, red spotted lunulae
Antimalarials	Retinopathy	—	Blue lunulae
Apert	Hypertelorism, exophthalmos	Craniosynostosis	Brittle nails, fusion of nails
Argyria	Blue/gray sclera	Blue/gray gums	Azure lunulae
Arsenic	—	Garlic breath, intra-abdominal radio-opacities (acute)	Mees lines
Ataxia-Telangiectasia (Louis–Bar)	Bulbar telangiectasia, strabismus, nystagmus	—	—
Behçet	Retinal vasculitis, uveitis, hypopyon, optic disc hyperemia, macular edema	Arthritis, oral ulcers	—
Buschke–Ollendorff	—	Osteopoikolosis	—
Carbon monoxide poisoning, Polycythemia, CTD, CHF	—	—	Red lunulae
CHIME	Retinal colobomas	—	—
Cicatricial pemphigoid	Conjunctivitis, symblepharon, synechiae, ankyloblepharon	Oral ulcers, hoarseness, dysphagia	—
Cirrhosis, CHF	—	—	Terry nails
Cholesterol emboli	Hollenhorst plaque	—	—
Cockayne	Salt and pepper retinal pigmentary degeneration, optic atrophy, cataracts, strabismus, nystagmus, sunken eyes	Dwarfism, dental caries, osteoporosis, overcrowded mouth	—

	Ocular	Skeletal/oral	Nail
Coffin–Siris	Bushy eyebrows	Hypoplastic/ absent fifth distal phalanges, microcephaly	Hypoplastic/absent fifth nail
Congenital erythropoietic porphyria	Conjunctivitis, scleromalacia perforans	Erythrodontia, acro-osteolysis, osteoporosis	Nail dystrophy
Congenital syphilis	Keratitis	Osteochondritis, saddle nose, mulberry molars, Hutchinson teeth, saber shins	—
Connective tissue disease, Trauma	—	Pterygium inversum unguis	—
Conradi–Hünermann syndrome	Striated cataracts, microphthalmus, optic nerve atrophy	Asymmetric limb shortening, chondrodysplasia punctata – stippled epiphyses (also in CHILD)	—
Cooks syndrome	—	Absent/hypoplastic distal phalanges, brachydactyly fifth finger	Anonychia/ onychodystrophy
Darier–White	—	—	Longitudinal red and white bands and ridging, V-shaped notches, subungual hyperkeratosis
Dermochondrocorneal dystrophy (Francois)	Corneal dystrophy, central opacities	Acral osteochondro- dystrophy, contractures, subluxations, gingival hyperplasia	—
Drug (azidothymidine, tetracycline), Ethnicity, Laugier– Hunziker, Peutz– Jeghers	—	—	Longitudinal melanonychia
Dyskeratosis congenita	Blepharitis, conjunctivitis, epiphora	Dental caries, loss of teeth, premalignant leukoplakia, dysphagia	Longitudinal ridging, thinning, pterygium

continued p.60

	Ocular	Skeletal/oral	Nail
Ehlers–Danlos VI	Fragile sclerae/cornea, keratoconus, hemorrhage, retinal detachment, blue sclerae, angioid streaks	Kyphoscoliosis	—
Ehlers–Danlos VIII	—	Periodontitis, loss of teeth	—
Ehlers–Danlos IX	—	Occipital horns, elbow and wrist defects	—
Endocarditis, trauma, trichinosis, cirrhosis, vasculitis	—	—	Splinter hemorrhages
Epidermal vevus syndrome	Lipodermoids, colobomas, choristomas	Kyphoscoliosis, abnormal skull shape, limb hypertrophy/asymmetry, rickets	—
Fabry disease	Circular corneal opacities (cornea verticillata), tortuous vasculature, spoke-like cataracts	Oral angiokeratoma (tongue), osteoporosis	—
Fanconi anemia	Strabismus, retinal hemorrhages	Radius and thumb defects	—
Fever, stress, meds (chemo)	—	—	Beau lines
Gardner	Congenital hypertrophy of retinal pigmented epithelium	Osteomas, dental abnormalities	—
Gaucher	Pingueculae	Erlenmeyer flask deformity, osteopenia, osteonecrosis	—
Goldenhar (Facioauriculo-lovertebral sequence)	Epibulbar choristomas, blepharoptosis or narrow palpebral fissures, eyelid colobomas, lacrimal drainage system anomalies	Ipsilateral mandibular hypoplasia, ear anomalies, vertebral anomalies	—

	Ocular	Skeletal/oral	Nail
Goltz	Retinal colobomas, microphthalmia, nystagmus, strabismus	Osteopathia striata, lobster claw deformity, cleft lip/palate, hypo/oligodontia, oral papilloma, enamel hypoplasia	—
Gorlin	Cataracts, strabismus, iris colobomas	Odontogenic cysts, fused/bifid ribs, spina bifida occulta, kyphoscoliosis, calcified falx cerebri, frontal bossing	—
Hallermann–Streiff syndrome	Microopthalmia, congenital cataracts, strabismus	Bird-like facies, natal teeth, hypodontia	—
Hemochromatosis	Angioid streaks	—	Koilonychia
Homocystinuria	Ectopia lentis (downward)	Marfanoid habitus, genu valgum, osteoporosis	—
Huriez	—	Scleroatrophy of hands, sclerodactyly, lip telangiectasia	Hypoplasia, ridging, white, clubbing
Hyperimmunoglobulin E syndrome	—	Osteopenia, fractures, scoliosis, hyperextensible joints, candidiasis	Chronic candidiasis
Hypoalbuminemia	—	—	Muehrcke lines
HSV, varicella	Dendritis, keratitis	—	
Incontinentia pigmenti (Bloch-Sulzberger)	Strabismus, cataracts, optic nerve atrophy, retinal vascular changes, detached retina, retinal/iris colobomas	Peg/conical teeth, partial adontia, late dentition	Nail dystrophy, grooving, painful subungual dyskeratotic tumors
Iron deficiency, Syphilis, Thyroid Dz	—	—	Koilonychia
Iso-Kikuchi	—	Index finger hypoplasia, brachydactyly	Hypoplastic index finger nail
JXG	Ocular JXG, hyphema, glaucoma	—	—

continued p.62

61

	Ocular	Skeletal/oral	Nail
KID	Keratoconjunctivitis, blepharitis, photophobia, corneal defects	—	Nail dystrophy
Kindler	—	Cicatricial pseudosyndactyly (between MCP and PIP), leukoplakia, caries	Nail dystrophy
Lamellar Ichthyosis	Ectropion, corneal damage	Phalangeal reabsorption	—
LCH: Hand-Schuller-Christian	Exophthalmos	Bone lesions (esp. cranium)	—
LEOPARD	Hypertelorism	—	—
Leprosy	Madarosis, lagophthalmos, keratitis, episcleritis, corneal anesthesia, blindness	Digital resorption, malaligned fractures, diaphyseal whittling, saddle nose	Longitudinal melanonychia, longitudinal ridging, subungual hyperkeratosis, rudimentary nail
Lichen planus	—	—	Pterygium
Linear morphea	—	Melorheostosis (of Leri; "flowing candle wax")	—
Lipoid proteinosis (Urbach-Wiethe)	Eyelid beading/moniliform blepharosis	Calcifications in hippocampus (suprasellar, "bean-shaped"), thick tongue, hoarseness	—
Mafucci	—	Enchondromas, chondrosarcoma	—
Marfan	Ectopia lentis (upward)	Marfanoid habitus	—
McCune–Albright	—	Polyostotic fibrous dysplasia	—
MEN IIb	Conjunctival neuroma	Plexiform neuromas (oral mucosa, tongue), nodular lips, marfanoid habitus	—
MEN III	—	Marfanoid habitus	—
Menkes	Blue irides, strabismus, aberrant eyelashes, iris stromal hypoplasia	Wormian bones of skull, metaphyseal spurring of long bones	—

	Ocular	Skeletal/oral	Nail
Multicentric reticulohistiocytosis	—	Mutilating arthritis	—
Myxoid cyst, verruca vulgaris	—	—	Median canaliform dystrophy
Naegeli–Franceschetti–Jadassohn	Periocular hyperpigmentation	Syndrome enamel defects, perioral hyperpigmentation	Malaligned great toenails
Nail–Patella	Lester iris, heterochromia irides	Patella aplasia, posterior iliac horns, elbow arthrodysplasia	Triangular lunulae, micro/anonychia
Necrobiotic xanthogranuloma	Scleritis, episcleritis	—	—
NF-1	Lisch nodules, congenital glaucoma, optic glioma	Sphenoid wing dysplasia	—
NF-2	Cataracts, retinal hamartomas	—	—
Nicotine, chemotherapy, potassium permanganate, podophyllin, hydroxyurea (streaks)	—	—	Brown nails
Niemann–Pick	Cherry red spots, macular haloes	—	—
Noonan	Hypertelorism, ptosis, epicanthic folds, downward palpebral fissures, epicanthic folds, refractive errors, strabismus, amblyopia	Pectus carinatum superiorly, pectus excavatum inferiorly, scoliosis, short stature, cubitus valgus, joint hyperextensibility	—
Old age	—	—	Diminished or absent lunulae, longitudinal ridging, onychogryphosis
Olmsted	Corneal anomalies	Osteoporosis, joint laxity, leukoplakia, periorifical keratotic plaques	Nail dystrophy

continued p.64

	Ocular	Skeletal/oral	Nail
Orofaciodigital 1	Colobomas	Bifid tongue, accessory frenulae, lip nodules/ pseudoclefting, supernumerary teeth, frontal bossing, syndactyly	—
Osteogenesis imperfecta	Blue sclera	Brittle bones	—
Pachyonychia congenita	Corneal dystrophy	Oral leukokeratosis, natal teeth	Thickened nails, pincer nails, paronychia
Papillon–Lefévre	—	Dural calcifications, periodonitis, gingivitis (+ acro-osteolysis and onychogryphosis in Haim-Munk)	
Phenylketonuria	Blue irides	Osteopenia	—
Porphyria cutanea tarda	—	—	Photo-onycholysis
Progeria	—	Delayed/abnormal dentition, high-pitched voice, acro-osteolysis, short stature, osteoporosis, persistent open fontanelles	—
Pseudomonas (Pyocyanin)	—	—	Green nails
Psoriasis	—	—	Nail pits, oil spots
PXE (Gronblad–Strandberg)	Angioid streaks (also Paget's Dz of bone, sickle cell, thalassemia, Pb poisoning, HFE, ED6)	Oral yellow papules	
Refsum	Salt and pepper retinitis pigmentosa	Epiphyseal dysplasia	—
Relapsing polychondritis	Conjunctivitis, scleritis, uveitis, corneal ulceration, optic neuritis	Arthritis (truncal), aphthosis	—
Renal disease	—	—	Lindsay nails

	Ocular	Skeletal/oral	Nail
Retinoids, indinavir, and estrogen	—	Isotretinoin – DISH-like hyperostotic changes (bones spurs, calcified tendons, and ligaments)	Pyogenic granuloma
Richner–Hanhart	Pseudoherpetic keratitis	Tongue leukokeratosis	—
Rothmund–Thomson	Cataracts	Anomalies of radius and hands, hypodontia	Nail dystrophy
Rubinstein–Taybi	Long eyelashes, thick eyebrows, strabismus, cataracts	Broad thumb-great toe, clinodactyly of fourth toe and 4th–5th fingers, short stature	Racquet nails
SAPHO	—	Osteomyelitis	—
Schnitzler	—	Bone/joint pain (iliac/tibia), hyperostosis, osteosclerosis	—
Schopf–Schulz–Passarge	Eyelid hidrocystomas	Hypodontia	Nail hypoplasia, dystrophy
Sjögren–Larsson	Retinitis pigmentosa, glistening dots	Short stature	—
Sturge–Weber	Glaucoma, retinal malformations	Tram-track calcifications (skull X-ray)	—
Sweet syndrome	Conjunctivitis, episcleritis, iridocyclitis	Arthritis, arthralgias	—
Tricho-dento-osseus	—	Caries, periodontitis, small teeth, enamel defects, tall stature, frontal bossing	Brittle nails
Trichorhinophalangeal	—	Cone-shaped epiphyses, shortened phalanges and metacarpals, thin upper lip	Nail dystrophy
Trichothiodystrophy	Cataract, conjunctivitis, nystagmus	Osteosclerosis, short stature	Koilonychia, ridging, splitting, leukonychia

continued p.66

65

	Ocular	Skeletal/oral	Nail
Tuberous sclerosis	Retinal hamartomas (mulberry appearing), hypopigmented spots on iris	Dental pits, gingival fibromas, bone cysts, osteosclerosis	Koenen tumor
Vitamin A deficiency	Night blindness, unable to see in bright light, xerophthalmia, Bitot spots, keratomalacia	Growth retardation, excessive periosteal bone (decreased osteoclastic activity)	Brittle nails
Vitamin B$_2$ (Riboflavin) deficiency (Oral–ocular–genital)	Eye redness, burning, fatigue, sandiness, dryness, photosensitivity to light, cataracts	Cheilosis, red sore tongue	—
Vitiligo	Uveitis, depigmented retina	—	—
Von Hippel Lindau	Retinal hemangioblastoma	—	—
Waardenburg	Dystopia canthorum, heterchromia irides	Caries, cleft lip/palate, scrotal tongue	—
Werner	Cataract, glaucoma	Sclerodactyly, osteoporosis, high-pitched voice	—
Wilson	Kayser-Fleischer ring	—	Blue lunulae
Witkop	—	Retained primary teeth	Nail dystrophy (toe>finger)
X-linked chthyosis	Posterior comma-shaped corneal opacities (Descemet's membrane)	—	—
Yellow nail syndrome	—	—	Yellow nails, thick, slowed growth Yellow lunulae – consider insecticides/weed killers (dinitro-orthocresol, diquat, and paraquat), tetracycline, smoking

Source: Adapted from Benjamin A. Solky, MD and Jennifer L. Jones, MD. Boards' Fodder – Bones, Eyes, and Nails.

Genital ulcers

Infection	Organism	Incubation	Presentation	Treatment	Notes
Chancroid	Haemophilus ducreyi	3–10 d	Painful, soft, ragged edges; tender, and unilateral LAN	Azithromycin, ceftriaxone, ciprofloxacin, and erythromycin	"School of fish" gram stain
Primary syphilis (Chancre)	Treponema pallidum	2–4 wk	Painless, indurated, sharp, and raised edges; bilateral and nontender LAN	Penicillin	Rubbery, "ham-colored base"
Genital HSV	HSV	3–7 d	Painful, grouped	Antivirals	—
Lymphogranuloma venereum	Chlamydia trachomatis serovars L1–3	3–12 d	Painless, soft, tender LAN	Doxycycline	"Groove sign" – tender nodes around Poupart's ligament
Donovanosis/granuloma inguinale	Calymmatobacterium/ Klebsiella granulomatis	2–12 wk	Non- or mildly painful, beefy red, bleeding	TMP-SMX, doxycycline, erythromycin, and ciprofloxacin	"Safety pin" Donovan bodies

Other infectious causes of genital ulcers: EBV, Amebiasis, Candida, TB, and Leishmaniasis.

Non-Infectious causes of genital ulcers: Behcet/Apthous, Crohn, Lichen Planus, Tumor, Lichen Sclerosis, Contact, Trauma, Factitial, Fixed drug (NSAIDs, metronidazole, sulfonamide, acetaminophen, TCN, phenytoin, OCPs, phenolphthalein, and barbiturates), Other meds (all-trans-retinoic acid, foscarnet), MAGIC syndrome, Cicatricial/Bullous pemphigoid, Hemangioma, EM/SJS/TEN.

INFECTION AND INFESTATIONS

Fungal Disease / Mycoses

Laboratory tests
Direct microscopy:

KOH: softens keratin, clearing effect can be acclerated by gentle heating
DMSO: softens keratin more quickly than KOH alone in the absence of heat
Chlorazole Black E: chitin specific, stains hyphae green
Parker Black Ink: stains hyphae, not chitin specific
Calcofluor White: stains fungal cell wall (chitin) and fluoresces blue/white
    or apple/green using fluorescent microscopy
India Ink: capsule excludes ink (halo effect) – best for Cryptococcus
    neoformans
Gram Stain: stains blue
PAS: stains red
GMS: stains black
Mucicarmine: pink = capsule; red = yeast
AFB: + if nocardia
Lactophenol cotton blue: use for mounting and staining fungal colonies

Cultures
Sabouraud's Dextrose Agar: standard medium for fungal growth +
    chloramphenicol: inhibits bacteria
    + cycloheximide: use to recover dimorphic fungi and dermatophytes.
        Inhibits crypto, candida (not albicans), Prototheca, Scopulariopsis,
        Aspergillus
Dermatophyte test medium (DTM): use to recover dermatophytes
    Turns medium from yellow to red (pH indicator)

Superficial mycoses
White piedra: Trichosporon. Soft mobile nodules, face, axilla, pubic, and
tropical.
Tx: Shave hair. Systemic antifungal if relapse.

Black piedra: Piedraia hortae. Hard nonmobile nodules, face, scalp, pubic,
and temperate.
Tx: Shave hair. Systemic antifungal if relapse.

Tinea nigra: Phaeoannellomyces (Hortaea) werneckii. Brown macules on
the palms.
Tx: Topical iodine, azole antifungal, terbinafine for two to four weeks
    beyond resolution to prevent relapse. Resistant to griseofulvin.

Tinea versicolor: Malassezia furfur/Pityrosporum ovale. Hypo/
hyperpigmented macules on trunk and extremities.
KOH: "spaghetti and meatballs" – hyphae and spores
Tx: Topical ketoconazole cream, selenium sulfide shampoo, oral
ketoconazole.

DDx superficial bacterial infection
Erythrasma: Corynebacterium minutissima (coproporphyrin III)
Trichomycosis axillaris: Corynebacterium tenuis
Pitted keratolysis: Micrococcus sedentarius

Cutaneous mycoses
Dermatophytes by sporulation characteristics

	Trichophyton	Microsporum	Epidermophyton
Macroconidia	Rare	Many	Many, Grouped
Shape	Cigar/pencil	Spindled/tapered	Club/blunt
Wall	Thin/smooth	Thick/echinulate	Thin/smooth
Microconidia	Many	Few	None

Dermatophytes by mode of transmission
Zoophilic and geographic dermatophytes elicit significant inflammation

Anthrophilic	Humans	*T. rubrum, T. tonsurans, E. floccosum, T. concentricum, T. mentagrophytes* var. interdigitale
Zoophilic	Animals	*T. mentagrophytes var. mentagrophytes, M. canis, T. Verrucosum*
Geographic	Soil	*M. gypseum*

Most common dermatophytes

Tinea corporis, tinea cruris, tinea mannum, tinea pedis	*T. rubrum, T. mentagrophytes, E. floccosum*
Tinea pedis	**Moccasin**: *T. rubrum, E. floccosum*
	Vesicular: *T. mentagrophytes var. mentagrophytes*
Onychomycosis	**Distal subungual**: *T. rubrum*
	Proximal white subungual (HIV): *T. rubrum*
	White superficial: *T. mentagrophytes* (adults); *T. rubrum* (children). Also molds: Aspergillus, Cephalosporium, Fusarium, Scopulariopsis
Tinea barbae	Usually zoophilic dermatophytes (especially *T. mentagrophytes* var. mentagrophytes and *T. verrucosum*) or *T. rubrum*

continued p.70

Tinea capitis	**US**: *T. tonsurans > M. audouinii, M. canis*
	Europe: *M. canis, M. audouinii*
	Favus: *T. schoenleinii > T. violaceum, M. gypseum*
Tinea imbricata/Tokelau	*T. concentricum*
Majocchi granuloma	Often *T. rubrum > T. violaceum, T. tonsurans*

Dermatophytes invading hair

Ectothrix	Fluorescent (pteridine)	*M. canis, M. audouinii, M. distortum, M. ferrugineum,* and *M. gypseum*
	Nonfluorescent	*T. mentagrophytes, T. rubrum, T. verrucosum, T. megninii, M. gypseum,* and *M. nanum*
Endothrix (black dot)	*T. rubrum, T. tonsurans, T. violaceum, T. gourvilli, T. yaoundie, T soudanense,* and *T. schoenleinii* (fluoresces)	

M. gypseum may or may not fluoresce; T. rubrum may be ecto- or endothrix
E. floccosum and T. concentricum do NOT invade scalp hair

Fungal Disease - Clinical Presentation and Management

Disease	Etiology	In Vivo/KOH (Tissue phase)	Culture (Mold phase)	Clinical	Tx
Subcutaneous mycoses					
Sporotrichosis	Sporothrix schenckii	Cigar-shaped budding yeast, Splendore–Hoeppli phenomenon	Hyphae with daisy sporulation	Florist, gardener, farmer- (rose thorn, splinter), Zoonotic (cats) Sporotrichoid spread (fixed if prior exposure) DDx for sporotrichoid spread: leishmaniasis, atypical mycobacteria, tularemia, nocardia, and furunculosis	Itraconazole, SSKI
Chromoblastomycosis	Fonsecaea (most common), Cladosporium, Phialophora, Rhinocladiella	Copper pennies/ Medlar bodies/Sclerotic bodies	—	Small pink warty papule → expands slowly to indurated verrucous plaques with surface black dots	Itraconazole, surgical excision
Phaeohyphomycosis	Exophiala jeanselmei, Wangiella dermatitidis, Alternaria, Bipolaris, Curvularia, Phialophora	Like chromo but with hyphae	—	Solitary subcutaneous draining abscess	Surgical excision, itraconazole

continued p.72

Disease	Etiology	In Vivo/KOH (Tissue phase)	Culture (Mold phase)	Clinical	Tx
Lobomycosis (Keloidal Blastomycosis)	Loboa loboi (Lacazia loboi)	Lemon-shaped cell chains with narrow intracellular bridges Maltese crosses – polarized light	Not cultured	Bottle nose dolphins and rural men in Brazil Confluent papules/ verrucous nodules that ulcerates/crusts Fibrosis may resemble keloids	Surgical excision
Zygomycosis	Conidiobolus coronatus	–	–	Rhinofacial subcutaneous mass	–
Rhinosporidiosis (protozoan)	Rhinosporidium seeberi	Giant sporangia (raspberries) Stains with mucicarmine	Not cultured	Stagnant water, endemic in India and Sri Lanka Nasopharyngeal polyps – may obstruct breathing	Surgical excision
Protothecosis (algae)	Prototheca wickerhamii	Morula (soccer ball)	–	Olecranon bursitis	–
Actinomycotic mycetoma (bacterial)	Actinomadura pelletierii (red) Actinomadura madurae (white) Streptomyces (yellow) Actinomyces israeli Botryomycosis Nocardia (white-orange)	–	–	Volcano-like ulcer and sinus tracts Sulfur grains – yellow, white, red, or brown Tissue swelling Early bone and muscle invasion	Antimicrobial

	Organism	Histology	Clinical features	Treatment
Eumycotic mycetoma (fungal)	*Pseudallescheria boydii* (most common, white-yellow) *Madurella grisea* *Madurella mycetomi* (brown-black) *Exophila jeanselmei* *Acremonium spp.* (white-yellow)	—	Small ulcer with sinus tracts Sulfur grains (white or black) Tissue swelling Lytic bone changes occur late; rare muscle invasion	Antifungal rarely effective; surgical excision
Systemic mycoses				
Coccidiomycosis (San Joaquin Valley Fever)	*Coccidioides immitis/ C. posadasii*	Large spherules, Splendore–Hoepli phenomenon	Boxcars: barrel-shaped arthroconidia alternating with empty cells	
			Southwestern US, Mexico, Central America Primary pulmonary infection (60% asx) Dissemination to CNS, bone Skin lesions more verrucous. May develop EN or EM lesions	Itraconazole, fluconazole, amphoB

continued p.74

73

Disease	Etiology	In Vivo/KOH (Tissue phase)	Culture (Mold phase)	Clinical	Tx
Paracoccidiomycosis (South American Blastomycosis)	*Paracoccidioides brasiliensis*	Mariner's wheel (thin-walled yeast with multiple buds)	Oval microconidia indistinguishable from Blastomyces	South America, Central America Chronic granulomatous pulmonary disease Disseminates to liver, spleen, adrenals, GI, nodes Skin: granulomatous oral/ perioral lesions *Men ≫ women: estrogen may inhibit growth	Ketoconazole
Blastomycosis (Gilchrist disease, North American Blastomycosis)	*Blastomyces dermatitidis*	Broad-based budding yeast with thick walls	Lollipop spores	Southeast US and Great Lakes Primary pulmonary infection Disseminates to CNS, liver, spleen, GU, long bones Skin: verrucous lesion with "stadium edge" borders	Itraconazole, amphoB
Histoplasmosis (Darling disease)	*Histoplasmosis capsulatum*/ *H. duboisii*	Intracellular yeasts in macrophages (parasitized histiocytes, may see halo unlike Leish)	Tuberculate macroconidia	Mississippi/ Ohio river valley basin – bird/bat droppings Most common: pulmonary infection (80–95%) Dissemination to liver, BM, spleen, and CNS Skin: molluscum-like lesions in AIDS	Itrazconaozle, amphoB

74

Opportunistic mycoses

Candidiasis	Candida albicans	Pseudohyphae or true septate hyphae	Part of normal enteric flora	Topicals: nystatin, miconazole, clotrimazole
			Infection is due to predisposing factors: impaired epithelial barrier: burns, maceration, wounds, occlusion, foreign bodies (dentures, catheters), and antibiotics	Systemic: SAF
			Constitutional disorders: DM2, polyendocrinopathy, and malnutrition	
			Immunodeficiency: cytotoxic agents, neutropenia, agranulocytosis, HIV, and chronic granulomatous disease	

continued p.76

Disease	Etiology	In Vivo/KOH (Tissue phase)	Culture (Mold phase)	Clinical	Tx
Cryptococcosis	*Cryptococcus neoformans*	Encapsulated yeasts with surrounding clear halo, "tear drop budding" Stain with mucicarmine, PAS, GMS, or India ink	Bird droppings – usually via pulmonary infection then hematogenous spread to lungs, bones, and viscera. Predilection for CNS. Skin: nasopharygeal papules/pustules, subQ ulcerated abscess	AmphoB fluconazole	
Aspergillosis	*Aspergillus flavus* A. fumigatus A. niger	Phialides with chains of conidia (broom brush) Septate hyphae 45° branching	Infection from inhalation of conidia → pulmonary aspergillosis Allergic bronchopulmonary aspergillosis: hypersensitivity, no tissue invasion Invasive/disseminated aspergillosis: angioinvasive	Allergic: steroid Invasive: SAF	

Zygomycosis/ Mucormycosis	Hyphae broad ribbon like with 90° branching	Most commonly respiratory portal of entry → rhinocerebral infection	AmphoB, surgical excision
	Rhizopus	Rhizoid opposite sporangia	Associated with diabetic ketoacidosis
	Mucor	No rhizoids	
	Absidia	Rhizoids between sporangia	
Penicilliosis	*Penicillium marneffei*	Histo-like intracellular yeasts	Southeast Asia
			Umbilicated lesions, 85% of affected patients have skin lesions	AmphoB, fluconazole

SAF – systemic antifungal: amphoB, liposomal amphoB, fluconazole, itraconazole, voriconazole, and caspofungin.

77

Viruses and diseases

	Family	Examples	Replication site	Genome (+ sense; − antisense)
DNA	Poxviridae	Molluscipox: Molluscum	Cytoplasm	dsDNA
		Orthopox: Vaccinia, smallpox, and cowpox		
		Parapox: Orf, milker's nodule		
	Papillomaviridae	Human papilloma virus	Nucleus	dsDNA
	Herpesviridae	HHV1: HSV1	Nucleus	dsDNA for all
		HHV2: HSV2		
		HHV3: VZV		
		HHV4: EBV		
		HHV5: CMV		
		HHV6: Roseola infantum, reactivation increases drug-induced hypersensitivity syndrome severity		
		HHV7: associated with Pityriasis rosea		
		HHV8: Kaposi sarcoma		
	Hepadnaviridae	HBV	Nucleus w/ RNA intermediate*	Gapped dsDNA
	Adenoviridae	Human adenovirus	Nucleus	dsDNA
	Parvoviridae	Erythema infectiosum	Nucleus	ssDNA
RNA	Paramyxoviridae	Measles, Mumps	Nucleus	−ssRNA
	Togaviridae	Rubella, Chikungunya	Cytoplasm	+ssRNA
	Rhabdoviridae	Rabies	Nucleus	−ssRNA
	Retroviridae	HIV, HTLV	Nucleus	+ssRNA (dsDNA intermediate
	Picornaviridae	Enterovirus (coxsackie; HAV)	Nucleus	+ssRNA
	Flaviviridae	HCV, West Nile, Yellow fever, Dengue	Cytoplasm	+ssRNA
	Filoviridae	Ebola, Marburg	cytoplasm	−ssRNA
	Bunyaviridae	Hantavirus, Rift valley, Congo-Crimean	cytoplasm	−ssRNA
	Arenaviridae	Lassa	cytoplasm	−ssRNA

*Therefore HBV is susceptible to anti-HIV medications.

Human papilloma virus

Disease	Description	Associated HPV type
Verruca vulgaris	Common warts	1, 2, 4
Myrmecia	Large cup-shaped palmoplantar warts	1
Verruca plantaris/ palmaris	Plantar warts	1, 2, 27, 57
Butcher's wart	Warty lesions from handling raw meat	2, 7
Verrucous carcinoma, foot	Epithelioma cuniculatum	2, 11, 16
Verruca planae	Flat warts	3, 10
Epidermodysplasia verruciformis	Inherited disorder of HPV infection and SCCs	3, 5, 8, 12, many others
Buschke and Löwenstein	Giant condyloma	6, 11
Condyloma acuminata	Genital warts	LOW RISK: 6, 11 HIGH RISK: 16, 18, 31 Flat condyloma: 42 Oral condyloma: 6, 11
Oral florid papillomatosis (Ackermann)	Oral/nasal, multiple lesions, smoking/irradiation/chronic inflammation	6, 11
Recurrent respiratory papillomatosis	Laryngeal papillomas	6, 11
Heck disease (Focal epithelial hyperplasia)	Small white and pink papules in mouth	13, 32
Bowen's disease	SCCIS	16, 18
Bowenoid papulosis	Red-brown papules and plaques on the genital resembling genital warts. Histologically SCCIS/ high-grade squamous intraepithelial lesion	16, 18
Erythroplasia of queyrat	Velvety erythematous plaque on the genital. Histologically SCCIS	16, 18
Stucco keratoses	White hyperkeratotic plaques on legs	23b, 9, 16
Ridged wart	Wart with preserved dermatoglyphics	60

Other viral diseases

Viral disease	Description	Cause
Boston exanthem	Roseola-like morbilliform eruption on face and trunk, small oral ulcerations	Echovirus 16
Castleman disease (associated w/ POEMS and paraneoplastic pemphigus)	(Angio)lymphoid hamartoma: hyaline-vascular type, plasma cell, and multicentric/generalized types	HHV-8
Dengue fever (virus may cause Dengue fever, Dengue hemorrhagic fever, or Dengue shock syndrome)	Rash in 50% of **patients**, flushing erythema within 1–2 d of symptom onset, then 3–5 d later a generalized often asx maculopapular eruption with distinct white "islands of sparing," 1/3 mucosal lesions, may be ecchymotic or petechial, incubation 3–14 d	Dengue flavivirus
Eruptive pseudoangiomatosis	Fever, transient hemangioma-like lesions, usually children, often with halo	Echovirus 25 and 32
Erythema infectiosum (Fifth disease)	Children aged 4–10 yr, "slapped cheeks," reticular exanthem, usually extremities, arthropathy in adults, anemia/hydrops in fetus, persistent in Sickle Cell	Parvovirus B19
Gianotti–Crosti syndrome (Papular acrodermatitis of childhood)	Children (often ≤4 yo) with acute onset of often asymptomatic, lichenoid papules on face and extremities, less on trunk	Various: HBV most common worldwide, EBV most common in the United States
Hand-Foot-and-Mouth	Brief mild prodrome, fever, erosive stomatitis, acral and buttock vesicles, highly contagious, mouth hurts, skin asymptomatic	Various Coxsackie viruses, Coxsackie Virus A16, Enterovirus 71
Herpangina	Fever, painful oral vesicles/erosions, no exanthem	Coxsackie Groups A and B, various echoviruses
Hydroa vacciniforme	Vesiculopapules, photosensitivity, pediatric with resolution by early adulthood	EBV (when severe, EBV-associated NK/T-cell lymphoproliferative disorders)

Viral disease	Description	Cause
Infectious mononucleosis (Glandular fever)	Two peaks: 1–6 yo and 14–20 yo; fever, pharyngitis, (cervical) lymphadenopathy, HSM, eyelid edema, 5% rash, leukocytosis, elevated LFTs; 90% get maculopapular exanthema with ampicillin/amoxicillin	EBV (also causes nasopharyngeal carcinoma, posttransplant lymphoproliferative disorder, African Burkitt lymphoma)
Kaposi sarcoma	Vascular tumors	HHV-8
Kaposi varicelliform eruption (Eczema herpeticum)	Often generalized, crusted, vesiculopustular dermatitis; may be umbilicated*; fever, malaise, lymphadenopathy	HSV, may also occur with coxsackie, vaccinia, and other dermatitides
Lichen planus	Purple, Polygonal, Planar, Pruritic, Papules	HCV
Measles (Rubeola)	Prodrome – cough, coryza, conjunctivitis, Koplik spots. Then maculopapular rash spreads craniocaudally. Incubation 10–14 days	Paramyxovirus
Milker's nodules	Similar to Orf	Paravaccinia/ Parapoxvirus
	From infected cows	
Molluscum Contagiosum	Umbilicated papules in children and HIV, or as STD	Poxvirus; 4 MCV subtypes: MCV 1 is most common overall, MCV 2 in immunocompromised
Monkeypox	Smallpox-like but milder and lesions may appear in crops, with prominent lymphadenopathy, and without centrifugal spread	Monkeypox/ Orthopoxvirus (smallpox vaccination is protective)
Oral hairy leukoplakia	Nonpainful, corrugated white plaque on lateral tongue in HIV or other immunosuppressed patients, + smoking correlation	EBV
Orf (Ecthyma Contagiousum)	Umbilicated nodule after animal contact, six stages; sheep, goats, reindeer; self-limiting in ~5 weeks	Orf/Parapoxvirus
Papular/Purpuric stocking-glove syndrome	Young adults, mild prodrome, enanthem, edema, erythema, petechiae, purpura, burning, pruritus on wrists/ankles	Various: Parvovirus B19, Coxsackie B6, HHV-6

continued p.82

Viral disease	Description	Cause
Pityriasis rosea	Usually asymptomatic papulosquamous exanthem	Possibly HHV-7
Ramsey hunt	Vesicular lesions following geniculate ganglion on external ear, tympanic membrane, with ipsilateral facial paralysis and deafness, tinnitus, vertigo, oral lesions	VZV
Roseola infantum (Exanthum subitum, Sixth disease)	Infants with high fever (×3 days) followed by morbilliform rash, 15% have seizure	HHV-6B, rarely HHV-6A or HHV-7
Rubella (German measles)	Mild prodrome, tender LAN, pain with superolateral eye movements, morbilliform rash, spreads craniocaudally, petechial enanthem (Forschiemer spots), incubation 16–18 days	Togavirus
Smallpox	7–17 day incubation, 2–4 day prodrome (fever, HA, and malaise), then centrifugal vesiculopustular rash, lesions are all the same stage, respiratory spread	Variola/Orthopoxvirus
STAR complex	Sore throat, elevated Temperature, Arthritis, Rash	Various: HBV, Parvovirus B19, Rubella
Unilateral laterothoracic exanthem	Age <4 years, morbilliform or eczematous, often starts in axilla, unilateral then spreads	Various: EBV, HBV, Echovirus 6

*Umblicated lesions DDx: molluscum, pox viruses, HSV, histoplasmosis, cryptococcosis, penicilliosis, perforating disorders, leprosy, and GA.
Adapted from Benjamin A. Solky, MD and Jennifer L. Jones, MD. Boards' Fodder – Viruses.

Infections/Bugs

Vector-borne diseases

Disease	Cause	Vector/transmission	Treatment
Acrodermatitis chronica atrophicans (Pick-Herxheimer disease)	*Borrelia afzelii*, *Borrelia garinii*	*Ixodes ricinus*, *Ixodes hexagonus*, *Ixodes persulcatus*	Amoxicillin, doxycycline, cefotaxime, penicillin G
African tick-bite fever	*Rickettsia africae*	*Amblyomma hebraeum*, *Amblyomma variegatum*	Doxycycline
African trypanosomiasis (sleeping sickness)	*Trypanosoma brucei gambiense* (West Africa)	Tsetse fly (*Glossina morsitans*)	Pentamidine isethionate (hemolytic stage) Melarsoprol or eflornithine (CNS involvement)
–Winterbottom sign (posterior cervical LAN)			
–Kerandel's sign (hyperesthesia)	*Trypanosoma brucei rhodesiense* (East Africa)	Tsetse fly (*Glossina morsitans*)	Suramin (hemolytic stage) Melarsoprol (CNS involvement)
Bacillary angiomatosis	*Bartonella henselae*, *Bartonella quintana*	Cat flea (*Pediculus humanus*)	Erythromycin, doxycycline
Brazilian spotted fever	*Rickettsia rickettsii*	Ixodid tick *Amblyomma cajennense* RESERVOIR: Capybara	Doxycycline
Carrion disease (Bartonellosis, Oroya fever, Verruga peruana)	*Bartonella bacilliformis*	Sandfly (*Lutzomyia verrucarum*)	Chloramphenicol (due to frequent superinfxn with salmonella)

continued p.84

Disease	Cause	Vector/transmission	Treatment
Cercarial dermatitis (Swimmer's itch)	Cercariae of animal schistosomes	Snail	Topical corticosteroids
Chagas disease (American trypanosomiasis)	Trypanosoma cruzi	Reduviid bug (assassin bug, kissing bug)	Benznidazole, nifurtimox
Cutaneous larva migrans (Creeping eruption)	Ancylostoma braziliense, Ancylostoma caninum	Animal feces	Albendazole, ivermectin OR Thiabendazole topically
Cysticercosis	Taenia solium	Contaminated pork	Albendazole, praziquantel
Dengue fever	Flavivirus	Aedes aegypti or albopticus	Supportive Tx
Dracunculiasis	Dracunculus medinensis (Guinea fire worm)	Cyclops water flea ingestion	Slow extraction of worm + wound care
			Oral metronidazole facilitates removal
Ehrlichiosis, human monocytic (HME)	Ehrlicha chaffeensis	Amblyomma americanum	Doxycycline, rifampin (pregnancy)
Ehrlichiosis, human granulocytic (HGE), and human granulocytic anaplasmosis (HGA)	Ehrlicha ewingii (HGE), Anaplasma phagocytophilum (HGA)	Ixodes persulcatus and Dermacentor variabilis	Doxycycline, rifampin (pregnancy)
Elephantiasis tropica (Lymphatic filariasis)	Wucheria bancrofti, Brugia malayi, Brugia timori	Culex, Aedes, and Anopheles mosquitos	Diethylcarbamazine
Erysipeloid (of Rosenbach)	Erysipelothrix rhusiopathiae	Fish, shellfish, poultry, and meat	Penicillin G, Cipro, erythromycin/rifampin
Glanders (Farcy)	Burkholderia (Pseudomonas) mallei	Horses, mules, and donkeys	Augmentin, doxycycline, TMP-SMX
Kala-azar (Visceral leishmaniasis)	L. donovani, L. infantum (Old World)	Phlebotomus sand fly	Pentavalent antimony (sodium stibogluconate) or amphotericin
Leishmaniasis, New World (Muco) Cutaneous (Chiclero Ulcer, Uta, Espundia, Bay Sore)	L. chagasi (New World) L. mexicana, L. braziliensis	Lutzomyia sand fly Lutzomyia sand fly	Pentavalent antimony (sodium stibogluconate) or amphotericin

Disease	Organism	Vector / Reservoir	Treatment
Leishmaniasis, Old World Cutaneous (Oriental/Baghdad/Dehli Sore)	*L. tropica; L. major; L. aethiopia, L. infantum*	Phlebotomus sand fly RESERVOIR: Rodents	Pentavalent antimony (sodium stibogluconate)
Loiasis (Calabar, Fugitive swelling)	*Loa loa*	*Tabanid* (horse/mango) fly, *Chrysops* (red, deer) fly	Diethylcarbamazine
Lyme disease	US: *Borrelia burgdorferi* EUROPE: *B. garinii* and *B. afzelli*	NE/GREAT LAKES: *Ixodes scapularis/dammini* WEST US: *I. pacificus* EUROPE: *I. ricinus*	Doxycycline / Amoxicillin if pregnancy or <9 yo
Mediterranean spotted fever (Boutonneuse fever)	*Rickettsia conorii*	*Rhipicephalus sanguinous* (dog tick)	Doxycycline, chloramphenicol, and floroquinolone
Melioidosis (Whitmore disease)	*Burkholderia (Pseudomonas) pseudomallei*	Tropical soil, water	IV ceftazidime (high-intensity phase) then TMZ-SMX and Doxycycline
Myiasis	*Dermatobia hominis* (botfly), *Cordylobia anthropophaga* (tumbu fly), *Phaenicia sericata* (green blowfly)	Mosquito (for *Dermatobia hominis*)	Removal of larvae and treatment with abx for superinfection
Onchocerciasis (River blindness)	*Onchocerca volvulus*	*Simulium* species (black fly)	Ivermectin
Plague (Bubonic)	*Yersinia pestis*	*Xenopsylla cheopis* (rat flea)	Streptomycin, gentamicin
Q Fever	*Coxiella burnetii*	Dried tick feces inhalation	Doxycycline
Rat-bite fever (Haverhill, Sodoku)	*Spirillum minus* (Asia/Africa), *Streptobacillus moniliformis* (US)	Rat bite, scratch, excrement, contaminated food	Penicillin

continued p.86

Disease	Cause	Vector/transmission	Treatment
Relapsing fever – Louse-borne	*Borrelia recurrentis* (Africa, South America)	Pediculosis humanus,	Doxycycline
Relapsing fever – Tick-borne	*Borrelia duttonii, Borrelia hermsii* (Western US)	Ornithodorus genus (soft bodied ticks)	Doxycycline
Rickettsialpox	*Rickettsia akari*	Allodermanyssus (Liponyssoides) Sanguineus (house mouse mite) RESERVOIR: Mus musculus – domestic mouse	Doxycycline
Rift valley fever	*Phlebovirus, bunyavirus*	Aedes	Supportive Tx, ribavirin (investigational)
Rocky mountain spotted fever	*Rickettsia rickettsii*	*Dermacentor andersoni, Dermacentor variabilis*	Doxycycline
Schistosomiasis/Bilharziasis (Cercarial dermatitis, Katayama fever, late allergic dermatitis, perigenital granulomata, extragenital infiltrative)	*Schistosoma mansoni* (GI), *S. japonicum* (GI), *S. haematobium* (urinary system)	Snail	Praziquantel
Scrub typhus (Tsutsugamushi fever)	*Rickettsia/Orientia tsutsugamushi*	Larval stage of trombiculid mite (chigger, *Trombicula/Leptotrombidium akamush*)	Doxycycline
South African tick-bite fever	*Rickettsia conorii*	Rhipicephalus simus, Haemaphysalis leachii, Rhipicephalus mushamae	Doxycycline

Disease	Organism	Vector/Reservoir/Transmission	Treatment
Sparganosis	*Spirometra* (dog and cat tapeworm larvae)	Application/ingestion of infected frog, snake, or fish	Surgical removal
Toxoplasmosis	*Toxoplasma gondii*	Cat feces, undercooked meat, milk	Pyrimethamine and sulfadiazine. First trimester: spiramycin
Trench (Quintana) fever	*Bartonella quintana*	*Pediculus humanus corporis*	Doxycycline, erythromycin
Trichinosis	*Trichinella spiralis*	Undercooked pig, wild game	Steroids for severe symptoms and mebendazole or albenazole
Tularemia (Deer fly fever, Ohara disease)	*Francisella tularensis*	Rabbit, *Dermacentor andersonii*, *Amblyomma americanum*, *Chrysops discalis* (deer fly), domestic cats	Streptomycin
Typhus, endemic; Murine/Flea-borne typhus	*Rickettsia typhi*	*Xenopsylla cheopis* (rat flea)	Doxycycline
Typhus, epidemic; Brill-Zinsser disease/relapsing Louse-Borne typhus	*Rickettsia prowazekii*	*Pediculus humanus*, squirrel fleas RESERVOIR: *Glaucomys volans*-flying squirrel	Doxycycline
Weil disease (leptospirosis)	*Leptospira interrogans icterohaemorrhagiae*	Rat urine	Doxycycline, penicillin, ampicillin, and Amoxicillin
West Nile fever	Arbovirus	*Aedes, culex, and anopheles*	Supportive Tx
Yellow fever	Arbovirus	*Aedes aegypti*	Supportive Tx

Source: Adapted from Benjamin A. Solky, MD and Jennifer L. Jones, MD. Boards' Fodder – Bugs and their Vectors. Treatment adapted from The Medical Letter 2004; 46(1189).

Creatures in dermatology

Creature	Scientific name	Special features
Spiders		
Brown recluse spider	*Loxosceles reclusa*	• VENOM: Sphingomyelinase-D, hyaluronidase • Violin-shaped marking on back • Painless bite but with extensive necrosis • Red, white, and blue sign • Viscerocutaneous loxoscelism: fever, chills, vomit, joint pain, hemolytic anemia, shock, and death • Tx: steroid, ASA, antivenom. Avoid debridement
Black widow spider	*Latrodectus mactans*	• VENOM: A-lactotoxin • Hourglass-shaped red marking on abdomen • Painful bites but no necrosis • Neurotoxin causes chills, GI sxs, paralysis, spasm, diaphoresis, HTN, and shock • Tx: IV Ca gluconate, muscle relaxant, antivenom
Jumping spider	*Phidippus formosus*	• VENOM: Hyaluronidase • Dark body hairs and various white patterns • Very aggressive spider • Painful with toxin venom but no systemic sxs
Wolf spider	*Lycosidae*	• VENOM: Histamine • Lymphangitis, eschar
Sac spider	*Chiracanthium*	• VENOM: Lipase • Yellow colored
Hobo spider	*Tegenaria agrestis*	• Herringbone-striped pattern on abdomen • Painless bite with fast onset induration then eschar • Aggressive spider • Funnel-shaped web
Green lynx spider	*Peucetia viridans*	• Green with red spots • Painful bite with tenderness and pruritus
Tarantula	*Theraphosidae*	• Hairs cause urticaria • Ophthalmia nodosa – if hair gets into eyes→ chronic granuloma formation

Creature	Scientific name	Special features
Caterpillers *Lepidoptera* (urticaria after contact with hairs)		
Puss/Asp	*Megalopyge opercularis*	• Brown woolly flat • Checkerboard eruption
Iomoth	*Automeris io*	• Green with lateral white strip from head to toe
Gypsy/Tent moth	*Lymantria dispar*	• Histamine in lance-like hair • Windborne can cause airborne dermatitis
Saddleback	*Sibine stimulea*	• Bright green saddle on the back
Hylesia moth	*Hylesia metabus*	• Caparito/Venezuela itch
Lonomia caterpillar	*Lonomia achelous/ obliqua*	• Latin America moth, fatal bleeding diathesis
Flies		
Black fly	*Simulium*	• VECTOR: Onchocerciasis
Sand fly	*Phlebotomus*	• VECTOR: *L. donovani, L. tropica, L. infantum, L. major*, and *L. aethiopia*
	Lutzomyia	• VECTOR: *L. mexicana, L. braziliensis*, and *Bartonellosis*
Tsetse fly	*Glossina*	• VECTOR: African trypanosomiasis
Deer fly	*Chrysops*	• VECTOR: Loiasis, tularemia
Botfly larvae	*Dermatobia hominis, Callitroga americana* (US)	• Myiasis when larvae (maggot) infest skin • Other flies whose larvae cause myiasis: Cordylobia anthopophaga (tumbu fly, moist clothing) and Phaenicia sericata (green blowfly, US)
Mosquitoes *Culicidae*		
	Anopheles	• VECTOR: Malaria, filariasis
	Aedes	• VECTOR: Yellow fever, dengue, and filariasis, Chikungunya
	Culex	• VECTOR: Filariasis, West Nile
Fleas *Siphonaptera*		
Human flea	*Pulex irritans*	• May play role in plague, affects other mammals
Cat flea	*Ctenocephalides felis*	• VECTOR: Bartonella hensalae → cat scratch disease and bacillary angiomatosis • PARINAUD: oculoglandular syndrome – granulomatous conjunctivitis and preauricular LAN
Rat flea	*Xenopsylla cheopis*	• VECTOR: R. typhi → endemic typhus • Yersinia pestis → bubonic plaque
Sand/Chigoe flea	*Tunga penetrans*	• Tungiasis • Give tetanus px when tx (surgery or ivermectin)

continued p.90

Creature	Scientific name	Special features
Beetles		
Rove beetle	*Paederus eximius*	• Nairobi eye
		• TOXIN: Pederin
Blister beetle	*Lytta vesicatorial* Spanish fly	• Source of cantharadin
		• Blister if squished on skin
Carpet beetle	*Attagenus megatoma* and *A. scrophulariae*	• ACD with larvae
Lice		
Pubic (Crab)	*Pthirus pubis*	• Shortest and broadest body with stout claws
		• Maculae ceruleae (blue macules) on surrounding skin from louse saliva on blood products
Head lice	*Pediculus capitis*	• Six legs, long narrow body
Body lice	*Pediculus humanus corporis*	• Narrow, longest body
		• Lives in folds of clothing not directly on host
		• VECTORS: Bartonella quintana → trench fever
		• Borellia recurrentis → relapsing fever
		Rickettsia prowazekii → epidemic typhus
Mites		
Scabies	*Sarcoptes scabiei hominis*	• Classic burrows along webspaces, folds
		• Skin scraping for eggs, feces, and mites
		• Tx: Permethrin, lindane, and ivermectin
Straw itch mite	*Pyemotes tritici*	• Found on grain, dried beans, hay, and dried grasses
		• Salivary enzymes are sensitizing
		• May cause systemic sx: fever, diarrhea, and anorexia
Demodex	*Demodicidae*	• Associated with acne rosacea, demodex folliculitis
		• Lives in human hair follicles
Grain mite	*Acarus siro*	• Causes baker's itch
Cheese mite	*Glyciphagus*	• Causes grocer's itch
		• Papular urticaria or vesicopapular eruption
Grocery mite	*Tyrophagus*	• Papular urticaria or vesicopapular eruption
Harvest mite (Chigger)	*Trombicula alfreddugesi*	• Intense pruritus on ankles, legs, and belt line
		• VECTOR: *R. tsutsugamushi* → scrub typhus

Creature	Scientific name	Special features
Dust mite	*Dermatophagoides Euroglyphus*	• Atopy
House mouse mite	*Allodermanyssus sanguineus*	• VECTOR: *R. akari* → rickettsialpox
Walking dander	*Cheyletiella*	• Walking dandruff on dogs/cats • Pet is asx; human gets pruritic dermatitis
Fowl mite	*Ornithonyssus, Dermanyssus*	• Bird handlers most commonly bitten • VECTOR: Western equine encephalitis
Copra Itch	*Tyrophagus putrescentiae*	• Causes itching to dried coconut handlers • Resembles scabies on hand but no burrows
Others		
Scorpions	*Centruroides sculuturatus* and *C. gertschi*	• Neurotoxin causes numbness distally • Systemic: convulsion, coma, hemiplegia, hyper/hypothermia, tremor, restlessness • Arrhythmia, pulmonary edema, hypertension • Local wound care, ice packs, antihistamine
Bedbugs	*Cimex Lectularius*	• Flat with broad bodies, 4–5 mm in length
Bees, wasps, hornets, ants	*Hymenoptera*	• May cause angioedema • VENOM of honeybee: Phospholipase A
Fire ant	*Solenopsis*	• VENOM: Solenopsin D (piperidine derivative)
Reduviid bug	*Hemiptera*	• Kissing/Assassin bugs • VECTOR: Trypanosoma cruzi → Chagas disease • Primary lesion: chagoma • Romana's sign: unilateral eyelid swelling • Acute: 1–2 weeks, fever, LAN, arthralgia, and myalgia • Chronic: progressive heart, megacolon
Centipedes	*Chilopoda*	• Carnivores: venomous claws causes painful bites with two black puncture wounds 1 cm apart
Millipedes	*Deplopoda*	• Vegetarians, emit toxin which burns, blister

continued p.92

Creature	Special features

Water Creatures

Leeches	• Medicinal use associated with Aeromonas hydrophila wound infection
Sea urchin	• Foreign body reaction to spines, use hot water and vinegar for pain relief and inactivating toxins
	• Black sea urchin = Diadema setosa
Sea cucumber	• Toxin holothurin causes conjunctivitis
Dolphins	• Lobomycosis – keloidal blastomycosis, Loboa loboi
Schistosomes (Flukes)	• **Swimmer's itch/Clam Digger's itch (uncovered** skin)
– nonhuman host	• Cercarial forms of flatworm penetrates skin in fresh or salt water (Northern US/Canada), causes allergic reaction
	• Schistosomes of ducks and fowls (nonhuman)
Schistosomes (Flukes)	• *S. mansonii, S. japonicum, S. hematobium* → Schistosomiasis
– human host	• Cercarial forms penetrates skin and enters the portal venous system to the lungs, heart, and mesenteric vessels
Stronglyoides stercoralis (Threadworm)	• **Cutaneous larva currens**
	• Serpiginous **urticarial** burrow on buttocks, groin, and truck
	• May penetrate basement membrane to affect lungs and GI tract (chronic strongyloidiasis, Loefler's syndrome)
	• FAST migration (5–10 cm/h)
	• Tx: Ivermectin
Ancylostoma caninum, *A. braziliense* (Hookworm)	• **Cutaneous larva migrans**
	• Hookworm penetrates skin on foot on sandy beaches
	• Cannot penetrate basement membrane (dead-end host)
	• Larvae deposited by dogs and cat feces
	• Serpiginous **vesicular** burrow
	• SLOW migration (2–10 mm/h)
	• Tx: Thiabendazole or ivermectin

Cnidarian - Jellyfish, Portuguese man of war, sea anemone, coral, and hydroids. Stingers (nematocytes) break through skin causing pain and potential systemic symptoms. Use 3–10% acetic acid or vinegar to fix nematocytes to prevent firing and toxin release

Box jellyfish	• Toxic stings may lead to shock
Portuguese Man of War	• Painful stings may cause hemorrhagic lesions with vesicles
Sea anemone (*Edwardsiella lineate*)	• **Seabather's eruption** (prurituic papules in areas **covered** by swimwear)
Thimble jellyfish (*Linuche unguiculata*)	• Contact with **cnidarian larvae** in salt water (Southern US/Caribbean), larvae trapped beneath swimsuit

Creature	Special features
Exotic pets, others	
Iguana	• Salmonella, Serratia marcescens, and Herpes-like virus
Hedgehog	• Trichophyton mentagrophytes, Salmonella, and atypical mycobacteria
Cockatoo, Pigeon	• Cryptococcus neoformans, avian mites
Chinchilla	• Trichophyton mentagrophytes, Microsporum gypseum, Klebsiella, and Pseudomonas
Fish/Fish tank/ Swimming pool	• Mycobacterium marinum • Treat with TMP-SMX, Clarithromycin, and Doxycycline
Flying squirrel	• *Rickettsia prowazekii, Toxoplasma gondii, Staphylococcus*
Lambs (lambing)	• Lambing ears: farmers develop blistering, itching, painful rash at pinnae (resembles juvenile spring eruption/PMLE)

CONTACT AND PLANT DERMATITIS

Patch testing

- Allergaic contact dermatitis = Type IV delayed-type hypersensitivity
  - Common location of rash – hands, face, and neck
  - Sensitization process takes 10–14 days. Upon reexposure, rash appears in 12–48 hours
  - Contrast with **Irritant Contact Dermatitis –** can occur from single application (no prior exposure) or multiple repeated applications. Usually more painful and burning (rather than itchy with ACD). Combination of exogenous irritant and loss of host barrier function.
    - **Hand Dermatitis** frequently presents with BOTH irritant and allergic contact dermatitis.
  - Contrast with **Type I (immediate hypersensitivity)** – IgE mediated. RAST test.
- Product usage – can trigger even if rarely used. Secondary allergy is common (i.e. product used after rash started)
- Stop immunosuppressive meds:
  - Decrease prednisone < 20 mg/d, ideally stop systemic corticosteroid one to two weeks
  - Stop topical meds 7–14 days prior to patch testing to testing area
  - No sun exposure/phototherapy three weeks prior
  - MTX, TNF-a, mycophenolate mofetil may be ok to continue (limited data showing patients on these meds have positive patch test)
  - Ok to continue antihistamines (except if contact urticaria is suspected)

- Adminstration
  - Use uninvolved skin on the upper back if possible (avoid preexisting dermatitis)
  - Shave back hair prior to day of testing
  - Mark patch sites with surgical pen and highlighter
  - Secure with hypoallergenic adhesive tape
  - Take picture of patch test placement
- Remove patch at 48 hours. Allow transient erythema to subside for 10–15 minutes then mark initial reaction.
- Followup in three to seven days for final read. Must keep back dry until final reading
  - Early reactors: carba mix, thiuram, and balsam of Peru
  - Late reactors: metals (gold), topical corticosteroid, antibiotics, dyes, formaldehyde-releasing preservatives, PPD, cocamide diethanolamine
- Positive reaction does not mean pt's rash is due to that specific antigen (clinical relevance!)

Reactions

–	**Negative – no reaction**
?	**Doubtful reaction**: Macular erythema only
+	**Weak reaction**: Nonvesicular – erythema, infiltration, and possibly papules
++	**Strong reaction**: Edematous or vesicular, erythema and papules
+++	**Extreme reaction**: Spreading, bullous, and ulcerative
IR	**Irritant reaction**
NT	**Not tested**

T.R.U.E Test (Thin-layer Rapid Use Epicutaneous Test): 36 chambers

- 35 allergens (1 negative control #9)
- True test identifies approximately 70–75% of positive reactions in the NACDG screening series of 70 allergens (see below)

Panel 1.3	Panel 2.3	Panel 3.3
1 Nickel sulfate	**13** *p*-tert-Butylphenol formaldehyde resin (PTBP)	**25** Diazolidinyl urea
2 Wood alcohols	**14** Epoxy resin	**26** Quinoline mix
3 Neomycin sulfate	**15** Carba mix	**27** Tixocortal-21-pivalate
4 Potassium dichromate	**16** Black rubber mix	**28** Gold sodium thiosulfate
5 Caine mix	**17** Cl Me Isothizolinone	**29** Imidazolidinyl urea
6 Fragrance mix	**18** Quarterium 15	**30** Budesonide
7 Colophony	**19** Methydibromo-glutaronitrile	**31** Hydrocortison-17-butyrate

Panel 1.3	Panel 2.3	Panel 3.3
8 Paraben mix	**20** p-Phenylenediamine	**32** Mercaptobenzothiazole
9 Negative control	**21** Formaldehyde	**33** Bacitracin
10 Balsamof Peru	**22** Mercapto mix	**34** Parthenolide
11 Eithylenediamine dihydrocholoride	**23** Thimerasal	**35** Disperse Blue 106
12 Colbalt dichloride	**24** Thiuram mix	**36** 2-Bromo-2-nitro-propane-1-3-diol (bronopol)

Common contact allergens

Allergen (standard testing concentration)	Uses/products/cross-reactions (X-RXN)	T.R.U.E test	NACDG rank*
Metal			
Nickel (2.5% pet.)	– Jewelry, watches, alloys, coins, buttons and belt buckles, eyelash curlers, kitchen utensils, scissors, razors, canned food, and electronics (phones)	#1	1
	– Dietary nickel: legumes, dark leafy green vegetables, chocolate, and oat		
	Can have coexisting allergies to chromate and cobalt		
	*Dimethylglyoxime – to detect nickel (turns pink)		
Cobalt (1.0% pet.)	Mixed with metals for strength	#12	14
	– Cement, cosmetics, vitamin B12 injections, pigment in porcelain, paint, crayon, glass, pottery, and blue tattoos		
	X-RXN: nickel, chromate		
Potassium dichromate/ chromium (0.25% pet.)	– Tanned leather, cement, mortar, matches, anti-rust products, paint, plaster, GREEN dyes/ tattoos (pool/ card table felt), metal working, chromic surgical gut suture, and implants	#4	40
	X-RXN: nickel, cobalt		
Gold sodium thiosulfate (0.5% pet.)	– Jewelry, dental restorations, electronics, and glass frames	#28	—
	X-RXN: nickel, cobalt		

continued p.96

Allergen (standard testing concentration)	Uses/products/cross-reactions (X-RXN)	T.R.U.E test	NACDG rank*
Resin/plastics/glue			
2-Hydroxyethyl methacrylate/HEMA (2% pet.)	– Artificial nails, dental work	—	30
Epoxy resin/Bisphenol A (1% pet.)	Allergens: bisphenol A, epichlorohydrin USES: Resin for adhesive – Glues, plastics, adhesives, PVC products, electrical insulation, paints, and protective coatings	#14	35
Methyl methacrylate (2% pet.)	– Artificial nails, dental work, glue for surgical prostheses, and exterior latex house paint	—	46
Ethyl acrylate (0.1% pet.)	Resin, plastics, rubber, and denture	—	51
p-tert-Butylphenol formaldehyde resin (PTBP)	USES: adhesive – Glues, shoes/watchband/handbag (glued leather products), plywood, disinfectants, rubber, varnish, printer inks, and fiberglass may cause depigmentation X-RXN: formaldehyde	#13	62
Ethyl cyanoacrylate (10% pet.)	"Superglue" – Artificial nails glue, liquid bandage	—	66
Toulene-sulfonamide/ tosylamide formaldehyde resin (10% pet.)	Nail lacquer/hardener: eyelid, face, neck, and finger dermatitis	—	47
Rubber compound			
Carba mix (3% pet.)	USES: Rubber stabilizer, fungicides, and pesticides – Elastic bands, condoms, shoes, cements, erasers, health-care equipments (gloves, masks, and tubing) X-RXN: thiurams	#15	11
Thiuram mix (1% pet.)	USES: Rubber additives, prevents degradation of rubber products – Gloves, adhesive, latex, condoms, neoprene, fungi and pesticides, and Disulfiram X-RXN: carba mix, rubber additives	#24	18

Allergen (standard testing concentration)	Uses/products/cross-reactions (X-RXN)	T.R.U.E test	NACDG rank*
Black rubber mix (0.6%pet.)	Isopropyl PPD, cyclohexyl PPD, and diphenyl PPD	#16	45
	USES: Rubber stabilizer		
	– Black and gray rubber products: tires, rubber boots, eyelash curlers, scuba suits, and balls		
	X-RXN: disperse dyes, hydrochlorothiazide, ester anesthetic (PABA), and sulfonamides		
Mercapto mix (1% pet.)	USES: Rubber accelerator	#22	61
	– Rubber products: gloves, makeup sponges, undergarments, and tires		
Mercapto-benzothiazole/ MBT (1% pet.)	USES: Rubber accelerator	#32	58
	– Rubber shoes, tires, undergarments, shoes, and neoprene		
	Co-sensitizer: rubber additives such as dibutyl and diphenyl thiourea		
Mixed dialkyl thioureas (1% pet.)	Rubber antioxidant	—	48
	– Wet suits, shoe insoles, adhesives, copy paper, and photography		
Vehicle and cosmetic ingredients			
Lanolin/ Wool alcohol (50% pet.)	USES: Emulsifier	#2	9
	From: sheep sebum (amerchol, cholesterol, lanosterol, agnosterol, and alcohol)		
	– Cosmetics, soaps, adhesives, and topical agents		
	X-RXN: Aquaphor, Eucerin (cetyl or stearyl alcohols)		
Propylene glycol (30% aq.)	Dimer alcohol to increase drug solubility	—	15
	– Vehicle base in topical meds, valium, lubricant jelly; brake fluid, and antifreeze		
Cocamidopropyl Betaine (1% aq.)	Nonionic surfactant from coconut oil	—	24
	Antigens: amidoamine, DMAPA, and CAPB		
	– Shampoo ("no more tears"), liquid soaps		
	Usually facial pattern rash		

continued p.98

Allergen (standard testing concentration)	Uses/products/cross-reactions (X-RXN)	T.R.U.E test	NACDG rank*
Cocamide DEA (0.5% pet.)	Shampoos, soaps	—	37
Cocamidopropyl betaine (1% aq.)	Nonionic surfactant from coconut oil	—	24
	Antigens: amidoamine, DMAPA, and CAPB		
	– Shampoo ("no more tears"), liquid soaps		
	Usually facial pattern rash		
Benzyl alcohol (10% pet.)	Solvent, preservative, and anesthetic	—	57
	– Plants, essential oils, foods, cosmetics, medications, and paints/lacquers		
Ethylenediamine dihydrochloride (1% pet.)	Industrial stabilizer	#11	59
	– Topical antibiotic/steroid creams (Mycolog cream); dye, rubber, resin, waxes, fuel additive, corrosion inhibitors, and plastic lubricants		
	X-RXN: DETA, epoxy amines, hydroxyzine, aminophylline, and phenothiazine		

Medicaments

Bacitracin (20% pet.)	– Triple antibiotics	#33	10
	Risk groups: leg ulcers, post-op, chronic otitis externa		
	Co-sensitivity: neomycin		
Neomycin sulfate (20% pet.)	Aminoglycoside group	#3	17
	– Triple antibiotics, ear/eye drops		
	X-RXN: aminoglycosides		
	Co-sensitivity: bacitracin		
Chloroxylenol (1% pet.)	– Carbolated vaseline, personal-care products, EKG paste, and surgical scrubs	—	56
Lidocaine (15% pet.)	Amide anesthetic	—	49
	Usually allergy due to paraben preservative and not amide		

Allergen (standard testing concentration)	Uses/products/cross-reactions (X-RXN)	T.R.U.E test	NACDG rank*
Benzocaine (5% pet.)	PABA derivative, ester anesthetic X-RXN: procaine, cocaine, PABA, sulfa meds, thiazide, and PPD	#5: Caine mix	54
Dibucaine (2.5% pet.)	Amide anesthetic X-RXN: lidocaine, bupivicaine	#5: Caine mix	63
Tetracaine (2% pet.)	PABA derivative, ester anesthetic X-RXN: procaine, cocaine, PABA, sulfa meds, thiazide, and PPD	#5: Caine mix	—
Corticosteroids	Four groups based on structure: A – HC/Prednisone – most allergenic B – TMC acetonide (also budesonide, desonide) C – Betamethasone, dexamethasone D1 – Clobetasone-17-propionate D2 – Hydrocortisone-17-butyrate	—	—
Tixocortol pivalate (1% pet.)	Test for group A corticosteroids (Hydrocortisone and Prednisone) – Medicaments, nasal spray	#27	19
Budesonide (0.1% pet.)	Test for group B corticosteroids (TMC and budesonide) X-RXN: D2 steroids (hydrocortisone-17-butyrate)	#30	42
Desoximetasone (1% pet.)	Test for group C corticosteroids (Betamethasone) X-RXN: none – more hypoallergenic	—	69
Clobetasol-17-propionate (1% pet.)	Test for group D1 corticosteroids	—	65
Hydrocortisone-17-butyrate (1% pet.)	Test for group D2 corticosteroids X-RXN: group A steroids (hydrocortisone)	#31	68

continued p.100

Allergen (standard testing concentration)	Uses/products/cross-reactions (X-RXN)	T.R.U.E test	NACDG rank*
Fragrances			
Fragrance mix I – 8 fragrances (8.0% pet.)	1. α-Amyl cinnamic aldehyde	#6	2
	2. Cinnamic alcohol		
	3. Cinnamic aldehyde (toothpaste, gum, and lipstick)		
	4. Hydroxycitronellal – synthetic, floral		
	5. Isoeugenol		
	6. Eugenol – clove		
	7. Evernia prunastri – oak moss/lichen extract		
	8. Geraniol – geranium		
	Found in personal hygiene products (perfumes, flavoring agents, and soaps), household cleaners, air fresheners, paper products, foods and flavorings, and candles		
	X-RXN: colophony, wood tars, turpentine, propolis, benzoin, storax, and balsam of Peru		
Balsam of Peru – *Myroxylon pereirae* resin (25% pet.)	Cinnamic acid, cinnamyl cinnamate, benzyl benzoate, benzoic acid, vanillin, and eugenol	#10	3
	– Fragrances, spices (cloves, cinnamon, and Jamaican pepper), flavoring agent (wine, tobacco, vermouth, and cola), mild antimicrobial properties, and candles		
	X-RXN: Colophony, benzoin, propolis, and fragrance mix		
Fragrance mix II (14% pet.)	1. Citronellol	—	8
	2. Hexyl cinnamal		
	3. Citral		
	4. Coumarin		
	5. Farnesol		
	6. Hydroxyisohexyl 3-cyclohexene carboxaldehyde (Lyral)		
	Found in personal hygiene products		

Allergen (standard testing concentration)	Uses/products/cross-reactions (X-RXN)	T.R.U.E test	NACDG rank*
Cinnamic aldehyde (1.0% pet.)	Oral hygiene products (toothpaste)	—	13
	Allergen is component of Frag mix I and balsam of Peru		
Colophony – rosin, abietic acid	– Adhesives, cosmetics, epilation wax, polish, paint, chewing gum, instrument rosin (violin), topical salves, paper products, wood products (sawdust, wood fillers); from conifer	#7	29
	X-RXN: wood tars, fragranes, spices, and rosin esters		
Limonene (2% pet.)	– Citrus peels, fragrance additive, sanitizers, cleansers, and degreasers	—	70
Preservatives – formaldehyde releasing			
Quaternium-15 (2% pet.)	Sensitivity may be to formaldehyde	#18	5
	#1 cause of hand dermatitis		
	– topical medications, soaps, shampoos, moisturizers, industrial polishes, waxes, ink, latex paints, and adhesives		
Formaldehyde (1% aq.)	– Ubiquitous – fabric finishes (waterproof, anti-wrinkle), cosmetics, cleansers, paper products, paint, pressed wood construction material, and embalming fluids	#21	7
	X-RXN: Formaldehyde-releasing preservatives: quaternium-15, imidazolidinyl urea, diazolidinyl urea, and DMDM-hydantoin		
Diazolidinyl urea (1% pet.)	Germall II	—	20
	– cosmetics, personal-care products		
	X-RXN: Formaldehyde-releasing preservatives		
DMDM hydantoin (1% pet)	• Cosmetics and personal-care products	—	23
	X-RXN: Formaldehyde-releasing preservatives		

continued p.102

Allergen (standard testing concentration)	Uses/products/cross-reactions (X-RXN)	T.R.U.E test	NACDG rank*
Bronopol/2-Bromo-2-nitropropane-1,3-diol (0.5% pet.)	– Topical medications, cosmetics, and personal-care products X-RXN: Formaldehyde-releasing preservatives	#36	26
Imidazolidinyl urea/ Germall 115/Tristat (2% pet.)	– Topical medications, cosmetics, skin/hair products, adhesive, and latex emulsions X-RXN: Formaldehyde-releasing preservatives	#25	28
Preservatives – non-formaldehyde releasing			
MCI/MI (Methyl-choloro-isothiazinolone)/ Kathon CG (0.01% aq.)	USES: biocide and preservative – Personal-care products, cosmetics, hair/skin products (Eucerin), household products (toilet paper, baby wipes), permanent waves, and latex emulsions	#17	4
Iodopropyl butyl carbamate (0.1% pet.)	– Personal-care products, baby wipes, and cosmetics	—	12
Methyldibromo glutaronitrile/MDBGN/ Euxyl K400 (1.0 % pet.)	USES: Preservative to prevent chemical change or microbial action – Cosmetic/personal-care products, paper towels, cutting oils, and adhesives	#19	16
Paraben mix (12% pet.)	Methyl, Ethyl, Propyl, Butyl, Benzyl p-hydroxybenzoate USES: preservatives in personal-care products, cosmetics, and medication X-RXN: PABA, PPD *paraben paradox – may only react on involved skin, patch test to normal skin is negative	#8	22
Thimerosal (0.1% pet.)	Components: thiosalicylic acid and ethyl mercuric chloride – Preservative/antiseptic/vaccine/ eye drops X-RXN: piroxicam, mercury *Frequently allergen is not relevant	#23	—

Allergen (standard testing concentration)	Uses/products/cross-reactions (X-RXN)	T.R.U.E test	NACDG rank*
Quinoline mix	Components: Clioquinol and Chlorquinaldol	#26	—
	– Preservative in antifungals, antibacterial medications, and paste bandage		
	X-RXN: vioform, diiodoquin, and quinoloar		
Hair care			
PPD/p-Paraphenylenediamine (1% pet.)	Blue-black aniline dye	#20	6
	– Permanent hair dyes, henna tattoos, photography solutions, printer inks, oils, gasoline, and black rubber products		
	X-RXN: pro/benzocaine, PABA, azo- and aniline dyes, sulfas, and para-aminosalicylic acid		
Ammonium persulfate (2.5% pet.)	Bleaching agent	—	—
	– Hair bleach, flour		
	Contact urticaria, anaphylactoid rxn		
Glyceryl thioglycolate/ GTG (1% pet.)	Acidic perming/permanent wave solutions	—	—
	Chemical remains in hair shaft for months		
Others			
Disperse Blue 106 (1% pet.)	Fabrics colored dark blue, brown, black, purple, and green	#35	43
	X-RXN: Disperse blue 124, para-phenylenediamine		
Latex	Sap from the rubber tree *Hevae brasiliensis*	RAST test, prick test	—
	– Gloves, condom, and balloon		
	High risk: children with spina bifida, health-care workers		
	X-RXN: avocado, banana, chestnut, kiwi, and papaya		
Gluteraldehyde (1% pet.)	Cold sterilizing solution	—	53
	Health-care workers, embalming fluid, electron microscopy, and hand cleansers		
	X-RXN: formaldehyde		

continued p.104

Allergen (standard testing concentration)	Uses/products/cross-reactions (X-RXN)	T.R.U.E test	NACDG rank*
Propolis (10% pet.)	Dimethylallyl ester of caffeic acid	—	32
	— Bee glue, lipstick, ointments, and mascara		
	— Organic cosmetics		
Parthenolide (3 mcg/cm²)	Plants: daisies, feverfew, and magnolia	#34	—
	— Natural remedies		

Source: Adapted from Goldenberg A, et al. Boards' Fodder – Contact Dermatitis Allergens Summer 2015 and Washau EM et al. Dermatitis. 2015 Jan–Feb;26(1):49–59.

*NACDG Rank Based on Table 8 Significance-Prevalence Index Number from Warshaw et al. *Dermatitis*, 2015; 26:56–57.

Allergic vs. irritant contact dermatitis

	Allergic contact	Irritant contact
Frequency	Less common (20%)	More common (80%)
Reaction	Immunologicl/Type IV delayed-type hypersensitivity (Th1)	Non-immunologic/Local toxic effect
Symptoms	Itchy, common on the hands, face, and neck	More painful and burning (rather than itchy)
Presentation	Hands, face, and neck	Erythema, edema, desquamation, and fissures
	Erythema, edema, vesicles, papules, and lichenification	
Onset	Hours to days	Usually minutes to hour
Distribution	May be focal or spread beyond area of exposure, appear in ectopic	Lesions restricted to areas where irritant damages the skin
Sensitization	Required. Usually takes 10–14 days. Upon reexposure, rash appears in 12–48 hours.	No sensitization. Can occur from single application without prior exposure or with multiple repeated applications. Affects everyone
Risk if atopic	Decreased	Increased
Cross-reaction	Can occur	No cross-reaction
Antigen	Requires lipophilic, low-molecular weight haptens	N/A
		Allergen-specific lymphocytes not involved
Concentration	Independent – can be low dose	Dependent (dose response)
Diagnosis	Patch testing	History and physical
		Negative patch test

Allergens – location specific

Location	Tips	Allergens
Hands/arms	Common to be combination of ICD and ACD 25–40% Irritant 25–75% ACD	• Quarternium-15 • Nickel sulfate • Fragrances, Balsam of Peru • Neomycin/Bacitracin • Rubber accelarators
Periorbital/ eyelids	Most common – cosmetics	• Nickel, gold – transfer from hands • Cobalt (blue eye makeup) • Fragrance, Balsam of Peru • Thimerasol, Neomycin • Nail products
Lip (cheilitis)/ perioral	Should get eval for ACD 85% in females	• Fragrance, Balsam of Peru • Nickel (transfer from hands) • Toothpastes, mouthwash, and flavors (spearmint, cinnamal) • Lipstick, lip balms – Propolis
Scalp and neck	Frequently personal-use products	• Fragrance, Balsam of Peru • PPD (hair dye and black henna) • Glycerol thioglycolate (perm. wave solutions) • Nail products • Shampoos – fragrances, isothiazolinones, Formaldehyde releasers (preservatives), Cocamidopropylbetaine
Axillary	Usually deodorants, textile Or systemic contact derm when feet and groin are also involved Antiperspirant rarely cause ACD	• Fragrance in deodorants (Hydroxyisohexyl-3-cyclohexene, Carboxaldehyde, Isoeugenol, Cinnamicaldehyde) • Natural botanicals • Texile: Disperse blue 106, 124, Urea formaldehyde – (permanent press)
Anogenital	Topically applied products 44% ACD 21% Irritant to soap and cleansers	• Cinnamicaldehyde, • Dibucaine, benzocaine, • Hydrocortisone-17-butyrate, budesonide

continued p.106

Location	Tips	Allergens
Feet	Consider patch test in patients with unexplained chronic dermatitis in lower extremities, feet, and/or sole Feet: Rubber chemicals, adhesives, leather in shoes	• Phenol formaldehyde resin (in adhesives), potassium dichromate, and cobalt chloride • Rubber chemicals – carbamates, thiurams, and mercaptobenzothiazole • Dialkylthioureas(adhesive)
Legs	Consider patch test in patients with unexplained chronic dermatitis in lower extremities, feet, and/or sole Legs: topically applied products	• Fragrance/ Balsam of Peru, • Neomycin, bacitracin • Corticosteroids • Lanolin

Features suggestive of specific irritant/toxin

Acne/folliculitis	Arsenic, oils, glass fibers, asphalt, tar, chlorinated naphthalenes, and polyhalogenated biphenyls
Miliaria	Occlusion, aluminum chloride, UV, and infrared
Alopecia	Borax, chloroprene dimers
Granulomatous	Silica, beryllium, keratin, talc, and cotton

Plants and Dermatoses

Plants causing non-immunologic contact urticaria
Urticaceae family (nettle):
• *Urtica* spp. (dioica) – stinging nettle
• *Dendrocnide* spp. – Australian stinging nettle, may be fatal
Euphorbiaceae family (spurge):
• *Acidoton* and *Cnidosculus* spp.
• Croton plant
Hydrophyllaceae family (water-leaf)

Plants causing mechanical irritant dermatitis
Hedera helix – Araliaceae – common ivy
Opuntia spp. – Cactaceae – prickly pear
Tulipa spp. – Liliaceae – tulip
Ficus and *Morus* spp. – Moraceae – fig, mulberry

Carduus and *Cirsium* spp. – Asteraceae – thistle
Bidens tripartita – Asteraceae – bur marigold
Other Asteraceae – dandelion, lettuce, chicory (irritant latex)

Plants causing chemical irritant dermatitis

Chemical	Plant	Scientific name
Calcium oxalate	Daffodil	*Narcissus* spp. (Amaryllidaceae)
	Century plant	*Agave americana* (Agavaceae)
	Dumb cane	*Dieffenbachia picta* and *Philodendron*
	Philodendrom	spp. (Araceae)
	Pineapple	*Ananas cosmosus* (Bromeliaceae)
	Hyacinth	*Hyacinthus orientalis* (Liliaceae)
	Rubarb	*Rheum rhaponticum* (Polygonaceae)
Thiocyanates	Garlic	*Allium sativum* (Alliaceae)
	Black mustard	*Brassica nigra* (Brassicaceae)
	Radish	*Raphanus sativus* (Brassicaceae)
Cashew nut shell oil	Cashew tree	*Anacardium occidentale* (Anacardiaceae)
Bromelin	Pinapple	*Ananas cosmosus* (Bromeliaceae)
Phorbol esters, diterpenes (latex)	Poinsetta	*Euphorbia pulcherrina* (Euphorbiaceae)
Protoanemonin	Buttercup	*Ranunculus* spp. (Renunculaceae)
Capsaicin	Chili pepper	*Capsicum anuum* (Salanaceae)

Phytophotodermatoses
Apiaceae: hogweed (*Heracleum sphondylium*), celery (*Apium gaveolens*), parsley (*Petroselinum*), parsnips, fennel (*Foeniculum vulgare*)
Rutaceae: lime, orange, lemon, garden rue, Hawaiian lei, gas plant/burning bush
Moraceae: mulberry, fig tree
Fabaceae/Leguminosae: bavachee/scurf-pea (vitiligo tx)

Plant allergic contact dermatitis

Allergen	Family	Plant (Scientific name)
Urushiol	Anacardiaceae	Poison ivy/oak/sumac (*Toxicodendron vernix*)
		Cashew nut tree (*Anacardium occidentale*)
		Mango (*Mangifera indica*)
	Cross-reactions: Ginko biloba, Grevillea	Brazilian pepper tree (*Schinus terebinthifolius*, Florida Holly)
		Indian marking tree nut (*Semecarpus anacardium*)
		Japanese lacquer tree (*Toxicodendron verniciflua*)
		Rengas tree (*Gluta* spp.)
		Poisonwood tree (*Metopium toxiferum*)
Sesquiterpene lactones	Asteraceae (Compositae)	Feverfew (*Tanacetum parthenium*)
		Chrysanthemum (*X Dendranthema*)
		Dandelion *(Taraxacum officinale)*
		Sunflower (*Helianthus annuus*)
		Scourge of India (*Parthenium hysterophorus*, wild feverfew)
		Daisy (*Leucanthemum* spp.)
		Ragweed (*Ambrosia* spp.)
		Marigold (*Tagetes* spp.)
		Artichoke (*Cynara scolymus*)
		Lettuce (*Lactuca sativa*)
		Endive (*Cichorium endiva*)
		Chicory (*Cichorium intybus*)
		Chamomile, mugwort (*Artemisia* spp.)
		Yarrow (*Achillea millefolium*)
Diallyl disulfide	Alliaceae	Onion (*A. cepa*)
		Garlic (*A. sativum*)
		Leek (*A. porrum*)
		Chive
Tuliposide A	Alstromeriaceae and Lillaceae	Tulip, Peruvian lily (*A. auriantiaca* and *A. ligtu)*
Primin	Primulaceae	Primrose (*Primula obconica*)
	Lamiaceae	Peppermint (menthol), spearmint (carvone), lavender, thyme
D-limonene	Myrtaceae	Tea tree (*Melaleuca* spp.)
Colophony and turpentine/carene	Pinaceae	Pine tree (*Pinus* spp.)
		Spruce tree (*Picea* spp.)
Ricin	Castor bean	*Ricinus communis*
Abrin	Jequirity bean	*Abrus precatorius*
Usnic acid, evenic acid, atronorin	Lichens	

TUMORS AND INFILTRATES

Cutaneous T Cell Lyphoma

CTCL WHO-EORTC Classification – Relative Frequency and 5-year Survival

	Relative Frequency (%)	5-Year Survival (%)
Indolent cutaneous T-cell and NK-cell lymphoma		
Mycosis fungoides	44	88
Follicular MF	4	80
Pagetoid reticulosis	<1	100
Granulomatous slack skin	<1	100
Cutaneous anaplastic CD30+ large cell lymphoma	8	95
Lymphomatoid papulosis	12	100
Subcutaneous panniculitis-like T-cell lymphoma	1	82
CD4+ small/medium pleomorphic T-cell lymphoma	2	75
Aggressive cutaneous T-cell and NK-cell lymphoma		
Sézary syndrome	3	24
Cutaneous aggressive CD8+ T-cell lymphoma	<1	18
Cutaneous γ/δ T-cell lymphoma	<1	—
Cutaneous peripheral T-cell lymphoma unspecified	2	16
Cutaneous NK/T-cell lymphoma, nasal-type	<1	—

Source: Modified from Willemze R, et al. WHO-EORTC classification for cutaneous lymphoma. *Blood.* 2005;105: 3798. Based on 1905 patients with primary cutaneous lymphoma registered at the Dutch and Austrian Cutaneous Lymphoma Group 1986–2002.

Mycosis Fungoides Variants
Alibert-Bazin – classic type of MF

Follicular MF – 10% of MF, folliculotropic infiltrates, follicular mucinosis, favors head and neck (esp eyebrow), alopecia, mucinorrhea, pruritic, stage as if classical tumor stage. Less responsive to skin-directed therapies due to the deep follicular localization of MF infiltrate.
- Primary localized – pediatric, H/N, upper trunk, usu resolve within several mos-yrs

- Primary chronic, generalized – adults, concerning for malignant progression
- Secondary – benign (lupus, LSC, ALHE, drug – adalimumab, imatinib), malignant (MF, KS, Hodgkin)

Woringer-Kolopp/Pagetoid Reticulosis – <1% of CTCL, localized, solitary hyperkeratotic patch/plaque, slowly progressive. Good prognosis – No reports of extracutaneous dissemination or disease-related deaths.

Ketron-Goodmann – disseminated pagetoid reticulosis, aggressive.

Granulomatous Slack Skin – pendulous atrophic lax skin, esp. axillae and groin. Associated with MF or Hodgkin lymphoma in 1/3 of cases. Usually indolent, very rare.

Sezary – 5% of MF cases, triad of exfoliative erythoderma, lymphadenopathy, and atypical circulating ("Sezary," "Lutzner," or "mycosis") cells. MF-like immunophenotype but characteristically CD26- and CD3+ but diminished. Change from Th1 to Th2 profile may drive progression to Sezary.

Clonality studies

- Suspected B-cell lymphomas: Flow cytometry (provides kappa:lambda ratio, requires fresh tissue in cell culture), immunoglobulin heavy chain gene rearrangement studies (can use paraffin-embedded tissue), immunohistochemistry for kappa or lambda restriction has low sensitivity (normally κ:λ ratio ~ 3).
- Suspected T-cell lymphomas: $\alpha\beta$ TCR gene rearrangement studies (more sensitive than $\gamma\delta$ TCR gene rearrangement studies, can use paraffin-embedded tissue), flow cytometry (less useful for suspected T-cell lymphomas).
- For detecting CTCL, specificity can be increased by performing TCR rearrangement studies on biopsy specimens from ≥2 anatomic locations looking for a shared clone.

CTCL Workup

1. Complete skin exam: patch, plaque vs. tumor, % skin involvement, check lymph nodes.
2. Skin biopsy of most indurated area: immunophenotype CD2, CD3, CD4, CD5, CD7, CD8, CD20, CD30, CD25, CD56, TIA1, granzyme B, βF1, TCR-CγM1, and TCR gene rearrangement.
3. Blood tests: CBC with diff, Sezary Prep, LFTs, LDH, CMP.

4. Optional for T1: Flow cytometry (CD3, CD4, CD7, CD8, CD26 to assess for expanded CD4+ cells with increased CD4/CD8 ratio or with abnormal immunophenotype, including loss of CD7 or CD26).

5. Radiology: CXR for Stage I and IIa. PET CT chest, abd, pelvis for Stage IIb and above.

CTCL (TNMB) staging

T (Skin)	N (Nodes)	M (Viscera)	B (Blood)
T1 = Patch/plaque < 10%	N0 = None	M0 = None	B0 = <5% Sezary cells
T1a = patch only	N1 = Palpable nodes, path (−)	M1 = Visceral involvement	B1 = >5% Sezary cells, low blood tumor burden
T1b = plaque ± patch	N2 = Palpable nodes, path (+), nodal architecture unaffected		B2 = high blood burden (1000/ ml Sezary cells and positive clone)
T2 = Patch/plaque > 10%			
T3 = Tumor(s)			
T4 = Erythroderma >90%	N3 = Palpable nodes, path (+), nodal architecture effaced		
	Nx = Palpable nodes, no histologic confirmation		

*Adapted from Kim YH. Mycosis fungoides and the Sezary syndrome. *Semin Oncol* 1999;26:276–289. Kim YH et al. Long-term outcome of 525 patients with mycosis fungoides and Sezary syndrome. *Arch Dermatol.* 2003;139:857–866. Amin, Mahul, et al. AJCC Cancer Staging Manual, 8th Ed. Springer International Publishing, 2017. NCCN Guidelines Version 4.2018.

Stage	Clinical involvement	Clinically enlarged nodes	Histologically + nodes	TNMB	5-year survival (%)*
IA	Patch/plaque < 10%			T1 N0 M0	96
IB	Patch/plaque > 10%			T2 N0 M0	73
IIA	Patch/plaque	+Nodes	−Path	T1–2 N1 M0	73
IIB	Tumor(s)	±Nodes	−Path	T3 N0-1 M0	44
IIIA	Erythroderma	−Nodes	−Path	T4 N0 M0	44
IIIB	Erythroderma	+Nodes	−Path	T4 N1 M0	
IVA	Any skin	+Nodes	+ Path	T1–4 N2–3 M0	27
IVB	Visceral involvement			T1–4 N0–3 M1	

CTCL Treatment Algorithm

Stage	First line	Second line	Experimental
IA	SDT or no therapy		
IB, IIA	SDT	TSEB	Cytokines (i.e. Il-2,
	PUVA, NB/BB UVB	Radiotherapy	IL-12, and IFN-γ)
		IFN-α	Pegylated
		PUVA + IFN-α, Retinoids,	liposomal
		or Baxarotene	doxorubicin
		Low-dose MTX	Chlorodeoxy-
		HDAC-inhibitors	adenosine
		(vorinostat, romidepsin)	
IIB	TSEB + Superficial	Denileukin Diftitox	Autologous PBSCT,
	radiotherapy	Baxarotene	mini-allograft
	Combination (2 of 3) tx w/	IFN-α	Zanolimumab
	IFN-α, PUVA, or Retinoids	Chemotherapy	
	HDAC-inhibitors (vorinostat,	Brentuximab vedotin	
	romidepsin)		
III	PUVA ± IFN-α or Retinoids	TSEB	Autologous PBSCT,
	ECP ± IFN-α	Denileukin diftitox	mini-allograft
	MTX	Bexarotene	Zanolimumab
	IFN-α	Chemotherapy	
	HDAC-inhibitors (vorinostat,	Alemtuzumab	
	romidepsin)	Brentuximab vedotin	
IVA, IVB	TSEB or radiotherapy,	IFN-α	Autologous PBSCT,
	chemotherapy	Bexarotene	mini-allograft
	HDAC-inhibitors (vorinostat,	Denileukin diftitox	Zanolimumab
	romidepsin)	Low-dose MTX	
		Alemtuzumab	
		Brentuximab vedotin	
		Palliative	

*Source: Modified from: Whittaker SJ, et al. Joint British Association of Dermatologists and U.K.
Cutaneous Lymphoma Group guidelines for the management of primary cutaneous T-cell lymphomas.
Br J Dermatol 2003 Dec;149(6):1095–1107 and Trautinger F, et al. EORTC Consensus Recommendations
for the Treatment of Mycosis Fungoides/Sézary Syndrome. Eur J Cancer 2006 May; 42(8):1014–1030*

SDT: Skin-directed therapy: Emollients, Topical steroids, Nitrogen mutard
(Mechlorethamine/HN$_2$, Carmustine/BCNU), Bexarotene gel, Imiquimod,
Topical MTX.
ECP: Extracorporeal photopheresis
TSEB: Total skin electron beam
PBSCT: Peripheral blood stem cell transplant
Denileukin diftitox = IL-2/Diptheria toxin fusion.

Acitretin = Retinoic acid receptor. 25–50 mg/d

Baxarotene = Retinoid X receptor specific. 300 mg/m^2/d

Vorinostat = Suberoylanilide hydroxamic acid, SAHA. Histone deacetylase inhibitor. 400 mg po qd with food. May decrease to 300 QD if intolerant.

Alemtuzumab (Campath) = anti-CD52

Zanolimumab = HuMax-CD4

Cutaneous B-cell lymphoma

Type	Clinical	Immunophenotype	5-year survival
Marginal zone	Often solitary lesions on trunk or extremities, possible Borrelia association, tattoo association	BCL2+ BCL6– CD10– IRTA1+	>95%
Primary follicle center	Often solitary/grouped plaques on scalp/forehead or trunk	BCL2– BCL6+ CD10± *	>95%
Diffuse large B-cell	80% on leg of elderly patients, F>M	BCL2+ BCL6+ CD10– MUM1/IRF4+	50%

Other B-cell lymphomas – Intravascular large B-cell lymphoma, Lymphomatoid granulomatosis, CLL (ZAP-70+), Mantle cell lymphoma, Burkitt lymphoma, and B-lymphoblastic lymphoma.

*Secondary cutaneous follicle center lymphoma – BCL2+ BCL6+ CD10+ with t(14;18)

PREVALENCE: 20–25% of primary cutaneous lymphomas are B-cell lymphomas, each of the three major types representing ≤10% of cutaneous lymphomas.

Leukemia cutis

- Affects children > adults
- Skin involvement rarely precedes systemic *dz*
- Except for congenital leukemia, leukemia cutis is a poor prognostic sign, especially with myeloid leukemia
- Frequently associated with extramedullary involvement
- Usually p/w asx papules and nodules
- Other presentations – CLL and HTLV-1-associated leukemia may be pruritic; greenish tumors = chloromas, aka granulocytic sarcomas (due to myeloperoxidase); gingival hypertrophy in AML-M4 and AML-M5; rarely leonine facies
- Histologically, often grenz zone (grenz zone DDx = granuloma faciale, lepromatous leprosy, lymphoma/leukemia/pseudolymphoma, acrodermatitis chronica atrophicans, AFX)
- Common types:
  - AML – 10% of affected **patients** develop leukemia cutis (especially w/ AML-M4 and -M5)

- CLL and Hairy cell leukemia – 5–10% of affected **patients** develop leukemia cutis
- HTLV-1-associated leukemia – very rare type of leukemia (except in Caribbean and Japan) but ~50% of patients may develop leukemia cutis (also get "infective dematitis")

Monoclonal Gammopathies in Dermatology

- Types of monoclonal gammopathies by frequency: monoclonal gammopathy of undetermined significance (MGUS) (65%), multiple myeloma (15%), AL amyloidosis (10%), others (10%): plasmacytoma, Waldenstrom, and lymphoma
- Ig produced by monoclonal gammopathies: IgG (60%), IgM (20%), IgA (15%), extremely rarely IgD or IgE

Disease	Ig type
Direct cutaneous infiltration of cells causing monoclonal gammopathy or depostion of cell products	
Waldenstrom	IgM
AL amyloidosis	IgG
Multiple myeloma	IgG
Plasmacytoma	IgA
Cryoglobulinemia	IgM
Disorders associated with monoclonal gammopathies	
Scleromyxedema	IgG λ
Schnitzler	IgM κ
POEMS	IgA > IgG
Scleredema	IgG κ
Plane xanthoma	IgG
EED	IgA
NXG	IgG κ
Pyoderma gangrenosum	IgA
Sneddon–Wilkinson	IgA
IgA pemphigus	IgA
Sweet	IgG

Source: Daoud et al. Monoclonal gammopathies and associated skin disorders. *J Am Acad Dermatol.* 1999;40(4):507–535.

Tumors and gene associations

Tumor	Gene	Protein	Comment
Anaplastic large cell lymphoma, primary systemic	NPM-ALK fustion	Nucleophosmin-anaplastic lymphoma kinase fusion protein	T(2:5)l(p23;q35); ALK+ systemic anaplastic large cell lymphomas have better prognosis than ALK− systemic large cell lymphomas (primary cutaneous cases are ALK−)
Basal cell carcinoma	PTCH2	Patched	Somatic and BCNS
Clear cell sarcoma	EWS-ATF1	Fusion of Ewing sarcoma and activating transcriptions factor 1	aka "malignant melanoma of the soft parts"
Dermatofibrosarcoma protuberans	COL1A	Collagen 1A	t(17;22)(q22;q13), may have supernumerary ring chromosome
	PDGF	Platelet-derived growth factor	
Hypereosinophilia syndrome	FIP1L1-PDGFRA	F/P fusion	~Chronic eosinophilic leukemia
Mantle cell lymphoma	T(11;14)	Fusion of Bcl-1/Cyclin D1 and immunoglobulin heavy chain	Tumor cells originate from the "mantle zone" of the lymph node; associated with men over the age of 60
Mastocytosis	KIT	C-kit	Adult but not childhood forms
Melanoma*	CDKN2A/p16-INK4A/p14-ARF, BRAF, KIT, NRAS, MITF, PTEN, AKT, MC1R, APAF-1		BRAF often mutated in melanoma and benign melanocytic nevi but unusual in Spitz nevi (similar to NRAS but reverse w/ HRAS); BRAF and NRAS mutations are reciprocal; BRAF phosphorylates ERKs/MAPKs; MC1R mutations impair cAMP synthesis; p16-INK4A inhibits Rb; p14-ARF inhibits p53 degradation

continued p.116

Tumor	Gene	Protein	Comment
Merkel cell carcinoma	Trisomy 6		
Mycosis fungoides	CDKN2A, TNFRSF6 (Fas), JUNB	P16 (INK4a), P14 (ARF)	Largely tumor suppressors
Pilomatricoma	CTNNB1	B-Catenin	Activating mutation; wnt signaling pathway
Seborrheic keratosis	FGFR3, PIK3CA	FGF receptor 3, Phosphatidylinositol kinase 3, catalytic, alpha	Same genes as epidermal nevi
Spitz nevi	11p amplifications	HRAS	Minority of Spitz have HRAS mutations, but much more often than in melanoma

*Melanomas from skin *without* chronic photodamage – BRAF and NRAS mutations but nl CDK4 and CCND1 vs. Melanomas from skin *with* chronic photodamage – increase in number of CDK4 and CCND1 but nl BRAF and NRAS vs. Melanomas from *non-sun-exposed* skin (acral, mucosal) – KIT mutations but nl BRAF and NRAS; Acral MMs have higher degrees of chromosomal aberrations; p53 mutations uncommon in MM except LMM or MM associated with XP-C or Li-Fraumeni. *CDKN2A* mutations also found late in sporadic tumors. *BRAF*-positive mutated melanomas can be treated with vemurafenib, dabrafenib, and other agents that may increase survival.

SYSTEMIC AND METABOLIC DISEASES

Amyloidoses

Stains: PAS +/diastase resistant. + Thioflavin T. Purple with crystal violet.

Birefringence with Congo red (absent after treating with potassium permanganate in AA subtype).

Classification	Type	Symptoms/Subtypes
Primary systemic	AL ≫ AH	40% have skin involvement: waxy skin-colored papules (nose, eyes, and mouth), alopecia, carpal tunnel, pinch purpura, shoulder pad sign. Also may deposit in heart, GI tract, and tongue.
Secondary/reactive systemic	AA	Skin NOT INVOLVED. Deposits in liver, spleen, adrenals, and kidney. Associated with chronic disease: especially TB, leprosy, Hodgkin, RA, and renal cell cancer.
Primary cutaneous	AL	Nodular amyloid: nodule(s) on extremities, trunk
	Keratin	Macular amyloid: pruritic macules interscapular region, associated with nostalgia paresthetica
	Keratin	Lichen amyloid: discrete papules on shins
Secondary cutaneous/tumor associated	Keratin	Following PUVA and in neoplasms
Familial syndromes	AA	Hereditary periodic fever syndromes: Familial Mediterranean fever and TNF receptor-associated periodic syndromes (but not Hyper-IgD)
	AA	Cryopyrin-associated periodic syndromes: Familial cold autoinflammatory, Muckle–Wells, CINCA/NOMID

Amyloid subtype		Association
AL	Ig light chain	Primary systemic, myeloma, plasmacytoma, nodular
AH	Ig heavy chain	Primary systemic, myeloma
AA	(apo) serum AA (SAA)	Reactive systemic, TRAPS, FMF, Muckle–Wells, familial cold autoinflammatory
ATTR	Transthyretin (prealbumin)	Familial amyloid polyneuropathy 1 and 2, Familial amyloid cardiomyopathy, Senile systemic
A β_2M	β_2-microglobulin	Hemodialysis
A β	A β precursor protein (AβPP)	Alzheimer, Down, Hereditary cerebral hemorrhage with amyloidosis (Dutch)

continued p.118

Amyloid subtype	Association
Keratinocyte tonofilaments	Macular and Lichen, MEN IIa, Secondary cutaneous (PUVA, neoplasms)
Apolipoprotein I	Familial amyloid polyneuropathy 3
Atrial natriuretic factor	Isolated atrial
Calcitonin	Medullary thyroid cancer associated
Cystatin	Hereditary cerebral hemorrhage (Icelandic)
Fibrinogen α chain	Familial fibrinogen associated
Gelsolin	Familial amyloid polyneuropathy 4 (Finnish)
Islet amyloid polypeptide	Diabetes mellitus II/Insulinoma associated
Lactoferrin	Corneal lactoferrin associated
Lysozyme	Familial lysozyme associated
Medin/Lactadherin	Aortic medial
Prion Protein/ Scrapie	Creutzfeld-Jacob

Histiocytosis

Histiocytosis	Onset	Clinical features	Associations	Pathology
Langerhans Cell Histiocytosis 2/3 children age 1–3 yo; 1/3 adults – usually pulmonary, often smokers. New classification by organ of involvement:				
1. Restricted LCH:	a. Skin only			
	b. Monostotic lesions ± diabetes insipidus (DI), LN, rash			
	c. Polyostotic lesions ± dDI, LN, rash			
2. Extensive LCH:	a. Visceral organ involvement w/o dysfunction ± dDI, LN, rash			
	b. Visceral organ involvement with dysfunction +/- DI, LN, rash			
Letterer–Siwe	0–2 yo	• Acute, disseminated, and multisystem form	ALL, solid tumors	• CD1a+, S100+, Placental Alk Phos+
		• Resembles seb derm		• Reniform, "coffee-bean" nuclei
		• Fever, anemia, LAN, osteolytic lesions, and HSM		• Birbeck granules
Hand-Schuller-Christian	2–6 yo	• Chronic, multisystem (skin lesions in 1/3)		
		• Classic triad: bone lesions (80%, esp. cranium), DI, and exophthalmos		
Eosinophilic granuloma	Older children/ adults	• Localized, benign		
		• May present with spontaneous fracture or otitis		
Hashimoto–Pritzker	Congenital	• aka Congenital self-healing reticulocytosis		
		• Widespread, red-brown papules or crusts		

continued p. 120

Histiocytosis	Onset	Clinical features	Associations	Pathology
Non-Langerhans Cell Histiocytosis w/o Malignant Features				
Juvenile xanthogranuloma	Early childhood	• **Most common histiocytosis, self-limiting** • Solitary lesion in 25–60% of cases • Head/neck > trunk > extremities • May be systemic (CNS, liver/spleen, lung, eye, and oropharynx) • Eye = most common extracutaneous site, unilateral	• NF1 • Leukemia • NF and juvenile CML	• Small histiocytes, Touton and foreign body giant cells, and foam cells • CD68+, factor XIIIa+, and vimentin+
Benign cephalic histiocytosis	0–3 yo	• 2–5 mm, yellow-red papules on face/neck of infant • Self-limiting • Spares mucous membranes and viscera	Probably same as JXG	aka Histiocytosis w/ intracytoplasmic worm-like bodies (on EM)
Generalized eruptive histiocytoma	Adults > children	• Crops of small, red-brown papules. Widespread axial distrib. • Spontaneous resolution		
Indeterminate cell histiocytosis	Adults > children	• Clinically identical to generalized eruptive histiocytoma		Antigenic markers of both LCH and non-LCH

Multicentric reticulohistiocytosis	Adults (F > M) 30–50 yo	• Joints, skin, mucous membranes (50%) • Papules/nodules – head, hand, elbow, and periungual "coral beads" • Often misdiagnosed as RA • Waxes/wanes, spontaneously remits in 5–10yr Giant cell reticulohistiocytoma = isolated, cutaneous tumor version of MRH	• 25% internal malignancies (gastric, breast, and GU) • 6–17% autoimmune conditions • 30–60% hyperlipidemia	• Histiocytes w/ "ground glass" appearance, oncocytic histiocytes • Mutinucleate giant cells • CD45+, CD68+, CD11b+, HAM56+, and vimentin+ • Usually S100-, Factor XIIIa-, and CD34-
Necrobiotic xanthogranuloma	Sixth decade	• Usu head/neck or trunk: esp. periorbital • Scleritis, episcleritis → possible blindness May have anemia, leukopenia, elevated ESR, and 20% HSM • Often chronic, progressive	• 90% IgG paraproteinemia • 40% cryoglobulinemia	• Hyaline necrobiosis, palisaded granuloma (cholesterol cleft) • Touton and foreign body giant cells • "Touton cell panniculitis" • CD15+, CD4+ • CD1a-, S100-
Xanthoma disseminatum	Any	• Proliferation of foamy histiocytes despite normal serum lipids • Flexors, skin folds, an dmucous membranes (eyes, URT, and meninges → leads to DI) • Usually benign, self-limiting		• Unique scalloped histiocytes in early lesions • Histiocytes, foam cells, chronic infl cells, and Touton and foreign body giant cells • CD68+, Factor XIIIa+ • CD1a-, S100-

Histiocytosis	Onset	Clinical features	Associations	Pathology
Rosai–Dorfman Dorfman aka Sinus histiocytosis with massive lymphadenopathy	10–30 yo, M > F	• Generally benign, self-limiting • Painless, cervical LAN • 40% have extranodal involvement (poor prognosis) • Skin is most common extranodal site		• Expansion of LN sinuses by large foamy histiocytes, plasma cells, and multinucleate giant cells • Emperipolesis • S100+, Factor XIIIa+ • CD1a−
Erdheim–Chester	Middle age	• Similar to XD, but 50% mortality • Symmetric sclerosis of metaphyses/diaphyses of long bones (virtually pathognomonic) → chronic bone pain • DI, renal and retroperitoneal infiltrates, xanthoma-like skin lesions (esp eyelids), pulmonary fibrosis, CNS		• Histiocytes, foam cells • CD68+, Factor XIIIa+ • CD1a− • Usu S100−
Hemophagocytic lymphohistiocytosis	Children	• Rare, life-threatening, rapidly progressive • Dx criteria: F, splenomegaly, cytopenia, hyperTG, hyper-fibrinogenemia, hemophagocytosis on tissue bx • Nonspecific rashes in ~60% • Median survival: 2–3 mo (BM failure, sepsis) • Two types – Primary and Familial HLH – in both cases, triggered by infection, esp. EBV	• CTD, malignancies, HIV *Familial HLH:* • FHL1 – HPLH1 • FHL2 – PRF1 (cytolytic granule content) • FHL3 – UNC13D (cytolytic granule secretion) • FHL4 – syntaxin-11 (membr-associated, SNARE family, docking/fusion)	

Sea-blue histiocytosis	Inherited	• Rare • BM, HSM – also lungs, CNS, eyes, and skin • Nodular lesions; eyelid infiltration	• APOE mutations • One of the manifestations of Niemann–Pick type B • Common (<1/3) in BM bx's of MDS	Large, azure blue, cytoplasmic granules with May-Gruenwald stain (yellow-brown on H&E, dark blue with toluidine or Giemsa)

Non-Langerhans Cell Histiocytosis with Malignant Features

Malignant histiocytosis	M > F 2:1	• Very rare, life-threatening • Liver, spleen, LN, and BM • p/w painful LAN, HSM, fever, and night sweats • Pancytopenia, DIC, and extranodal extension • 10–15% skin involvement (esp. lower legs, buttocks)		Variable

Xanthomas

Type	Distribution/ appearance	Associations
Xanthelasma palpebrarum	Polygonal papules esp. near medial canthus	May be associated with hyperlipidemia (50%) including any primary hyperlipoproteinemia or secondary hyperlipidemias such as cholestasis
Tuberous xanthomas	Multilobulated tumors, pressure areas, extensors	Hypercholesterolemia (esp. LDL), familial dysbetalipoproteinemia (type 3/broad beta dz), familial hypercholesterolemia (type 2), secondary hyperlipidemias (nephrotic syndrome, hypothyroidism)
Tendinous xanthomas	Subcutaneous nodules esp. extensor tendons of hands, feet, Achilles, and trauma	Severe hypercholesterolemia (esp. LDL), particularly type 2a, apolipoprotein B-100 defects, secondary hyperlipidemias (esp. cholestasis, cerebrotendinous xanthomatosis, and beta sitosterolemia)
Eruptive xanthomas	Crops of small papules on buttocks, shoulders, extensors, and oral	Hypertriglyceridemia (esp. types 1, 4, and 5 hyperlipidemias), secondary hyperlipidemias (esp. DM2)
Plane xanthomas	Palmar creases	Familial dysbetalipoproteinemia (type 3), secondary hyperlipidemia (esp. cholestasis)
Generalized plane xanthomas	Generalized, esp. head and neck, chest, flexures	Monoclonal gammopathy, hyperlipidemia (esp. hypertriglyceridemia)
Xanthoma disseminatum	Papules, nodules, and mucosa of upper aerodigestive tract	Normolipemic
Veruciform xanthomas	Solitary, oral or genital, adults	Normolipemic

Hyperlipoproteinemias: Fredrickson classification

Type	Name	Defect, AR/AD	Lipid profile	Xanthomas	Other clinical
I	Hyperlipoproteinemia	Lipoprotein lipase, AR	↑ Chylomicrons, chol, TG ↓ LDL, HDL	Eruptive xanthomas (2/3), lipemia retinalis	↑ CAD, HSM, and pancreatitis
IB	Apolipoprotein C-II deficiency	APOC2 AR	Similar to lipoprotein lipase deficiency		
IIA*	Familial hypercholesterolemia, LDL receptor disorder	LDL receptor, AD	↑ LDL, chol, TG	Tuberous, intertriginous, tendinous, planar xanthomas, xanthelasma, and corneal arcus	↑ CAD
	Familial hyper-cholesterolemia, type B	APOB, AD	Same as IIA		
IIB	Combined hyperlipoproteinemia	Heterogeneous	↑ LDL, VLDL, chol, TG	Xanthomas rare	↑ CAD

continued p.126

Type	Name	Defect, AR/AD	Lipid profile	Xanthomas	Other clinical
III	Familial dysbetalipoproteinemia, Broad betalipoproteinemia	APOE, AR	↑ Chylomicron remnants/VLDL, chol, TG	Planar palmar crease, tuberous xanthomas, and xanthelasma	↑ CAD, DM2
IV	Carbohydrate-inducible lipemia	AD	↑ VLDL, TG ↓ HDL	Tuberoeruptive xanthomas	↑ CAD, DM2, obesity, etoh, hypothyroidism, pancreatitis, uremia, myeloma, nephrotic, hypopituitarism, and glycogen storage type I
V	Mixed hyperprebeta-lipoproteinemia and chylomicronemia	APOA5, AR/AD	↑ Chylomicrons, VLDL, TG, chol ↓ LDL, HDL	Eruptive xanthomas, lipemia retinalis	Abd pain, pancreatitis, DM2, HTN, hyperuricemia, OCPs, etoh, and glycogen storage type I

Source: Susan B. Mallory. An Illustrated Dictionary of Dermatologic Syndromes, Second Edition, Taylor & Francis, 2006.

*Other familial hypercholesterolemia syndromes – AR hypercholesterolemia (ARH/LDLR adaptor protein mutations), AD hypercholesterolemia type 3 (PCSK9/PROTEIN CONVERTASE, SUBTILISIN/KEXIN-TYPE, 9 mutations).

Vitamin Deficiencies/Hypervitaminoses

Vitamin A
Vitamin A supplementation helpful in rubeola

Deficiency = Phrynoderma (toadskin)

- Due to fat malabsorption, diet; found in animal fat, liver, and milk
- Night blindness, poor acuity in bright light, Bitot spots, keratomalacia, xerophthalmia, xerosis, follicular hyperkeratosis, fragile hair, apathy, mental and growth retardation

Hypervitaminosis A
- Similar to medical retinoid treatment: dry lips, arthralgias, cheilitis, alopecia, onychodystrophy/clubbing, hyperpigmentation, impaired bone growth, hyperostosis, pseudotumor cerebri, lethary, anorexia

Vitamin B_1 – Thiamine
Deficiency = Beriberi

- Due to diet (polished rice), pregnancy, alcoholism, and GI disease
- Glossitis, edema, glossodynia, neuropathy, Wernicke–Korsakoff, CHF

Vitamin B_2 – Riboflavin
Deficiency

- Alcoholics, malabsorption, neonatal phototherapy, and chlorpromazine
- Oral-ocular-genital syndrome: cheilts, seborrheic dermatitis-like rash, tongue atrophy, belpharitis, conjunctivitis, photophobia, genital and peri-nasal dermatitis, and anemia

Vitamin B_3 – Niacin/Nicotinic acid
Deficiency = Pellagra

- May be due to precursor (tryptophan, Hartnup) deficiency, alcoholism, carcinoid tumor, INH, 5-FU, azathioprine, GI disorders, and anorexia
- Casal necklace eruption, photosensitivity, shellac-like appearance, acral fissures, perineal rash, cheilitis, diarrhea, and dementia
- Below granular layer (stratum malphighii): vacuolar changes

Vitamin B_6 – Pyridoxine
Deficiency

- Due to cirrhosis, uremia, isoniazid, hydralazine, OCP, phenelzine, and penicillamine
- Rash resembling seborrheic dermatitis, intertrigo, cheilitis, glossitis, conjunctivitis, fatigue, neuropathy, disorientation, N/V

Vitamin B$_{12}$ – Cyanocobalamin

Deficiency

- Due to diet (found in animal products), pernicious anemia, and malabsorption
- Glossitis, hyperpigmentation, canities, and neurologic symptoms

Vitamin C

Deficiency = Scurvy

- Alcoholics, diet
- Water-soluble, fruits/vegetables
- Perifollicular hyperkeratosis and petechiae, corkscrew hairs, hemorrhagic gingivitis, epistaxis, hypochondriasis, subperiosteal hemorrhage (pseudoparalysis), soft teeth, gingivitis, hematologic changes, and weakness

Vitamin D

Physiology:

- Vit D$_2$ and D$_3$ in the diet are transported to the liver in chylomicrons and Vit D$_3$ from the skin and Vit D$_2$ and D$_3$ from fat cell stores are bound to Vit D-binding protein for transport to the liver
- In the liver, Vit D-25-hydroxylase turns Vit D into 25-hydroxyvitamin D, or 25(OH)D, the main circulating form of Vit D
- 25(OH)D is biologically inactive until it is converted to 1,25-dihydroxyvitamin D, or 1,25(OH)$_2$D, by 25-hydroxyvitamin D-1α-hydroxylase in the kidneys
- 1,25(OH)$_2$D is inactivated by 25-hydroxyvitamin D-24-hydroxylase and turned into the calcitroic acid, which is excreted in bile
- In osteoblasts, 1,25(OH)$_2$D increases RANKL which bind RANK on preosteoclasts, leading to activation
- In intestinal cells, 1,25(OH)$_2$D binds VDR-RXR, leading to increased calcium channel TRPV6 and calcium-binding protein calbindin 9K60 mg^2/dl^2; between 42 and 52 mg^2/dl^2 is desirable in the ESRD population 60 mg^2/dl^2; between 42 and 52 mg^2/dl^2 is desirable in the ESRD population

Deficiency

- Poor diet (Vit D is fat soluble – found in oily fish, eggs, butter, liver, cod-liver oil), insufficient sun (need UVB to convert 7-dehydrocholesterol to previtamin D$_3$, which is quickly turned into vitamin D$_3$), anticonvulsants, fat malabsorption, old age, chronic kidney disease, breast feeding (human milk has low Vit D)

- Requirements: controversial, ~800 IU/d of vitamin D_3
- Alopecia, rickets/osteomalacia, osteoporosis, cancer (colon, breast, prostate, and hematologic), autoimmune disease, muscle weakness

Hypervitaminosis D
- Hypercalcemia, calcinosis, anorexia, headache, N/V

Vitamin K
Deficiency

- Due to diet (fat-soluble, meat, green leafy vegetables; GI flora produces 50% of requirements), anorexia, CF, liver dz, malabsorption, coumadin, cephalosporins, salicylates, cholestyramine
- Hemorrhage

Zinc deficiency
- Due to AR genetic defect, diet (low zinc, excess fiber), malabsorption, CRF, alcoholism, TPN, cancer
- Typically when wean breastfeeding but zinc in human breastmilk does have lower bioavailability than cowmilk and may sometimes be low; premature infants have reduced zinc stores, poor GI absorbance, and higher zinc needs
- Acrodermatitis enteropathica (acral, periorificial, periungual, and cheilitis), diarrhea, alopecia, candida/staph superinfection, paronychia, irritable, photophobia, blepharitis, and failure to thrive
- Resembles biotin deficiency, essential fatty acid deficiency, CF, Crohn, necrolytic migratory erythema
- Low alkaline phosphatase
- Histo: epidermal pallor ± psoriasiform hyperplasia, necrosis, subcorneal/intraepidermal vesicle (similar to necrolytic migratory erythema, necrolytic acral erythema, genetic deficiency of M subunit of LDH)
- Zinc-responsive diseases: necrolytic acral erythema, amicrobial pustulosis of the flexures and scalp

Biotin deficiency
- Due to short gut (gut bacteria make biotin), malabsorption, avidin (raw egg white) consumption, biotinidase deficiency (infantile), multiple carboxylase synthetase, or holocarboxylase synthetase defects (neonatal)
- Rash-like zinc deficiency, alopecia, conjunctivitis, fatigue, and paresthesias

Essential fatty acid deficiency
- Due to GI abnormalities/surgery, diet, chronic TPN

- Rash resembling biotin and zinc deficiencies, alopecia, leathery skin, intertrigo
- Eicosatrienoic acid: Arachidonic acid ratio > 4

Copper
- Deficiency in Menkes, Wilson
- Local, exogenous excess – green hair (copper in water)

Selenium deficiency
- Component of glutathione peroxidase
- Due to TPN, low soil content
- Weakness, cardiomyopathy, elevated transaminases and CK, hypopigmentation (skin/hair), leukonychia

Lycopenemia
- Excess consumption of red fruits/vegetables (tomatoes, papaya) → reddish skin

Carotenemia
- Carotene-containing foods: carrots, squash, oranges, spinach, corn, beans, eggs, butter, pumpkins, papaya, and baby foods
- Yellow soles/palms, central face (sebaceous area)

Kwashiorkor
- Protein deficiency
- Due to diet, GI surgery, and HIV
- Dyschromia, pallor, flaky paint desquamation, sparse, hypopigmented hair, flag sign, potbelly, edema, moon facies, cheilitis, soft nails, irritable, infections

Marasmus
- Protein and caloric deficiency
- Due to diet, neglect, anorexia, malabsorption, HIV, and liver/kidney failure
- Xerotic, lax, thin skin, follicular hyperkeratosis, broken lanugo-like hair, monkey/aged facies, and no edema/hypoproteinemia

PEDIATRIC AND PREGNANCY DERMATOLOGY

Vascular tumors and malformation

| | Vascular tumor | | | Vascular malformation |
	Infantile hemangioma	Congenital hemangioma	Kaposiform hemangioendothelioma; tufted angioma	Arterial/capillary/venous/lymphatic combined lesions (see below)
Presentation	10–15 d after birth 30% present as red macul	Commonly large at birth	At birth or few days after birth	Present at birth
Growth	Rapid growth till 6 mo then slow growth till 1 yr of age Superficial, deep, or mixed	No growth	Slow growth during childhood, can be locally aggressive	Growth proportional to child's growth
Involution	Slow, spontaneous involution 30% by age 3, 50% by age 5, 70% by age 7, 90% by age 9	Rapidly involuting congenital hemangioma (RICH) – usually regress completely by age 2. Non-involuting congenital hemangioma (NICH)- No involution	No involution	No spontaneous regression
Histology	GLUT-1: positive	GLUT-1: negative	GLUT-1: negative; KMS: positive	GLUT-1: negative

Vascular malformation

	Slow flow	Fast flow	Combined
Presentation	Capillary (Port wine stain, salmon patch, nevus flammeus)	Arterial AV malformation (congenital)	Capillary-venous Lymphatic-venous
	Venous	AV fistula (acquired)	Capillary lymphatic venous Capillary arterivenous
	Lymphatic		Capillary lymphaticarteriovenous

Infantile Hemangioma (IH) Management

(From Cheng CE, Friedlander, SF. *Semin Cut Med Surg* 2015;35: 108–116)

Diagnosis: made based on medical history and clinical features

A. **Proliferating phase (<one year of age)**
   1. **Asymptomatic, inconspicuous lesions** – clinical observation
   2. **Endangering/symptomatic (ulceration, bleeding, rapid growth, functional impairment) or disfigurement**
      a. Propranolol – First line treatment (see Section "**Propranolol treatment for infantile hemangioma**")
      b. Corticosteroid – Second line treatment, for patients with complicated IH who do not respond to propranolol
      c. Topical therapy
         a) Timolol 0.5% gel forming (ophthalmic) solution BID – can be used for small, superficial IH. Potential for systemic absorption (higher risk in premies on scalp)
         b) Intralesional corticosteroid – potential systemic aborption and skin atrophy
         c) Intralesional propranolol – lack of efficacy
      d. PDL– for superficial lesions
      e. Surgical excision – for pedunculated IH
   3. **Multifocal (>5–10)**
      a. Consider liver US
      b. If + intrahepatic hemangioma – consider TSH for hypothyroidism and ECHO for high output cardiac failure if large
      c. Propranolol can work in hepatic hemangiomas – esp. in multifocal disease (Verasso *et al. Hepatology* 2017, Jan)
   4. **Special location and situations**
      a. **Large subcutaneous lesions** – may need ECHO due to risk of high-output cardiac failure
      b. **Segmental hemangioma/extensive hemangioma of the face/neck** – risk of PHACE(S)

P	Posterior fossa malformation	Dandy–Walker, cerebellar hypoplasia/dysplasia
H	Hemangioma	Facial or neck hemangioma >5 cm
A	Arteriral anomalies	Dysplasia or hypoplasia of the large cerebral arteries
C	Cardiac defects	Coarctation of the aorta, cardiac defects
E	Eye abnormalities	Optic nerve hypoplasia, posterior segment abnormalities
S	Sternal clefting and supraumbilical raphe	Sternal defect/cleft. Supraumbilical raphe

Need MRI head and neck (including aortic arch) and ECHO prior to starting propranolol

c. **Periocular IH** – risk of compromising vision, needs eye exam

d. **Beard/airway IH** – can lead to airway obstruction

e. **Intertrigious areas** (neck, axillary, and diaper area) – risk of ulceration.

f. **Lumbosacral IH** – can be associated with tethered cord, spinal defects, GU anomalies, and anorectal malformations. Look for asymmetric gluteal crease, tufts of hair, sacral pits, and masses. Needs MRI of spine.

g. **Ulcerated IH**

  a) Ddx: hemangioma, HSV, and perineal groove (self-resolving)

  b) First line: local wound care: topical antibiotics (topical metronidazole gel + mupirocin), barrier creams, nonstick dressings, oral propranolol.

  c) Second line: becaplermin, pulsed dye laser

  d) Analgesia: oral acetaminophen or topical lidocaine 2–5% (risk for systemic absorption)

B. **Involuting phase (12–18 months of age)**

  1. **Asymptomatic, involuting lesions – clinical observation**

  2. **Symptomatic or large lesions** – may consider treatment with propranolol to shrink lesion

C. **Involuted phase (>three years of age)**

  1. **Risk of scarring** (Baselga E et al. *JAMA Derm* 2016;152(11):1239–1243)

    a. Mixed > superficial > deep

    b. Sharp step off border

    c. Cobblestone > smooth

  2. **Atrophic scar** – fractionated or ablative erb:yag or CO_2 laser

  3. **Residual redness** – pulsed dye laser

  4. **Redundant or fibrofatty skin** – surgical excision

  5. **May still consider propranolol in older patients**

Propranolol Treatment for Infantile Hemangioma

(From Hoeger PH, Harper JI, Baselga E. et al. *Eur J Pediatr* 2015;174: 855.)

- Propanolol has been used since 1964 at doses up to 6–8 mg/kg/d in infants and children for treatment of hypertension.
- First report of propranolol in treatment of hemangioma in 2008
- FDA approved for treatment of proliferating IH
- Response rate of oral propranolol at 2–3 mg/kg/d × 6 mo = 96–98%
- More efficacious and safer than steroid

> Propranolol oral solution: generic supplied as 20 mg/5 ml
>
> Brand name (Hemangeol) supplied as 4.28 mg/ml
>
> Target dose: 2–3 mg/kg/d, divided BID or TID

Side effects of oral propranolol for treatment of IH

- Common (1–10%)
  - Sleep disturbances/night terror – consider changing to atenolol (does not cross blood–brain barrier – 1 mg/kg/d, similar efficacy)
  - Asymptomatic hypotension – HR is good proxy for BP
  - Somnolence
  - Cold extremties/acrocyanosis
  - Bronchospasm– stop if pt has bronchospasm and initiating beta agonist
- Uncommon (<1%)
  - Hypoglycemia – administer during the day with feeds, avoid fasting, discontinue if intercurrent illness
  - AV block
  - Bradycardia
- Does not cause long-term neuropsychiatric problems (Moyakine AV. *JAAD* 2017;2)

Pretreatment Evaluation

- Check for contraindications (see below)
- Baseline history (cardiac and pulmonary history), medications
- Clinical exam – check HR and BP (HR is pretty good proxy for BP), listen for arrhythmias. Baseline glucose level for preterm or small infants
- Consult pediatric cardiology and ECG if bradycardia, hypotension, or concern for arrhythmia

Reference values – lower limits of normal for age

Age (mo)	Heart rate (bpm)	Blood pressure (mm Hg)	Blood glucose
0–3	100	65/45	<2.6
3–6	90	70/50	
6–12	80	80/55	

Contraindications for propranolol therapy for IH

- Neonates zero to four weeks: except in rapidly growing, life-threatening IH
- Potential drug interactions: i.e. Ca+ blocker, antiarthyrmic agents, digitalis, dihydropyridines, NSAID, lipid-lowering agents, phenobarbital, corticosteroids
- Brochial asthma and concurrent beta agonist use
- Propranolol does not cause wheezing/asthma (no difference in # of respiratory episodes in pt with hemangioma treated with and without propranolol) Mei-Zahav et al. *Pediatri Pulm* 2017;52(8): 1071–1075
- Underlying cardiac issues: AV block, cardiac failture
- Baseline bradycardia or hypotension, or prone to hypoglycemia

Initiation of Propranolol Therapy and Dosage
(From Hoeger PH, Harper JI, Baselga E. *et al. Eur J Pediatr* 2015;174: 855 and Leaute-Labreze C *et al. N Eng J Med* 2015;372:735–746.)

A. Hospital admission

   1. For selected infants to monitor HR, BP, and glucose

      a. <Eight weeks of age (age corrected for prematurity)

      b. Weighing less than 3.5 kg

      c. Inadequate social support

      d. Life-threatening subglottic hemangioma

      e. Infant with PHACE syndrome

      f. Significant comorbities requiring cardiovascular, respiratory, or blood glucose monitoritng

   2. Start at 1.0 mg/kg/d = 0.33 mg/kg po TID.

   3. Increase **daily** by 1 mg/kg/d until final dose of 2–3 mg/kg/d

B. Outpatient therapy

1. Start at 1.0 mg/kg/d = 0.33 mg/kg po TID
2. Increase **weekly** by 1 mg/kg/d until final dose of 2–3 mg/kg/d
3. Common now to do BID dosing rather than TID

C. Monitoring

1. Baseline HR and BP. Check HR and BP at one and two hours after each dose increase.
2. Routine screening of blood glucose not indicated since timing of hypoglycemic event is variable. Recommend administration of propranolol with feeding. Hold dose if infant has poor oral intake, vomiting, diarrhea, or has episode of bronchitis.
3. Adjust dose every four weeks (due to increase in body weight).

Duration of therapy

Standard duration = 6 months, though best to treat till infant is 12 months of age

Relapse rate: 6 months of treatment = 17–20%

12 months of treatment = 5%

Neonatal vesiculopustular eruptions

Condition	Population	Onset	Duration	Description	Diagnostic	Treatment
Non-infections						
Erythema toxicum neonatorum	1/3–2/3 of fullterm	Usually 1–2 d	1 wk–1 mo	Erythematous macules, papules, (subcorneal or intraepi) pustules, wheals, usually on trunk, spares palms/soles	Smear – eos	None needed
Transient neonatal pustular melanosis	4% of Black, <1% in White; Fullterm	Birth	Pustules – days; PIH – months	Fragile (subcorneal) pustules at birth → resolve with collarette of scale → PIH	Smear — PMNs	None needed
Neonatal cephalic pustulosis/neonatal acne	10%	Variable w/i first month	Within 6 mo	Inflammatory papules/pustules on head/neck, no comedones, may scar, controversial pathogenesis – may be 2/2 hormones and/or malassezia	Smear – malassezia, PMNs	Self-limited, topical imidazole or BP/ erythromycin
Miliaria crystallina	4%; high in tropics	Birth or first few weeks	Resolves w/i days when precipitants removed	Superficial clear noninflammatory vesicles; forehead, upper trunk (sub/ intracorneal eccrine duct obstruction)	Smear – negative	Avoid overheating and swaddling

continued p.138

Condition	Population	Onset	Duration	Description	Diagnostic	Treatment
Miliaria rubra	4%; high in tropics	Usually after first week	Resolves w/i days when precipitants removed	Pruritic, erythematous papules and pustules usually on forehead, upper trunk (eccrine duct obstruction at the malphigian layer)	Smear – negative	Avoid overheating and swaddling
Infantile acropustulosis	<1%, increased in Black males	Up to 18 mo, usually 3–6 mo	Until 2–3 yr	Pruritic acral (subcorneal) pustules/vesicles in crops (q2–4 wk), eosinophilia, no burrows	Smear – eos (early), PMNs (late); Scabies prep neg	Midpotency topical steroids, antihistamines
Eosinophilic pustular folliculitis/Ofuji's	M>F	Birth or first few weeks	Several years	Pruritic, crusted, erythematous follicular papules/pustules/vesicles in crops (q2–4 wk), mainly on scalp, eosinophilia	Smear – eos	Topical steroids, systemic abx
Congenital self-healing langerhans/Hashimoto–Pritzker	Unknown, likely underreported	Birth or days	Weeks–months	Widespread red-brown nodules, skin-limited	Bx – CD1a+, S100+	None needed
Incontinentia pigmenti/ Blochh–Sulzberger	1:300 000, XLD	Birth or days	Linear and whorled; Stages: Vesicular/Bullous (birth–1 yr) → Verrucous (months–3 yr) → Hyperpigmented (1–20 yr) → Hypopigmented/ Atrophic (adulthood)	Bx: Bullous – eos spong, Verrucous – eos dysk, Hyperpig – dermal melanin, Hypopig – epi atrophy, no appendages	Referrals: ophtho, audiology, neuro, and dental

Viral

HSV – congenital/intrauterine	5% of newborn HSV	Birth	—	Generalized vesicles, pustules, scars, erosions, microcephaly, choriotretinitis, hydranencephaly, and microphthalmia	Tzank – multinucleated giant cells; DFA, PCR, Cx and IgG serology	IV acyclovir
HSV – primary neonatal	95% of newborn HSV (usually peri-not postnatal infxn); ~1:3 200 deliveries	Birth (30%) to several weeks	30–50% mortality if disseminated	40% Skin-eye-mucosal dz, 35% CNS, 25% disseminated (sepsis, hepatitis, resp, coag); Primary maternal infxn has 10× the risk of perinatal infxn vs. recurrent maternal infxn	Tzank – multinucleated giant cells; DFA, PCR, Cx and IgG serology	IV acyclovir
VZV – congenital	~10% risk with exposure (<20 wk gestation)	Birth	—	LBW, scars, limb hypoplasia, microcephaly encephalitis, cortical atrophy, optho, MSK, GI, GU	Tzank – multinucleated giant cells; DFA, Cx	VZIG/acyclovir w/i 5 d to exposed mom
VZV – neonatal	20–60% risk with maternal exposure 5 d before or 2 d postpartum	Birth to 2 wk	30% mortality	Pustules, vesicles → may ulcerate, necrose; pneumonitis, encephalitis, and hepatitis	Tzank – multinucleated giant cells; DFA, Cx	VZIG/acyclovir w/i 5 d to exposed mom and to neonate

continued p.140

Condition	Population	Onset	Duration	Description	Diagnostic	Treatment
VZV – infantile zoster	2% of patients w/ intrauterine exposure by 20 wk gestation	First year	—	Dermatomal papules, vesicles	Tzank – multinucleated giant cells; DFA, Cx	Consider IV acyclovir
Fungal						
Candidiasis – congenital/ intrauterine	<1%	Birth	Several weeks	Widespread erythematous papules/ pustules, thrush, rarely systemic; Risk factors – prematurity, cervical/ uterine foreign bodies	KOH: budding yeast, pseudohyphae	Topical nystatin or imidazole unless severe or disseminated
Candidiasis – neonatal	5%	Few days or weeks	Several weeks	Red plaques, satellite papules/ pustules, more common and may disseminate in LBW babies	KOH: budding yeast, pseudohyphae	IV fluconazole if preterm/LBW
Aspergillosis	Premature/LBW/ immunodef	Days or weeks	—	Necrotic papules, pustules, and ulcers	Bx: branching hyphae at 45°; Cx	Debridement, ampho
Parasites						
Scabies	Rare in neonates	—	—	Excoriated vesicles, pustules, papules, nodules, burrows	KOH/Mineral oil – mites, feces/scybala, eggs	Permethrin 5% 1 week apart, treat linens/family; Sulfur; Lindane contraindicated

Bacterial

	Onset	Clinical features	Diagnosis	Treatment
Impetigo neonatorum	Anytime	Erythematous pustules, vesicles, tense bullae, honey-colored crust, oozing, glazed, central clearing, satellite lesions, fever, adenopathy, and diarrhea	Gram stain and cx; Staph – Gram + cocci in clusters; Strep – Gram + cocci in chains	Mupirocin, oral abx, and nursery isolation
Rare, life-threatening bacterial infxns: Listeria monocytogenes, Chlamydia trachomatis, E. coli, H. influenzae, Pseudomonas	Onset: Birth, days, or weeks	Systemic involvement; Risk factors: prematurity, LBW, immunodeficiency, and maternal fever	Gram – rods: *Pseudomonas, H. influenzae, E. coli* Gram + rods: *Listeria monocytogenes*	

Source: Adapted from Van Praag MC *et al.* Diagnosis and treatment of pustular disorders in the neonate. Pediatr Dermatol. 1997 March–April; 14(2):131–43; Johr RH and Schachner LA. Neonatal dermatologic challenges. Pediatrics in Review. 1997; 18:86–94. Pauporte M and Frieden I. Vesiculobullous and erosive diseases in the newborn,
In: Bolognia Jorizzo JL, Rapini RP. Dermatology, Vol. 1. London: Mosby, 2003.
Other neonatal vesiculopustular eruptions: Pustular leukemoid rxn in Down syndrome, HyperIgE, Neonatal Behçet, Pustular Psoriasis, Zygomycetes, and Syphilis.

Genodermatoses

Disease	Gene	Protein		Comment
Acral peeling skin syndrome	TGM5	Transglutaminase-5	AR	Defective cornified cell envelope
Acrodermatitis enteropathica	SLC39A4	Intestinal zinc-specific transporter	AR	Defective zinc absorption from the gut
Acrokeratosis verruciformis of Hopf	ATP2A2	ATPase, Ca2+ transporting	AD	Allelic to Darier
AEC	P63	P63	AD	Tumor suppressor; Allelic to EEC, Rapp-Hodgkin, limb-mammary syndrome, split-hand and split-foot malformation type 4, and acro-dermatoungual-lacrimal-tooth (ADULT)
Albright hereditary osteodystrophy	GNAS1	G protein, alpha stimulating	AD	G protein subunit of adenylate cyclase; Allelic to McCune-Albright and progressive osseus heteroplasia
Alagille	JAG1	Jagged-1 NOTCH2	AD	Jagged-1 is a ligand for NOTCH
Alkaptonuria	HGO	Homogentisate 1,2-dioxygenase	AR	Deficient homogentisic acid oxidase causes homogentisic acid to accumulate in tissues
Alport	COL4A3 COL4A4 COL4A5	Colagen 4	AR AR XL	Associated with kidney disease, hearing loss, and eye abnormalities

Anhidrotic ectodermal dysplasia (Christ–Siemens–Touraine; Hypohidrotic)	EDA	Ectodysplasin-A	XLR	Similar to AD form due to ectodysplasin anhidrotic receptor (EDAR) mutation; Similar to AR form due to either EDAR or EDAR-associated death domain (EDARADD) mutations
Anhidrotic ectodermal dysplasia with immune deficiency ± osteoporosis and lymphedema	NEMO	NF-κB essential modulator/ IKK-gamma	XLR	Allelic to IP
Anonychia congenita	RSPO4	R-spondin 4	AR	Wnt/β-catenin signaling pathway (no bone hypoplasia unlike Cooks)
Apert	FGFR2	Fibroblast growth factor receptor 2	AD	Allelic to Beare–Stevenson and Crouzon
Argininosuccinic aciduria	ASL	Argininosuccinate lyase	AR	Urea cycle defect
Arrhythmogenic right ventricular dysplasia/Cardiomyopathy	DSP	Desmoplakin	AR	
	PLK2	Plakophilin-2		
	DSG2	Desmoglein-2		
	DSC2	Desmocollin-2		
Atrichia with papular lesions	HR	Hairless	AR	Zinc finger protein
Ataxia–Telangiectasia	ATM	Ataxia telangiectasia mutated	AR	Phosphatidyl inositol 3 kinase-like domain
Autoimmune polyendocrinopathy	AIRE	Autoimmune regulator	AD	Candidiasis, ectodermal dysplasia
			AR	
Bannayan–Riley–Ruvalcaba	PTEN	Phosphatase and tensin homolog	AD	Tumor suppressor; Allelic to Cowden and Lhermitte–Duclos

continued p.144

Disease	Gene	Protein		Comment
Bart–Pumphrey	GJB2	Connexin 26	AD	Knuckle pads, leukonychia, and sensorineural deafness; Allelic to KID and classic Vohwinkel
Basal cell nevus syndrome (Gorlin)	PTCH1	Patched	AD	Tumor suppressor, SHH transmembrane receptor, inhibits SMOH
Beare–Stevenson cutis gyrata	FGFR2	Fibroblast growth factor receptor 2	AD	Allelic to Apert and Crouzon
Beckwith–Wiedemann	CDKN1C/KIP2/P57; NSD1; 11p15 imprinting	Cyclin-dependent kinase inhibitor 1C	Sp > AD	Deregulation of imprinted growth regulatory genes; 11p15 imprinting region also involved in Russell–Silver
Birt–Hogg–Dube	FLCN	Folliculin	AD	Interacts with AMPK and FNIP1 in mTOR signaling
Bloom	RECQL3	RecQ protein-like 3	AR	DNA helicase
Brooke–Spiegler	CYLD	Cylindromatosis	AD	Tumor suppressor
Bruton agammaglobulinemia	BTK	Bruton agammaglobulinemia tyrosine kinase	XLR	Tyrosine kinase
Bullous congenital ichthyosiform	KRT 1, 10	Keratin 1, 10	AD	Intermediate filaments
Erythroderma (epidermolytic hyperkeratosis)				
Buschke–Ollendorff	LEMD3/MAN1	LEM domain-containing protein 3	AD	Inner nuclear membrane protein; Allelic to familial cutaneous colagenoma syndrome

Capillary malformation–arteriovenous malformation	RASA1	RAS family, GTPase-activating protein	AD	Allelic with Parkes Weber and associated with basal cell carcinomas
Cardiofaciocutaneous	KRAS BRAF MEK1 MEK2	Kirsten rat sarcoma virus oncogene homolog	Sp	All proteins in RAS-ERK pathway
Carney complex (NAME, LAMB)	PRKAR1A	Protein kinase A regulatory subunit 1α	AD	Increased risk for cardiac myxomas, PPNAD, psammomatous melanotic schwannoma, and lentigines
Carney complex with distal arthrogryposis	MYH8	Myosin heavy chain 8	AD	Variant associated with trismus and pseudocamptodactyly
Cartilage hair hypoplasia	RMRP	Mitochondrial RNA-processing endoribonuclease	AR	Metaphyseal dysplasia without hypotrichosis
Carvajal	DSP	Desmoplakin	AR	Dilated cardiomyopathy with woolly hair and keratoderma; Allelic to keratosis palmaris striata II, lethal acantholytic EB, skin fragility-wolly hair syndrome
CEDNIK (cerebral dysgenesis, neuropathy, ichthyosis, PPK)	SNAP29	Synaptosomal-associated protein 29	AR	Vesicle fusion; major psychomotor retardation in the first year
Cerebral capillary malformations, Familial	CCM1/KRIT1	Krev-interaction trapped 1	AD	Hyperkeratotic AVMs

continued p.146

145

Disease	Gene	Protein		Comment
Cerebrotendinous xanthomatosis	CYP27	Cytochrome p450, subfamily 27A, polypeptide 1 (sterol-27-hydroxylase)	AR	Breakdown of cholesterol to form bile acids
Chédiak–Higashi	LYST	Lysosomal trafficking regulator	AR	Lysosomal transport – transfer of melanosomes
CHILD	NSDHL	NADP steroid dehydrogenase-like	XLD	Cholesterol biosynthesis (aka 3β-hydroxysteroid dehydrogenase)
Chondrodysplasia punctata 1	ARSE	Arylsulfatase E	XLR	—
Chondrodysplasia punctata 2 (Conradi–Hünermann)	EBP	Emopamil-binding protein	XLD	Sterol isomerase – cholesterol biosynthesis
Chondrodysplasia punctata, Rhizomelic, Type 1	PEX7	Peroxisomal type 2 targeting signal receptor (PTS2)	AR	Allelic to Refsum
Chondrodysplasia punctata, Rhizomelic, Type 2	DHAPAT	Acyl–CoA:dihydroxyacetone phosphate acyltransferase	AR	Allelic with Refsum disease
Chronic granulomatous Dz Cytochrome, X-linked	CYBB	p91–Phagocyte oxidase (Cytochrome b-245 beta subunit)	XLR	Cytochrome b is part of NADPH oxidase – need oxidative burst to kill catalase+ bacteria
Chronic granulomatous Dz Cytochrome b-negative	CYBA	p22–Phagocyte oxidase	AR	Subunit of NADPH oxidase, essential role in phagocytes and neutrophils

Disease	Gene	Protein	Inheritance	Notes
Chronic granulomatous Dz Cytochrome b-positive type 1	NCF1	p47–Phagocyte oxidase	AR	Allelic with Williams syndrome
Chronic granulomatous Dz Cytochrome b-Positive Type 2	NCF2	p67–Phagocyte oxidase	AR	Increases the risk for systemic lupus erythematosus
Cleft lip-palate with ectodermal dysplasia	PVRL1	Poliovirus receptor-like 1	AR	Cell adhesion molecule/herpes virus receptor; Margarita Island ED, Rosselli–Giulienetti, Zlotogora–Ogur
Cockayne	ERCC6 ERCC8	Excision repair cross-complementing group 6 or 8	AR	Extreme photosensitivity; gene products associated with DNA repair
Congenital adrenal hyperplasia	CYP21A2 CYP11B1 CYP17A1 STAR	21-hydroxylase 11-β-hydroxylase 17-α-hydroxylase Steroidogenic acute regulatory protein	AR	21-hydroxylase = most common; STAR = lipoid variant, most severe
Congenital contractural arachnodactyly (Beals)	FBN2	Fibrillin 2	AD	Similar to Marfan syndrome
Congenital generalized lipodystrophy (Berardinelli–Seip)	AGPAT2 BSCL2	1-Acylglycerol-3-phosphate O-acyltransferase-2 (Lysophosphatidic acid acyltransferase) Seipin	AR	Converts LPA to PA

continued p.148

147

Disease	Gene	Protein		Comment
Congenital ichthyosiform Erythroderma (Nonbullous)	TGM1	Transglutaminase-1	AR	Allelic variants of TGM1 include lamellar ichthyosis and self-healing collodion baby
	ALOXE3	Lipoxygenase-3		
	ALOX12B	12R-Lipoxygenase		
	CGI58/ABHD5	Abhydrolase domain-containing 5 (Dorfman–Chanarin)		
Corneal dystrophy of Meesmann	KRT3	Keratin 3	AD	Structural framework in the corneal epithelium
	KRT12	Keratin 12		
Cornelia de Lange	NIPBL	Nipped-β-like	Sp>AD	Components of cohesin complex
	SMC1A (x-linked)	Structural maintenance of chromosomes 1A and 3		
	SMC3			
Costello	HRAS	Harvey and Kirsten Rat Sarcoma virus Oncogene homolog	Unk	Oncogene
	KRAS			
Cowden	PTEN	Phosphatase and tensin homolog	AD	Tumor suppressor; Allelic to Bannayan–Riley-Ruvalcaba and Lhermite-Duclos
Crohn's disease susceptibility	CARD15/NOD2	Caspase recruitment domain-containing protein 15 Nucleotide-binding oliogomerization domain protein 2	Cplx	CED4/APAF family of apoptosis regulators Allelic to Blau syndrome and early-onset sarcoidosis

Crouzon	FGFR2	Fibroblast growth factor 2	AD	Allelic to Apert and Beare–Stevenson
Crouzon with Acanthosis Nigricans	FGFR3	Fibroblast growth factor 3	AD	Allelic to severe achondroplasia with developmental delay and acanthosis nigricans (SADDAN)
Cutaneomucosal venous malformation	TIE2/TEK, VMCM1	Tyrosine kinase, endothelial	AD	Endothelial cell-specific receptor tyrosine kinase
Cutis Laxa (x-linked variant = Ehlers–Danlos 9, Occipital Horn Syndrome)	FBLN5	Fibulin 5	AR, AD	
	FBLN4	Fibulin 4	AR	
	ELN	Elastin	AD	Copper ion-binding ATPase
	ATP7A	ATP7A	XLR	ATP7A allelic to Menkes.
Darier	ATP2A2	SERCA2 – Sarcoendoplasmic reticulum Ca2+ ATPase isoform 2	AD	Ca2+ ATPase; Allelic to Acrokeratosis verruciformis
Dowling–Degos–Kitamura	KRT5	Keratin 5	AD	Allelic to EBS
Drug hypersensitivity (anticonvulsant hypersensitivity syndrome, DRESS)	EPHX	Epoxide hydrolase	AR/AD	Detoxifies reactive intermediates called arylamines generated during aromatic anticonvulsant metabolism
Dyschromatosis symmetrica hereditaria	ADAR1	Double-stranded RNA-specific adenosine deaminase	AD	Viral inactivation via dsRNA editing
Dyskeratosis congenita	DKC1	Dyskerin	XLR AD	Ribosomal assembly chaperone
	TERC	Telomerase RNA candidate 3		
Ectodermal dysplasia–skin fragility	PKP1	Plakophilin 1	AD	Desmosomal component

continued p.150

Disease	Gene	Protein	Comment
Epidermolysis bullosa (EB), Dominant dystrophic (Cockayne–Touraine)	COL7A1	Collagen 7	AD 290 kD, Anchoring fibrils
EB, recessive dystrophic (Hallopeau–Siemens)	COL7A1	Collagen 7	AR 290 kD, Anchoring fibrils
EB Simplex	KRT5, 14	Keratin 5, 14	AD Intermediate filaments
EB Simplex, Koebner type	KRT5	Keratin 5	AD Allelic to Dowling–Degos–Kitamura
EBS with muscular dystrophy, Also EBS Ogna variant	PLEC1	Plectin	AR In hemidesmosomes, intermediate filament-binding protein
GABEB (generalized atrophic benign epidermolysis bullosa) – junctional	COL17A1 LAMA3 LAMB3 LAMC2	Collagen 17 Laminin A3 Laminin B3 Laminin C2	AR Structural protein – BP Ag 2 Laminin subunits
EB, junctional – Herlitz type	LAMA3 LAMB3 LAMC2	Laminin 5 subunits	AR In lamina lucida, anchoring filaments
EB, junctional – Non-Herlitz	LAM5 COL17A1	Laminin 5 Collagen 17	AR Laminin 5 or type 17 Collagen

EB, junctional with pyloric atresia	ITGA6 ITGB4	Alpha 6 Beta 4 Integrin	AR	Hemidesmosome transmembrane protein complex
Ectodermal dysplasia, skin fragility	PKP1	Plakophilin 1	AR	Desmosomal plaque protein
Ehlers–Danlos, severe classic/ Gravis 1	COL5A1 COL5A2 COL1A1	Collagen 5α1 Collagen 5α2 Collagen 1α1	AD	Allelic to Ehlers–Danlos 2 (COL5A1/2) Allelic to Ehlers–Danlos 7 and osteogenesis imperfecta (COL1A1)
Ehlers–Danlos, mild classic/Mitis 2	COL5A1 COL5A2	Collagen 5α1 Collagen 5α2	AD	Allelic to Ehlers–Danlos 1
Ehlers–Danlos, hypermobility 3	COL3A1 TNXB	Collagen 3α1 Tenascin XB	AD	Allelic to Ehlers–Danlos 4 TNXB = extracellular membrane protein
Ehlers–Danlos, vascular 4	COL3A1	Collagen 3A1	AD, AR	Allelic to Ehlers–Danlos 3
Ehlers–Danlos, X-linked 5	Unknown		XLR	
Ehlers–Danlos, Kyphoscoliosis/ Ocular 6	PLOD	Lysyl hydroxylase	AR	Produces hydroxylysine which cross-links collagen molecules
Ehlers–Danlos Arthrochalasis 7a, 7b	COL1A1 COL1A2	Collagen 1α1 Collagen 1α2	AD	Defective conversion of procollagen into type I collagen
Ehlers–Danlos Dermatosparaxis 7c	ADAMTS-2	Procollagen N-peptidase	AR	—
Ehlers–Danlos, Periodontosis 8	Unknown		AD	—
Ehlers–Danlos, Occipital Horn 9	ATP7A	ATP7A	XLR	X-linked cutis laxa; Allelic to Menkes; copper transporter

continued p.152

Disease	Gene	Protein		Comment
Ehlers–Danlos, Fibronectin-deficient 10	Fibronectin		AR	Involved in blood clotting
Ellis–Van Creveld–Weyers Acrodental dysostosis complex (Chondroectodermal dysplasia)	EVC1 EVC2	Ellis–Van Creveld 1, 2	EVC = AR WAD = AD	EVC2 = Limbin
Epidermodysplasia verruciformis	EVER1 EVER2	Epidermodysplasia Verruciformis 1, 2	AR	Susceptible to HPV 3, 5, 8
Erythrokeratoderma variabilis (Mendes de Costa)	GJB3 GJB4	Connexin 31 Connexin 30.3	AD	GAP junction protein
Erythromelalgia	SCN9A/Nav1.7	Sodium channel, voltage-gated, type 9, subunit α	AD	Involved in action potential in peripheral neurons
Fabry	GLA	α-galactosidase A	XLR	Lysosomal hydrolase; buildup of glycosphingolipids in the body – ceramide trihexose
Familial dysautonomia (Riley Day)	IKBKAP	Inhibitor of Kappa light polypeptide gene enhancer in B cells, Kinase complex-associated protein	AR	Ashkenazi Jews
Familial GIST with hyperpigmentation	C-KIT	= Mast cell growth/Stem cell factor	AD	±mastocytosis; Activating mutations unlike piebaldism
Familial mediterranean fever	MEFV	Pyrin	AR	PMN inhibitor

Familial partial lipodystrophy 1 (Köbberling)	Unknown	Fat loss confined to lower portions of arms and legs. Affected individuals have increase fat distribution on the face and neck
Familial partial lipodystrophy 2 (Dunnigan)	LMNA	Nuclear lamins A/C	AD	Intermediate filament proteins; allelic with Charcot–Marie–Tooth disease, Emery–Dreifuss muscular dystrophy and familial dilated cardiomyopathy
Familial partial lipodystrophy 3	PPARG	Peroxisome proliferator-activated receptor-gamma		Subfamily of nuclear receptors; associated with obesity, DM type II, carotid internal medial thickness
Farber lipogranulomatosis	AC/ASAH	Acid ceramidase/N-acylsphingosine amidohydrolase	AR	Ceramide accumulates
Gardner	APC	Adenomatous polyposis coli	AD	Tumor suppressor, cleaves β-catenin
Gaucher	GBA	Acid-β-glucosidase	AR	Decreased glucocerebrosidase activity
Giant axonal neuropathy with curly hair	GAN1	Gigaxonin	AR	Protein degradation, neuronal survival
Glomuvenousm malformations	GLMN	Glomulin	AD	
Griscelli 1	MYO5A	Myosin 5A	AR	Melanosome transport to keratinocytes
Griscelli 2	RAB27A	RAB27A	AR	Ras-related GTP-binding protein
Griscelli 3	MLPH	Melanophilin	AR	Melanosome transportation
	MYO5A	Myosin 5A		

continued p.154

153

Disease	Gene	Protein		Comment
Hailey–Hailey	ATP2C1	ATPase, Ca²⁺ transporting	AD	Calcium ATPase
Haim–Munk	CTSC	Cathepsin C	AR	Allelic to Papillon–Lefévre
Harlequin Ichthyosis	ABCA12	ATP-binding cassette, subfamily A, member 12	AR	ABC transporter superfamily; Allelic to lamellar ichthyosis 2
Hartnup	SLC6A19	System B(0) neutral amino acid transporter-1	AR	Failure to transport tryptophan; Pellagra-like photosensitive rash, cerebellar ataxia, emotional instability, and aminoaciduria
Hemochromatosis 1	HFE	Hemochromatosis	AR	Increased intestinal Fe absorption
Hemochromatosis 2A	HJV	Hemojuvelin	AR	Juvenile type
Hemochromatosis 2B	HAMP	Hepcidin antimicrobial peptide	AR	Juvenile type
Hemochromatosis 3	TFR2	Transferrin receptor 2	AR	Helps iron enter hepatocytes
Hemochromatosis 4	SLC40A1	Ferroportin	AD	Transports iron from small intestines into the bloodstream; also transports iron out of reticuloendothelial cells
Hereditary angioedema 1, 2	C1INH	C1 esterase inhibitor	AD	Serine protease inhibitor (serpin)
Hereditary angioedema 3	F12	Coagulation factor 12	AD	Involved in coagulation
Hereditary hemorrhagic telangiectasia 1 (Osler–Weber–Rendu)	ENG	Endoglin	AD	TGF-β-binding protein Higher incidence of pulmonary AVMs

Hereditary hemorrhagic telangiectasia 2	ALK1/ACVRL1	Activin receptor-like kinase	AD	TGF-β receptor-like
Hereditary hemorrhagic telangiectasia with juvenile polyposis	SMAD4	Mothers against decapentaplegic, drosophila, homolog of 4	AD	Higher incidence of hepatic AVMs and GI bleed; Tumor suppressor; intracellular TGFb receptor signal transducer
Hereditary lymphedema 1 (Nonne–Milroy)	FLT4	Vascular endothelial growth factor receptor 3 (VEGFR-3)	AD	Gene is FMS-like tyrosine kinase
Hereditary lymphedema 2 (Meige, Late-onset, Praecox)	MFH1/FOXC2	Forkhead box C2	AD	Transcription factor; allelic to lymphedema-distichiasis, lymphedema and ptosis,a nd lymphedema and yellow nail syndrome
Hermansky–Pudlak syndrome 1	HPS1, 3-8	Hermansky–Pudlak	AR	Lysosome, melanosome, and platelet dense body formation; HPS7 = DTNBP1, HPS8 = BLOC1S3
Hermansky–Pudlak syndrome 2	AP3B1	Adaptin β-3a subunit	AR	Type 2 has immunodeficiency
Hidrotic ectodermal dysplasia (Clouston)	GJB6	Connexin 30	AD	Gap junction β-6, more commonly known as connexin 30; same gene that causes nonsyndromic hearing loss
Holt–Oram syndrome (Heart–Hand)	TBX5	T-box 5	AD	Thumb anomaly and atrial septal defect
Homocystinuria	CBS	Cystathionine β-synthetase	AR	Condensation of homocysteine and serine; homocystine builds up
Howel–Evans syndrome (Tylosis with esophageal cancer)	TOC	Tylosis with esophageal cancer	AD	High lifetime risk for esophageal cancer

continued p. 156

Disease	Gene	Protein		Comment
Hypereosinophilic syndrome	FIP1L1-PDGFRA fusion	Fusion of FIP1-like-1 and PDGF receptor-α		4q12 deletion; constitutively activated tyrosine kinase
Hyper-IgD	MVK	Mevalonate kinase	AR	Allelic to mevalonic aciduria
Hyper-IgE	STAT3	Signal transducer and activator of transcription 3	AD	Downstream target of IL-6
	TYK2	Tyrosin kinase 2		
Hyperlipoproteinemia Type 1A	LPL	Lipoprotein lipase	AR	Increased chylomicrons
Hyperlipoproteinemia Type 1B	APOC2	Apolipoprotein C2	AR	Increased chylomicrons
Hyperlipoproteinemia Type 2A	LDLR	Low-density lipoprotein receptor	AD	Familial hypercholesterolemia
				High LDL and cholesterol
Hyperlipoproteinemia Type 2B	APOB	Apolipoprotein B-100	AD	Mutation in LDL receptor-binding domain of this apolipoprotein
Hyperlipoproteinemia Type 3 (Dysbetalipoproteinemia)	APOE	Apolipoprotein E2	AR	Defective clearing of intermediate density lipoproteins and chylomicrons
Hypotrichosis with Juvenile macular dystrophy	PCAD/CDH3	P-cadherin	AR	Membrane glycoprotein, calcium-dependent cell-cell adhesion; Allelic to ectodermal dysplasia, ectrodactyly, macular dystrophy, monilethrix-like
Hypotrichosis, localized, AR	DSG4	Desmoglein 4	AR	Overlap with AR monilethrix
	LIPH	Lipase H		
Hypotrichosis-lymphedema-telangiectasia	SOX18	SRY-box 18	AD, AR	HMG box-containing transcription factor

Hypotrichosis simplex	CDSN	Corneodesmosin	AD	Corneodesmosome component (desquamation of corneocytes), psoriasis susceptibility gene
Ichthyosis bullosa of Siemens	KRT2A	Keratin 2A (2e)	AD	Expressed in upper spinous layer with keratin 9
Ichthyosis, Congenital, AR	NIPAL4	Ichthyin	AR	Diagnosis is based on skin findings at birth
Ichthyosis Hystrix Curth–Macklin	KRT1	Keratin 1	AD	Tonofibril defect, resembles EHK
Ichthyosis, Lamellar 1	TGM1	Transglutaminase 1	AR	Abnormal epidermal cross-linking; Allelic to NCIE and self-healing collodion baby
Ichthyosis, Lamellar 2	ABCA12	ATP-binding cassette, subfamily A, member 12	AR	ABC transporter superfamily; Allelic to harlequin ichthyosis
Ichthyosis vulgaris	FLG	Filaggrin	AD	Creates structure to the outermost skin cells and hydrates skin; same gene that causes atopic dermatitis
Ichthyosis, X-linked	STS	Aryl sulfatase C	XLR	Steroid sulfatase
Incontinentia pigmenti	NEMO	NF-κB essential modulator/ IKK-gamma	XLD	Allelic to AED with immune deficiency ±osteoporosis and lymphedema
Immunodysregulation, Polyendocrinopathy, and Enteropathy, X-linked	FOXP3	Forkhead Box P3	XLR	Forkhead family transcription factor
Insensitivity to pain, congenital, with anhidrosis	NTRK1	Neurotrophic tyrosine kinase receptor 1	AR	Signal transduction of nerve growth factor

continued p.158

Disease	Gene	Protein		Comment
Juvenile hyaline fibromatosis (systemic juvenile hyalinosis)	CMG2/ANTXR2	Capillary morphogenesis protein-2/Anthrax toxin receptor 2	AR	Involved in formation of capillaries
Kallman 1	ANOS1	Anosmin	XLR	Involved in the movement of nerve cells and outgrowth of olfactory neurons in the brain during embryonic development
Kallman 2	KAL2 (FGFR1)	Fibroblast growth factor receptor 1	AD	Migration of olfactory neurons; allelic with 8p11 myeloproliferative syndrome, osteoglophonic dysplasia, Pfeiffer syndrome
Keratosis palmoplantaris striata Type 1 (Brunauer–Fohs–Siemens)	DSG1	Desmoglein 1	AD	Calcium-binding transmembrane desmosomal glycoprotein; PF antigen
Keratosis palmoplantaris striata Type 2	DSP	Desmoplakin	AD	Desmosomal plaque protein
Keratosis palmoplantaris striata Type 3	KRT1	Keratin 1	AD	Suprabasal expression
KID syndrome (Keratitis–Ichthyosis–Deafness)	GJB2	Connexin 26	AD or AR	Allelic to Bart–Pumphrey and Classic Vohwinkel
Kindler	KIND1	Kindlin-1	AR	Focal contact for keratinocyte
Klippel–Trenaunay–Weber	VG5Q (AGGF1)	Angiogenic factor with G patch and FHA domains 1	Sp	This defect in some cases only
Leiomyomata, multiple cutaneous, and uterine	FH	Fumarate hydratase	AD	Enzyme in Krebs cycle. Defect also causes hereditary leiomyomatosis and renal cell cancer

LEOPARD-1	PTPN11	Protein–tyrosine phosphatase, nonreceptor	AD	Same gene as Noonan-1
Leprechaunism	INSR	Insulin receptor	AR	Allelic to Rabson–Mendenhall
Lesch–Nyhan	HGPRT	Hypoxanthine guanine phosphoribosyltransferase	XLR	Purine salvage pathway
Lhermitte–Duclos	PTEN	Phosphatase and tensin homolog gene	AR	Allelic to Bannayan–Riley–Ruvalcaba and Cowden
Lipoid proteinosis	ECM1	Extracellular matrix protein 1	AR	Anti-ECM1 antibodies in lichen sclerosis
Loeys–Dietz	TGFβR1,2	TGFβ receptors 1 and 2	AD	Marfan-like but short – arterial aneurysms and tortuosity, hypertelorism, bifid uvula, cleft palate
Lymphedema and ptosis, Lymphedema–Distichiasis, Hereditary lymphedema 2	FOXC2 (MSH1)	Forkhead box C2	AD	Transcription factor
Mal de Meleda	SLURP1	Ly6/uPar-related protein 1	AR	Keratoderma palmoplantaris transgrediens
Marfan	FBN1	Fibrillin 1	AD	Elastic fibers fragmented
Marinesco–Sjögren	SIL1	BIP-associated protein (BAP)	AR, AD	Endoplasmic reticulum glycoprotein, interacts with BIP, involved in nucleotide exchange
McCune–Albright	GNAS1	Guanine nucleotide-binding protein alpha subunit	Som	Stimulates G protein, increases cAMP by regulating adenylate cyclase

continued p.160

Disease	Gene	Protein		Comment
Melanoma	CDKN2A	Cyclin-dependent kinase inhibitor 2a	AD	Hereditary melanoma; Defective MC1R cannot convert eumelanin to pheomelanin
	CDK4	Cyclin-dependent kinase 4		
	MC1R	Melanocortin 1 receptor		
Menkes Kinky hair syndrome	ATP7A	ATPase, Cu²⁺ transporting, alpha subunit	XLR	Allelic to occipital horn syndrome and X-linked cutis laxa Wilson disease = ATP7B
MIDAS	HCCS	Holocytochrome C synthase	XLD	Mitochondrial
Monilethrix	KRTHB1	Keratin hair, basic 1, 3, and 6	AD	Intermediate filaments; human hair keratins
	KRTHB3			
	KRTHB6			
	DSG4	Desmoglein-4	AR	Hair shaft "blebs"
Muckle wells	CIAS1	Cryopyrin	AD	Alllic to chronic infantile neurologic cutaneous and articular (CINCA) syndrome and familial cold autoinflammatory syndrome
Mucopolysaccharidosis 1 (Hurler syndrome)	IDUA	α-L-iduronidase	AR	Buildup of glycosaminoglycans due to lack of degradation
Mucopolysaccharidosis 2 (Hunter syndrome)	IDS	Iduronate 2-sulfatase	XLR	Buildup of glycosaminoglycans due to lack of degradation

Muir–Torre	MLH1	MutL homolog 1, colon cancer, nonpolyposis type 2	AD	DNA mismatch repair genes; also seen in lynch cancer family syndrome (Hereditary nonpolyposis colorectal cancer)
	MSH2	MutS homolog 2, colon cancer, nonpolyposis type 1		
Multiple Carboxylase Deficiency	BTD	Biotinidase	AR	Decreased free serum biotin; metabolic acidosis
	HLCS	Holocarboxylase synthetase		
Multiple cutaneous and uterine leiomyomas	FH	Fumarate hydratase	AD	Krebs cycle enzyme
Multiple endocrine neoplasia 1 (Werner)	MEN1	Menin	AD	Binds nuclear GUND
Multiple endocrine neoplasia 2a (Sipple), 2b	RET	Receptor tyrosine kinase	AD	Protooncogene, encodes a tyrosine kinase receptor
Multiple familial trichoepithelioma	CYLD	Cylindromatosis	AD	Same gene as Brooke–Spiegler Tumor suppressor
Naegeli–Franceschetti–Jadassohn	K14	Keratin 14	AD	Allelic to EBS and dermatopathia pigmentosa reticularis; NFJ/DPR – mutations in nonhelical head (E1/V1) domain EBS – mutations in central alpha-helical rod domain
Nail–Patella	LMX1B	LIM homeobox transcription factor 1β	AD	

continued p. 162

161

Disease	Gene	Protein		Comment
Naxos	JUP	Junction plakoglobin	AR	PPK with woolly hair and RV cardiomyopathy
Netherton	SPINK5 (LEKT1)	Serine protease inhibitor, Kazal-type 5	AR	Serine protease inhibitor
Neurofibromatosis 1	NF1	Neurofibromin	AD	Inhibits Ras, Allelic to NF-1-Noonan overlap syndrome, similar to NF1-like syndrome due to SPRED1 defects
Neurofibromatosis 2	NF2	Neurofibromin 2 (Schwannomin, merlin)	AD	Crucial to cell shape, cell movement, and communication between cells by having merlin associate with cytoskeleton; also a tumor suppressor protein
Niemann–Pick disease A,B	SMPD-1	Sphingomyelin phosphodiesterase-1	AR	Sphingomyelinase deficiency
Niemann–Pick disease C1, D	NPC1	Niemann–Pick C1	AR	Cholesterol esterification
Niemann–Pick disease C2	NPC2/HE1	Niemann–Pick C2	Ar	Cholesterol binding
Noonan 1	PTPN11 (SHP2)	Protein tyrosine phosphatase, non-receptor type 11	AD, Sp	Allelic to LEOPARD-1
Noonan 3	KRAS	Kirsten rat sarcoma virus oncogene homolog	AD	Allelic to CFC and Costello
Noonan 4	SOS1	Son of sevenless, drosophila homolog		Guanine nucleotide exchange factor; Allelic to gingival fibromatosis
Noonan 5	RAF1	V-RAF-1 murine leukemia viral oncogen homolog 1	AD	Serine–threonine kinase, activates MEK1/2; Allelic to LEOPARD-2
Oculocutaneous albinism 1	TYR	Tyrosinase	AR	Melanin pathway
Oculocutaneous albinism 2	P gene	Mouse pink-eyed dilution gene	AR	Regulation of melanosome pH

Oculocutaneous albinism, Rufous, and OCA 3	TYPR1	Tyrosinase-related protein 1	AR	Stabilizes tyrosinase
Omenn syndrome	RAG1 RAG2 DCLRE1C	Recombinase-activating Artemis	AR	Omenn = SCID with hypereosinophilia; RAG1 and RAG2 mutations may also cause a more severe T-B-NK+ SCID; DCLRE1C mutations may also cause SCID with sensitivity to ionizing radiation
OrofacioDigital 1 (Papillon–Leage)	CXORF5	Chromosome X open reading frame 5	XLD	Associated with cleft tongue, cleft palate, hypertelorism, brachydactyly, clinodactyly; same gene that causes Joubert syndrome and primary ciliary dyskinesia
Osteogenesis imperfecta I–IV	COL1A1 COL1A2	Collagen 1α1 Collagen 1α2	AD or AR	Allelic to Ehlers–Danlos 7
Pachyonychia congenita 1 (Jadassohn–Lewandowsky)	KRT6A KRT16	Keratin 6a Keratin 16	AD	Intermediate filaments; KRT16 mutations also associated with nonepidermolytic palmoplantar keratoderma (nonepidermolytic Unna–Thost)
Pachyonychia congenita 2 (Jackson–Lawler)	KRT6B KRT17	Keratin 6b Keratin 17	AD	Intermediate filaments; KRT17 version allelic to SCM
Palmoplantar keratoderma, Epidermolytic (Vörner)	KRT9	Keratin 9	AD	Expressed in upper spinous layer

continued p.164

Disease	Gene	Protein		Comment
Palmoplantar keratoderma, Nonepidermolytic (Unna–Thost)	KRT1 KRT16	Keratin 1 Keratin 16	AD	KRT1 mutations also associated with epidermolytic hyperkeratosis, BCIE, ichthyosis hystrix; KRT16 mutations also associated with PC1
Papillon–Lefèvre	CTSC	Cathepsin C	AR	Lysosomal protease; Allelic to Haim–Munk
Peutz–Jeghers	STK11	Serine threonine kinase 11	AD	Tumor suppressor
Phenylketonuria	PAH	Phenylalanine hydroxylase	AR	Phenylalanine and metabolites buildup
Piebaldism	KIT	C-KIT	AD	Inactivating mutations; Protooncogene, tyrosine kinase
	SNAI2	Snail, drosophila homolog of 2		Neural crest transcription factor
Popliteal pterygium	IRF6	Interferon regulatory factor 6	AD	Allelic to Van der Woude
Porphyria, Acute intermittent	PBGD	Porphobilinogen deaminase	AD	PBGD also referred to as hydroxymethylbilane synthase (HMBS)
Porphyria, Congenital erythropoietic (Gunther)	UROS	Uroporphyrinogen III synthase	AR	UROS also referred to as hydroxymethylbilane hydrolyase
Porphyria, Hepatoerythropoietic	UROD	Uroporphyrinogen decarboxylase	AD	Cytosolic
Hereditary coproporphyria	CPOX	Coproporphyrinogen oxidase	AD	Mitochondrial gene
Erythropoietic protoporphyria	FECH	Ferrochelatase	AD/R	Mitochondrial gene
Porphyria cutanea tarda	UROD	Uroporphyrinogen decarboxylase	AD	Increased skin uroporphyrin causes photosensitivity to light at 400–410 nm
Porphyria, Variegate	PPOX	Protoporphyrinogen oxidase	AD	Mitochondrial gene
Progeria (Hutchinson–Gilford)	LMNA	Lamin A	AD	Nuclear envelope

Progressive symmetric erythrokeratodermia (PSEK)	LOR	Loricrin	AD	Allelic to Vohwinkel and EKV
Prolidase deficiency	PEPD	Peptidase D	AR	Splits iminodipeptides
Pseudofolliculitis barbae	K6hf	Keratin 6, hair follicle		Susceptibility gene
Pseudoxanthoma elasticum	ABCC6	ATP-binding cassette subfamily C, member 6	AR	Transmembrane transporter gene
			AD	
Psoriasis		HLA-Cw6, IL-15, SLC12A8, IL-23/IL-23R, HLA-B17		Susceptibility genes
PXE-like syndrome	GGCX	Gamma-glutamyl carboxylase	AD/AR	Gamma-carboxylation of gla-proteins; associated with cutis laxa and coagulation defects
Pyogenic arthritis-pyoderma gangrenosum-acne (PAPA)	PSTPIP1	Protein-serine-threonine phosphatase-interacting protein 1	AD	Cytoskeletal protein binds to and downregulates CD2; binds PTP and directs them to c-Abl kinase to mediate c-Abl dephosphorylation, thereby, regulating c-Abl activity. Also interacts with pyrin
Hereditary angioedema 1 and 2	C1NH/ SERPING1	C1 esterase inhibitor	AD	Inhibits first component of complement
Hereditary angioedema 3 (estrogen-related)	F12	Coagulation factor 12	AD	Allelic to Hageman trait (F12 deficiency)
Refsum	PAHX	Phytanoyl Co-A hydroxylase	AR	Phytanic acid builds up
	PEX7	Peroxin-7	>	
			AD	Receptor targets enzymes to peroxisomes

continued p.166

Disease	Gene	Protein	Comment
Refsum, Infantile form	PEX1 PEX2 PEX6	Peroxin-1, 2, and 6	Deficient and impaired peroxisomes, severe defects cause Zellweger syndrome
Restrictive dermopathy	ZMPSTE24 (FACE-1) LMNA	Zinc metalloproteinase STE24, Lamin A	AR — Cleaves prelamin A
Richner–Hanhart (Tyrosinemia II)	TAT	Tyrosine aminotransferase	AR — Tyrosine accumulates in all tissues
Rothmund–Thomson (Poikiloderma congenita)	RECQL4	RecQ protein-like 4	AR — DNA helicase
Rubinstein–Taybi	CREBBP EP300	CREB-binding protein E1A-binding protein, 300kd	AD — CREB = cAMP response element-binding protein / Transcriptional coactivators
SCID, X-linked	IL2Rγ	IL-2 receptor γ chain	XLR — T-B+NK-
SCID, Autosomal recessive	ADA	Adenosine deaminase	AR — T-B-NK-
	JAK3	Janus kinase 3	T-B+NK-
	IL7Rα		T-B+NK+
	CD3δ		T-B+NK+
	CD3ε		T-B+NK+
	CD3ζ		T-B+NK+
	CD45		T-B+NK+
	ZAP-70		T-B+NK+

SCID with sensitivity to ionizing radiation	DCLRE1C	DNA cross-link repair 1C (Artemis)	AR	T-B-NK+
SCID, T-B-NK+	RAG1 RAG2	Recombinase-activating gene	AR	Allelic to Omenn Allelic to Omenn
Self-healing collodion baby	TGM1	Transglutaminase	AR	Allelic to lamellar ichthyosis 1 and NBCIE
Sjögren–Larssen	ALDH3A2	Fatty aldehyde dehydrogenase	AR	Breaks down fatty aldehydes to fatty acids; associated with ichthyosis, neurological abnormalities, and eye problems
Steatocystoma multiplex	KRT17	Keratin 17	AD	In pachyonychia congenita 2
Striate PPK 1	DSG1	Desmoglein 1	AD	Cadherin-like transmembrane glycoprotein making up the desmosome
Striate PPK 2	DSP	Desmoplakin	AD	Allelic to skin fragility-woolly hair
Systemic sclerosis	CTGF	Connective tissue-growth factor	AR	Polymorphism in promoter region
T-cell immunodeficiency, Congenital alopecia, and Nail dystrophy	FOXN1 (WHN)	Forkhead box N1	AR	Transcription factor
Takahara (Acatalasemia)	CAT	Catalase	AR	Associated with ulcers and gangrene and may increase the risk for DM type II; single mutation causes hypocatalasemia
Tangier	ABCA1/CERP	ATP-binding cassette A1/Cholesterol efflux regulatory protein	AR	Allelic to familial HDL deficiency (which may also result from Apolipoprotein A-1 mutations)

continued p. 168

Disease	Gene	Protein		Comment
Thrombotic thrombocytopenic purpura, congenital (Schulman–Upshaw)	ADAMTS13/VWFCP	von Willebrand factor-cleaving protease	AR	Unprocessed vWF leads to abnormal blood clotting
Tietz (Albinism-Deafness)	MITF	Microphthalmia-associated transcription factor	AD	Allelic to Waardenberg 2A
TNF receptor-associated periodic fever (TRAPS)	TNFRSF1A	TNF receptor 1	AD	Binds TNF and two other TNFR1 proteins forming a trimer that can cause inflammation or apoptosis
Trichodentoosseous	DLX3	Distal-less homeobox 3	AD	Characterized by curly, kinky hair at birth, enamel hypoplasia, taurodontism, thickening of cortical bones and variable expression of craniofacial morphology
Trichorhinophalangeal 1 and 3	TRPS1	Trichorhinophalangeal syndrome 1	AD	Putative transcription factor
Trichorhinophalangeal 2	Continuous TRPS1 and EXT1 deletion	TRP1 and Exostosin	AD	TRP1 with multiple exostoses
Trichothiodystrophy (PIBIDS)	ERCC2 (XPD) ERCC3 (XPB)	Excision repair cross-complementing rodent repair deficiency, complementation groups 2 and 4	AR	ERCC2 same as XP group D; DNA helicase; most cases caused by mutations in XPD, a subunit of transcription factor IIH
TTD, Nonphotosensitive 1 (TTDN1/BIDS)	TTDN1/C7ORF11	Chromosome 7 open reading frame 11	AR	Helps regulate the cell cycle; associated with slow growth, intellectual disability, and brittle hair
Ullrich, Congenital scleroatonic muscular dystrophy	COL6A1/2/3	Colagen VI	AR	Located in the extracellular matrix surrounding skeletal muscle cells and connective tissue cells

Tuberous sclerosis	TSC1	Hamartin	AD	GTPase-activating protein domain
	TSC2	Tuberin		
Van de Woude	IRF6	Interferon regulatory factor 6	AD	Allelic to popliteal pterygium
Vitiligo, associated autoimmune/ inflammatory conditions	NALP1	NACHT leucine-rich-repeat protein 1	AD	Regulator of the innate immune system; SNPs related to susceptibility
Vohwinkel Syndrome, variant form (mutilating keratoderma with ichthyosis)	LOR	Loricrin	AD	Cornified cell envelope component; Allelic to PSEK
Vohwinkel syndrome, classic, with deafness	GJB2	Connexin 26	AD	Allelic to Bart–Pumphrey and KID
Von–Hippel Lindau syndrome	VHL	von Hippel–Lindau	AD	Tumor suppressor gene
Waardenburg 1	PAX3	Paired box gene 3	AD	Transcription factor, activates MITF promoter; dystopia
Waardenburg 2A	MITF	Microphthalmia-associated transcription factor	AD	Transactivates tyrosinase gene, no dystopia; Allelic to Tietz (Waardenburg 2D is due to SNAI2)
Waardenburg 3 (Klein–Waardenburg)	PAX3	Paired box gene 3	AD, AR	Directs the activity of genes that signal neural crest cells to form specialized tissues or nerve tissue, craniofacial bones, and melanocytes
Waardenburg 4 (Waardenburg–Shah)	EDNRB	Endothelin receptor B	AD	Involved in neural crest cell migration; Endothelin 3 is aligand for endothelin B receptor; SOX 10 is a transcription factor, activates MITF promoter
	EDN3	Endothelin 3		
	SOX10	SOX10		

continued p.170

Disease	Gene	Protein		Comment
Watson	NF-1	Neurofibromin	AD	Café-au-lait macules with pulmonic stenosis, ~ to NF-1
Werner	RECQL2	RecQ protein-like 2	AR	DNA helicase enzyme
	LMNA	Nuclear lamin A/C		Lamin defect – severe phenotype
White sponge nevus (Cannon)	KRT4	Keratin 4	AD	Forms intermediate filaments
	KRT13	Keratin 13		
Wilson	ATP7B	ATPase, Cu²⁺ transporting, beta subunit	AR	Defect in copper transport and biliary excretion of copper
Wiskott–Aldrich	WAS	Wiskott Aldrich syndrome protein	XLR	Binds GTPase and actin
Witkop	MSX1	Muscle segment, homeobox, drosophila, homolog of 1	AD	Critical for the development of teeth and other structures in the mouth; associated with cleft palate and cleft lip
Xeroderma pigmentosum		XPA – DDB1 (DNA damage-binding protein)	AR	50% will develop skin cancers by the age of 10
		XPB – ERCC3 (excision repair cross-complementing)		
		XPC – Endonuclease		
		XPD – ERCC2		
		XPE – DDB2		
		XPF – ERCC4		
		XPG – Endonuclease		
		XPV – Polymerase		

X-linked dominant disorders: Incontinentia Pigmenti, Goltz, CHILD, MIDAS, OFD–1, Conradi–Hunermann, Bazex

X-linked recessive disorders: Chad's Kinky Wife
CGD, Hunter, Anhidrotic Ectodermal Dysplasia, Dyskeratosis Congenita, SCID, Kinky (Menkes, Cutis Laxa, Occipital Horn), Wiskott–Aldrich, Ichythosis X-Linked, Fabry, Ehlers–Danlos 5,9; Also: Bruton's Agammaglobulinemia, Chondrodysplasia Punctata 1, Kallman 1, Lesch–Nyhan, X-linked SCID (IL2Rγ)

Chromosome abnormalities

Syndrome	Chromosome
Cri du Chat	5p-
Down	Trisomy 21
Edwards	Trisomy 18
Hypomelanosis of Ito	Various
Klinefelter	X aneuploidy – i.e. XXY
Pallister–Killian	Mosaic Tetrasomy 12p
Patau	Trisomy 13 (Phyloid pigmentation = mosaic trisomy 13)
Turner	XO monosomy
Warkany	Mosaic Trisomy 8 (nail/patella dysplasia)

Genodermatoses *in greater detail*

Disorders of cornification
Ichthyosis
Acquired ichthyosis: Neoplastic (Hodgkins, multiple myeloma, and MF), autoimmune (sarcoid, dermatomyositis, GVHD, and SLE), drugs (nicotinic acid), infections (HIV, leprosy), endocrine (hypothyroidism, hyperparathyroidism), and metabolic (chronic liver or kidney dz).

Atrophoderma vermiculatum: Reticular atrophy on cheeks, AD, may be seen in: Rombo, Nicolau–Balus (+ eruptive syringoma and milia) (atrophoderma vermiculatum is similar to atrophia maculosa varioliformis cutis of Tuzun).

Bullous CIE/epidermolytic hyperkeratosis: Rapidly resolving collodion baby→ diffuse erythema, scale, bullae, erosions, acantholysis, "gothic church" hyperkeratosis. AD, KRT1, or 10 defects.

CHILD: Congenital Hemidysplasia, Icthyosiform erythroderma, Limb Defects, >2/3 in females, cardiovascular (main cause of death, CNS, and renal defects, 2/3 right-sided involvement. XLD, NSDHL defects.

Collodion baby: Most often – lamellar or NBCIE; others – Sjögren–Larsson, Dorfman–Chanarin, EHK, self-healing, TTD, Netherton, ectodermal dysplasias, and rarely ichthyosis vulgaris.

Congenital ichthyosiform erythroderma/nonbullous CIE: Subtype of lamellar ichthyosis. AR, TGM1, ALOXE3, ALOX12B, and CGI58/ABHD5 defects.

Conradi–Hunerman/XLD chondrodysplasia punctata: Collodion-like presentation, large-scale, ichthyosiform erythroderma in Blaschko's lines → follicular atrophoderma ± hypo/hyperpigmentation, flat face, linear alopecia, stippled epiphyses, asymmetric limb shortening, scoliosis, hip dysplasia, and eye abnormalities. XLD, EBP defects.

Dorfman–Chanarin/neutral lipid storage disease with Ichthyosis: Lamellar ichthyosis, MR, cataracts, and lipid vacuoles in circulating leukocytes. AR, CGI58/ABHD5 defects.

Epidermal nevus syndrome: Sporadic, linear whorled verrucous plaques, MR, szss, hemiparesis, deafness, corneal opacities, assoc with syringocystadenoma papilliferum, Wilm's tumor, and astrocytoma.

Erythrokeratoderma variabilis/Mendes de Costa: Erythematous, hyperkeratotic, well-demarcated plaques in bizarre geographic, and figurate distributions with daily variations. AD, defects: GJB3/Connexin 31 and GJB4/Connexin 30.3.

Harlequin fetus: Massive hyperkeratosis, deep fissures, ectropion, eclabium, necrotic phalanges, absent lamellar granules, fatal without high-dose retinoids. AR, ABCA12 defects.

Icthyosis bullosa of Seimens: Collodion-like→ superficial, rippled hyperkeratosis, erosions, bullae in early childhood, PPK, mauserung = oval desquamation, minimal erythema,. AD, KRT2e defects.

Icthyosis follicularis with atrichia and photophobia: Alopecia, non-erythematous, follicular keratoses, atopy, epilepsy, recurrent respiratory infections, corneal vascularization, blindness, and retinal vascular tortuosity.

Ichthyosis hystrix – Curth Macklin: AD, KRT1 defects.

Icthyosis vulgaris: Onset: infancy, gray-brown, erythematous scales, may spare flexures and face, atopy, KP, hyperlinear palms, decreased stratum granulosum. AD, Filaggrin defects. (Mutated filaggrin is also a risk factor for atopic dermatitis and associated with disease severity. *Among* patients with atopic dermatitis, mutated filaggrin is associated with asthma, allergic rhinitis, and allergic sensitization. However, mutated filaggrin is not independently associated with asthma. Mutated filaggrin is not associated with psoriasis, keratosis pilaris, hand eczema, or contact allergy. Among **patients** with alopecia areata, filaggrin mutations predict more severe courses.)

KID: Keratitis, Ichthyosis, Deafness, spiny hyperkeratosis, sparse hair, absent eyelashes, follicular plugging, onychodystrophy, hypohidrosis, limbal stem cell deficiency, and SCC. AD, GJB2/Connexin 26 defects.

Lamellar ichthyosis: Collodion baby, ectropion, eclabion, everted ears, plate-like scale, PPK, erythroderma, phalangeal reabsorption. AR, TGM1, or ABCA12 defects.

Lipoid proteinosis: Skin and mucous membrane infiltrated with hyaline-like material, weak cry/hoarseness as infant, bullae, pustules, crusts, pitted scars, verrucous plaques on elbows and knees, sickle/bean-shaped calcification of temporal lobes, and szs. AR, ECM1 defects.

Netherton: Collodion baby, erythroderma, ichthyosis linearis circumflexa (serpiginous, double-edged, migratory erythema), atopy, trichorrhexis invaginata, asthenia. AR, SPINK5/LEKT1 defects.

Refsum: IV-like ichthyosis, retinitis pigmentosa, peripheral neuropathy, cerebellar ataxia, nerve deafness, ECG abnormalities/arrhythmias, increased tissue and plasma phytanic acid, eliminate dietary chlorophyll (animal fat/phytol, green vegetables/phytanic acid) and avoid rapid loss of weight (releases phytanic acid). AR, PAHX, or PEX7 defects.

Rud: Ichthyosis, hypogonadism, short stature, MR, epilepsy, and retinitis pigmentosa.

Sjögren–Larsson: Onset: birth or early infancy, generalized, pruritic ichthyosis, spastic paralysis, MR, szs, degenerative retinitis, maculopathy (white macular dots). AR, FALDH defects.

Pityriasis rotunda: Circular, hypopigmented, hyperkeratotic plaques, confluent and geometric, AD, South Africa, Sardinia, Japan, Type 1: Asians, Blacks, hyperpigmented, older, malignancies, Type 2: Whites, hypopigmented, younger.

Multiple minute digitate hyperkeratosis: Minute keratotic spikes on extremities and trunk.

Self-healing collodion baby: AR, TGM1 defects.

Ulerythema ophryogenes/KP atrophicans facei: Erythematous, follicular papules with scarring alopecia, KP, atopy, woolly hair, AD, loss of lateral 1/3 eyebrows, may be seen in: Noonan, CFC, and IFAP.

X-linked Ichthyosis: Onset: third to sixth months (never collodion baby!), widespread, dirty, brown scales, "dirty face," may spare flexures, delayed parturition, comma-shaped/flower-like (pre-Descemet) corneal opacities in posterior capsule, cryptorchidism, if broad deletion → hypogonadotropic hypogonadism with anosmia (Kallman) or chondrodysplasia punctata, neither hyperlinear palms nor KP, low maternal serum unconjugated estriol during pregnancy screening. XLR, ARSC!/ (steroid sulfatase or arylsulfatase C defects).

Keratodermas
Inherited Keratoderma

Transgrediens	Clouston, Mal de Meleda, Olmsted, Papillon–Lefévre, Greither
Non-transgrediens	Unna–Thost, Vorner, Howel–Evans

Acrokeratoelastoidosis of Costa: Asymptomatic, firm, translucent papules on lateral acral margins, starts at puberty, uncommon and controversial association with scleroderma, AD but F > M, if elastorrhexis is absent on biopsy then dx = focal acral hyperkeratosis, DDx includes keratoelastoidosis marginalis – due to chronic sun and trauma.

Carvajal: PPK, woolly hair, and LV cardiomyopathy. AR, Desmoplakin defects.

Disseminated superficial actinic porokeratosis (DSAP): 3rd-4th decade, F > M, lowest risk of malignant transformation among the porokeratosis syndromes (except punctate variety which has no risk; linear and long-standing lesions have the greatest risks). AD, SART3 defects.

Haim–Munk: PPK, periodontitis, onychogryphosis, and arachnodactyly. AR, Cathepsin C defects.

Howel–Evans: Tylosis, blotchy PPK, non-transgrediens, esophageal CA, and soles > palms. AD, TOC defects.

Huriez: Scleroatrophy, sclerodactyly, PPK, nail hypoplasia, nasal poikiloderma, lip telangectasia, hypohidrosis, fifth finger contractures, SCC, bowel cancer, and AD.

Mal de Meleda: Glove and sock PPK, transgradiens, hyperhidrosis, pseudoainhum, onychodystrophy, and high-arched palate. AR, SLURP1 defect.

Naxos: PPK, woolly hair, and RV cardiomyopathy. AR, Junctional Plakogobin defects.

Olmsted: Periorificial plaques, thick, transgrediens PPK, mutilating, pseudoainhum, and leukokeratosis.

Papillon–Lefévre: Transgrediens PPK, periodontitis, can involve knees/elbows, calcified dura mater, falx cerebri and pyogenic liver abscesses. AR, Cathepsin C defects.

Richner–Hanhart: Tyrosinemia Type 2, painful PPK, esp. weightbearing surfaces, plaques on elbows/knees, leukokeratosis, MR, and corneal ulceration. AR, Tyrosine aminotransferase defects.

Striate keratoderma/Brunauer–Fuchs: Linear keratotic plaques. AD, defects: DSG1, DSP.

Symmetric progressive erythrokeratoderma/Gottron: Non-migratory, hyperkeratotic, erythematous plaques, favors extremities and buttocks, PPK, and pseudoainhum. AD, Loricrin defects.

Unna–Thost/nonepidermolytic PPK: Thick, yellow, well-demarcated PPK, non-transgrediens, and hyperhidrosis. AD, KRT1 or 16 defects.

Vorner/epidermolytic PPK: Resembles Unna–Thost, non-transgrediens, may blister, and EH on histopath. AD, KRT9 defects.

Vohwinkel: Honeycomb hyperkeratosis, pseudoainhum, starfish keratoses, and scarring alopecia. AD, GJB2/Connexin 26 (Classic with deafness) or Loricrin (Mutilating variant with Ichthyosis) defects.

Acquired Keratoderma

Keratoderma climactericum: pressure-bearing acral area, peri-menopausal, associated with Psoriasis.

Porokeratosis plantaris discreta: Painful, sharply marginated, rubbery nodules on weight-bearing surface, adult females, and SCC.

Acantholytic disorders

Acrokeratosis verruciformis of Hopf: Verrucous papules on dorsal hands/feet, punctate pits on palms/soles, and onychodystrophy. AD, ATP2A2 defects.

Darier: Dirty, malodorous papules on face, trunk, flexural, punctate keratosis on palms/soles, V-shaped nicking, red/white nail bands, mucosal cobblestoning, guttate leukoderma, schizophrenia, and MR. AD, ATP2A2/SERCA2 defects.

Hailey–Hailey/Benign familial chronic pemphigus: Vesicles, crust, erosions in intertriginous areas, begins in adolescence. AD, ATP2C1 defects.

Peeling skin syndrome/keratolysis exfoliativa congenita: Exfoliation and scale ± erythema and pruritus, esp. palms/soles, AR.

Disorders of connective tissue

Adams–Oliver: Aplasia cutis, cutis marmorata, heart defects, limb hypoplasia, and AD

Bart: Aplasia cutis (esp. legs), DDEB > JEB

Aplasia cutis congenita: Group 1: solitary scalp ACC, Group 2: scalp ACC + limb defects, Group 3: scalp ACC + epidermal/sebaceous nevus, Group 4: scalp ACC overlying embryologic defect, Group 5: ACC + fetus papyraceous (linear/stellate, trunk or limb), Group 6: ACC + EB, Group 7: localized ACC on extremities, Group 8: ACC due to HSV, VZV, methimazole (imperforate anus), Group 9: ACC in trisomy 13 (Patau, large membranous scalp defects), 4p- (Wolf-Hirschhorn), Setleis, Johanson-Blizzard, Goltz, amniotic band, Delleman, Xp22 (Reticulolinear).

Buschke–Ollendorff: Osteopoikilosis, disseminated lenticular CT nevus, sclerotic bone foci. AD, LEMD3 defects

Cutis laxa: Elastolysis, sagging skin, hound dog appearance, deep voice, emphysema, diverticuli, hernia, hook nose, oligohydramnios, and CV anomalies. AR (FBLN4 or 5, or ATP6V0A2), AD (Elastin or FBLN5), and XL (ATP7A – EDS9 and Menkes)

Ehlers–Danlos: See Table below.

Francois/dermochondrocorneal dystrophy: Papulonodules on dorsal hands, nose, ears, gingival hyperplasia, osteochondrodystrophy, corneal dystrophy, and AR

Goltz/focal dermal hypoplasia: Cribiform fat herniations in Blaschko's lines, papillomas (genital, anal, and face), osteopathia striata, syndactyly, oligodactyly, and colobomas. XLD, PORCN defects

Juvenile systemic fibromatosis/infantile systemic hyalinosis: Nodules on H/N (ears/nose/scalp) and fingers, gingival hypertrophy, joint contractures, osteopenia, short stature, and myopathy. AR, Capillary morphogenesis protein-2 (CMG2/ANTXR2) defects

Marfan: Hyperextensible joints, arachnodactyly, aortic aneurysms, dissection/insufficiency, MVP, downward ectopia lentis, PTX, striae, xerosis, EPS, tall stature, long facies, and pectus excavatum. AD, Fibrillin-1 defects (Fibrillin-2 defects = Beals, Congenital Contractural Arachnodactyly – "crumpled ears")

Osteogenesis imperfecta: Brittle bones, thin translucent skin, EPS, bruising, hyperextensible joints, wormian bones, hearing loss, normal teeth, ~normal stature, hernias, arcus senilis, respiratory failure 2/2 kyphoscoliosis, Tx: bisphosphonates. Type 1: blue sclerae, Type 2: perinatal lethal/congenital, Type 3: progressively deforming with normal sclerae, Type 4: normal sclerae, Genetic basis – Type 1, 2A, 3, 4: AD defects in COL1A1 or COL1A2; Type 2B, 7: AR defects in CRTAP

Pachydermoperiostosis/Touraine–Solente–Gole: Thickening of skin and folds and creases on the face, scalp, and extremities, clubbing, AD

Pseudoxanthoma elasticum/Gronblad–Strandberg: Calcification/clumping/fragmentation of elastic fibers, "plucked chicken" skin, angoid streaks, tears in Bruch's membrane, ocular hemorrhage, retinal pigmentary changes, claudication, CAD/MI, GI hemorrhage, HTN, and EPS. AR, ABCC6 defects

PXE-like: PXE-like phenotype + cutis laxa, vit K-dep clotting factor deficiency, cerebral aneurysms, and minimal ocular sxs. AR, GGCX defects

Setlets: Bitemporal forcep-like lesions, leonine facies, absent eyelashes, low frontal hairline, periorbital swelling, fl at nasal bridge, upslanting eyebrows, large lips, bulbous nose (Brauer syndrome – isolated temporal lesions), AD or AR.

Ehlers–Danlos

	Type	Inhr	Defect	Characteristics
I	Gravis	AD	COL 5A1,2	Skin fragility, joint/skin hyperextensibility, bruising, "cigarette paper" scars, prematurity of newborn, molluscoid pseudotumors (at scars), and SQ spheroids
II	Mitis	AD	COL 5A1	Similar to Gravis but less severe
III	Hypermobile	AD	COL 3A1, Tenascin-XB	Marked small and large joint hypermobility and dislocation, *minimal* skin changes, and MSK pain
IV	Vascular/ ecchymotic/ sack	AD	COL 3A1	*Arterial, bowel, and uterine rupture*, bruising, thin, translucent skin with visible/ *varicose* veins, only mild small joint hyperextensibility, tendon/ muscle rupture, EPS, facies – thin nose, hollow cheeks, and staring eyes
V	X-linked	XLR	—	Similar to Mitis, bruising/ skin hyperextensibility > skin fragility
VI	Kyphoscoliotc/ ocular-scoliotic	AR	Lysyl hydroxylase, PLOD1	Skin and joint laxity, *corneal and scleral fragility*, keratoconus, intraocular hemorrhage, *muscle hypotonia* (neonatal), kyphoscoliosis, and arterial rupture, reduced urinary pyridinium cross-links
VII A,B	Arthrochalasia multiplex	AD	COL 1A1,2	*Congenital hip dislocation*, severe joint hypermobility, soft skin, abnormal scars, short, micrognathia
VII C	Dermatosparaxis	AR	ProCOL I N-proteinase/ ADAMST2	Skin fragility (dermatosparaxis = "*skin tearing*"), *sagging and redundant* skin, joint/skin hyperextensibility, bruising, short, micrognathia

continued p.178

	Type	Inhr	Defect	Characteristics
VIII	Periodontal	AD	—	Similar to types I/II + prominent *periodontal* disease, pretibial hyperpigmented (NLD-like) scars
IX	Occipital horn/ Cutis laxa	XLR	ATP7A	Occipital exostoses, abnormal clavicles, abnormal copper transport, joint hypermobility, GU abnormalities, malabsorption, and allelic to Menkes
X	Fibronectin	AR	Fibronectin	Bruising, abnormal clotting, defective platelet aggregation, skin laxity, and joint hypermobility
XI	Large joint hypermobile	AD	—	—

Collagen types

Type	Distribution	Diseases
I	Skin (85% of adult dermis), bone, tendon, and ECMs	Arthrochalasia multiplex, EDS Osteogenesis imperfecta
II	Vitreous humor, cartilage	Stickler arthro-ophthalmopathy, Kneist dysplasia, Spondyloepiphysela dysplasia, Achondrogenesis, Avascular necrosis of femoral head, Antibodies: Relapsing polychondritis
III	Skin (10% of adult dermis), fetal skin, GI/lung, and vasculature	Vascular (Type 4) > Hypermobile (Type 3) EDS types 4 (usu) or 3
IV	Basement membranes	Goodpasture, Alport, Benign familial hematuria, Porencephaly, Diffuse leiomyomatosis
V	Ubiquitous	EDS types 1 and 2
VI	Cartilage, skin, aorta, placenta, and others	Ullrich muscular dystrophy, Bethlem myopathy
VII	Anchoring fibrils, skin, cornea, mucous membranes, and amnion	DEB, Isolated toenail dystrophy, Transient bullous dz of the newborn, EB pruriginosa, Antibodies: CP and BLE
VIII	Endothelial cells, skin, and Descemet's membrane	Fuchs corneal dystrophy
IX	Cartilage	Stickler arthro-ophthalmopathy, Multiple epiphyseal dysplasia ± myopathy, and Intervertebral disc dz susceptibility

Type	Distribution	Diseases
X	Cartilage (hypertrophic)	Metaphyseal chondrodysplasia
XI	Hyaline cartilage	Stickler arthro-ophthalmopathy, Marshall skeletal dysplasia, Familial deafness, Otospondylomegaepiphyseal dysplasia
XVII	Skin hemidesmosomes	JEB, Generalized atrophic EB, Antibodies: BP

Fibril-forming: I, II, III, IV, V, and XI

Fibril-associated collagens with interrupted triple helices: IX, XII, XIV, XVI, XIX, XX, and XXI

Microfibrillar: VI

Network-forming: VIII, X

Transmembrane domains: XIII, XVII

Lysyl oxidase – crosslinking of collagen; cofactors – vitamin C, B6, and copper

Cystathionine synthase – crosslinking of collagen; homocytinuria

Tenascin-XB – EDS3 and EDS-like syndrome

Disorder of hair, nail, ectoderm
Hair
Acquired progressive kinking of the hair: Rapid, adolescent onset, curly, lusterless, frizzy hair, frontotemporal and vertex, may evolve into androgenetic alopecia

Bjornstad: Deafness, pili torti. AD, BCS1L defects

Cantu: Congenital hypertrichosis, osteochondrodysplasia, cardiomegaly, MR, short stature, macrocranium, hypertelorism, cutis laxa, wrinkled palms and soles, joint hyperextensibility, and AD

Citrullinemia: Pili torti, periorificial dermatitis. AR, defects: Argininosuccinate synthetase or SLC25A13

Congenital temporal triangular alopecia: Onset: birth to 6 years old, uni- or bilateral, nl number of follicles but all vellus, AD

Crandall: Deafness, hypogonadism, and pili torti

GAPO: Growth retardation, alopecia, pseudoanodontia, optic atrophy, cranial defects, frontal bossing, umbilical hernia, muscular appearance, and renal abnormalities

Generalized congenital hypertrichosis/hypertrichosis lanuginosa: "Werewolf," curly hairs, sparing palms/soles and mucosa, X-linked

Hallermann–Streiff: Beaked nose, microphthalmia, micrognathia, mandibular hypoplasia, dental abnormalities, congenital cataracts, hypotrichosis (following cranial sutures), dwarfism

Kinky hair: Menkes, woolly hair syndromes, woolly hair nevus, pili torti syndromes, pseudomonilethrix, uncombable hair, APKH, Tricho-Dento-Osseous, and oral retinoids

Klippel–Feil: Low posterior hairline, short webbed neck, fused cervical vertebra, scoliosis, renal anomalies, hearing impairment, torticollis, cardiac septal defects, cleft palate, increased in females, and AD or AR

Localized hypertrichosis: Becker nevi, casts, POEMS, and pretibial myxedema, cubiti, auricle

Marinesco–Sjögren: TTD + neonatal hypotonia, cerebellar ataxia, congenital cataracts, MR, thin brittle nails, short, hypogonadism, and myopathy, chewing difficulties. AR, SIL1 defects

Menkes: Steel wool-like hair, pili torti, monilethrix, trichorrhexis nodosa, epilepsy, hypothermia, and decreased copper and ceruloplasmin. XLR, ATP7A defects

Monilethrix: Beaded hairs, dry, fragile, sparse, associated with KP and brittle nails. AD or AR: type 2 hair keratins KRTHB1, 3, or 6 defects (AD), Desmoglein-4 (AR)

Naxos: PPK, RV cardiomyopathy, Junctional plakogobin

Pili annulati: Ringed hair, spangled, alternating bands (light bands to the naked eye = dark bands on light microscopy = air-filled cavities within the cortex of the hair shaft), associated with alopecia areata, AD

Pili Torti: Twisting, brittle hair, AD, syndromes: Menkes, Bjornstad, Crandall, TTD, hypohidrotic ED, and Bazex, anorexia nervosa, Laron

Trichothiodystrophy: Sulfur (cystine, cysteine)-deficient brittle hair, tiger-tail polarizing, trichoschisis, absent cuticle, immunodeficiency, and osteosclerosis; PIBIDS: Photosensitivity, ichthyosis, brittle hair, decreased intellect, decreased fertility, Short. AR, Defects in ERCC2/XPD, ERCC3/XPB, TFB5 – all TFIIH subunits – and TTDN1/C7ORF11 (nonphotosensitive TTD)

Trichorrhexis invaginata: Bamboo hair, Netherton

Trichorrhexis nodosa: Arginosuccinic aciduria (red fluorescence of hair), citrullinemia, Menkes, TTD, Netherton, isotretinoin, hypothyroidism, physical/chemical trauma, proximal in Blacks and genetic forms vs. distal in Whites and Asians

Uncombable hair: AR, spun glass hair, longitudinal groove, pili canaliculati et trianguli

Woolly hair: Onset: birth, "Afro in a non-African". Isolated forms secondary to LIPH and LPAR6 mutations. Syndromic forms have mutations in desmoplakin (DSP) (Naxos disease), plakoglobin (JUP) (Carvajal syndrome), and ATPase copper transporting alpha polypeptide (ATP7A) (Menkes disease). KANK2 mutations found in family with woolly hair and keratoderma without any accompanying heart defects.

Hair color

Chediak–Higashi: Silvery hair

Early graying: Familial, Hutchinson–Gilford, Werner, Book syndrome (premolar aplasia, hyperhidrosis, and canities premature)

Elejalde: Silvery hair, diffuse hypopigmentation, MR, psychomotor retardation, szs, hair shaft pigment inclusions, and no immunodeficiency. AR, MYO5A, may be same as GS1

Fe deficiency: Segmental heterochromia (Canities segmentata sideropaenica)

Gray patches: Piebaldism, Vitiligo, Vogt–Koyanagi–Harada, NF1, Tietze, Alezzandrini, TS

Griscelli: Silvery hair, diffuse hypopigmentation. AR, Type 1: MYO5A defect, CNS dysfunction, normal immunologically, no hemophagocytosis, Type 2: RAB27A/GTPase defect, immunodeficiency (lymph and NK cells cannot secrete cytotoxic granules), hemophagocytosis, Type 3: MLPH/Melanophilin or MYO5A defects

Homocystinuria: Bleached hair

Menkes: Light hair

PKU: Blonde hair

Nail and oral disorders

Cannon: White sponge nevus, not premalignant. AD, KRT4, and 13 defects

Cooks: Anoncyhia-onychodystrophy (fingers and toes) with absent or hypoplastic distal phalanges, AD

Dyskeratosis congenita/Zinsser–Cole–Engman: Nail thinning, longitudinal ridging, oral leukokeratosis (premalignant), neck – poikiloderma vasculare atrophicans, thin hair, hands/feet: dorsal atrophy/ventral hyperkeratosis, epiphora, aplastic anemia, caries, defects: DKC1 (XLR), TERC (AD) (**Hoyeraal–Hreidarsson** – DC + cerebellar hypoplasia)

Iso-Kikuchi: Congenital onychodysplasia of the index finger, brachydactyly, short hands, inguinal hernia, digital artery stenosis, and AD

Naegeli–Franceschetti–Jadassohn: Hyperkeratotic nails with congenital malalignment, reticulate pigmentation, punctate PPK, enamel hypoplasia, hypohidrosis, and abnormal dermatoglyphics. AD, KRT14 defects

Nail–Patella: Fingernails: hypo- or anonychia and triangular lunula, absent/hypoplastic patella, luxation, posterior iliac horns, renal dysplasia, GU anomalies, and Lester iris. AD, LMX1B defects

Oral–facial–digital-1/Papillon–Leage: Bifid tongue, accessory frenulae, cleft palate/lip, lip nodules, milia, alopecia, dystopia canthorum, syndactyly, brachydactyly, CNS anomalies, and polycystic kidneys. XLD, CXORF5/OFD1 defects

Pachyonychia congenita: Type 1 (Jadassohn–Lewandowsky): Thickened nails, yellow, pincer nails, PPK, follicular keratosis on elbows/knees, oral leukokeratosis, Type 2 (Jackson–Sertoli): 1 + steatocystoma multiplex, PPK may blister, hyperhidrosis, natal teeth, Type 3: 1 + 2 + ocular lesions, cheilosis, Type 4: 1 + 2 + 3 + thin, sparse hair, MR, laryngeal involvement, AD, Defects: KRT6A and 16 (type 1), KRT6B and 17 (type 2)

Rubinstein–Taybi: MR, broad thumbs/great toes, hypertrichosis, high arched palate, crowded teeth, beak-shaped nose, heavy eyebrows, capillary malformation, keloids, pilomatricomas (multiple pilomatricomas also reported with Steinert myotonic dystrophy, Turner, sarcoidosis), and cardiac abnormalities. AD or AR, CREBBP or EP300 defects

Yellow nail: Yellow nails, lymphedema, pleural effusions, and bronchiectasis. AD, FOXC2/MFH1 defects

Ectodermal dysplasia

Acral–dermato–ungual–lacrimal–tooth/ADULT: Ectrodactyly, freckling, onychodysplasia, lacrimal duct defects, and hypodontia

Ankyloblepharon–ectodermal dysplasia–clefting/AEC: Ankloblepharon, ectodermal dysplasia, clefting, chronic erosive dermatitis – especially scalp, patchy alopecia, hypotrichosis, lacrimal duct defects, hypospadias, includes CHAND syndrome

Ectrodactyly–ectodermal dysplasia–clefting/EEC: Lobster claw deformity, ectodermal dysplasia, sparse wiry blond hair, peg-shaped teeth, dystrophic nails, cleft lip, and lacrimal duct defects

Ellis–Van Creveld–Weyers/acrodental dysostosis: Hypoplastic nails, sparse hair, dwarfism (short distal extremities), cone-shaped epiphyses of hand bones, natal teeth, and septal heart defects

Hidrotic ectodermal dysplasia/Clouston: Hypotrichosis, nail dystrophy, keratoderma, normal teeth, and normal sweating. AD, GJB6/ Connexin 30 defects

Hypohidrotic/anhidrotic ectodermal dysplasia/Christ–Siemens– Touraine: Heat intolerance 2/2 decreased or absent sweating, hypodontia, fine sparse hair, brittle nails, thick lips, saddle nose, sunken cheeks, frontal bossing, depressed cell-mediated immunity, elevated IgE, rhinitis, no smell or taste, salivary abnormalities, decreased pulmonary/GI secretions, xerosis, and eczema. XLR: EDA, AD: EDAR, AR: EDAR, EDARADD

Hypohidrotic ectodermal dysplasia with immunodeficiency ± osteoporosis and lymphedema: AR, NEMO defects

Limb-mammary type 4: Aplastic nipples/mammary glands, limb defects, onychodysplasia, MR, and hair defects

P63 complex: EEC, AEC, Rapp-Hodgkin, Limb-Mammary type 4, ADULT, all are AR

Rapp–Hodgkin: Ectodermal dysplasia, clefting, onychodysplasia, dry wiry hair, hypodontia, and hypospadias

Tricho–Dento–Osseous: Whitish, curly hair, brittle nails, xerosis, taurodontism, **and** tall. AD, DLX3 defects

Witkop/tooth-and-nail: Onychodystrophy, toenails > fingernails, retained primary dentition. AD, MSX1 defects

Ectomesodermal dysplasia

Goltz: Cribiform fat herniations in Blaschko lines, perinasal red papules, papillomas in genital and folds, mosaic hypohidrosis, onychodysplasia, scarring alopecia, syndactyly, eye defects, delayed dentition, osteopathia striata, and coloboma. XLD, PORCN defects

MIDAS: Microphthalmia, dermal aplasia, sclerocornea, linear atrophic Blaschkonian plaques, MR, coloboma, strabismus, CNS lesions, and cardiac defects. XLD, Holocytochrome C Synthase/HCCS defects

Phakomatoses

NF1: Diagnosis: At least 2 of: >6 CALM, >2 neurofibromas, 1 plexiform neurofibroma, axillary/inguinal freckling, optic glioma, first degree relative, Lisch nodules, winged sphenoid, pheochromocytoma (1% of pts). Ad, AD, Neurofibromin defects

NF2: Neurofibromas, bilateral acoustic neuromas, schwannomas, and posterior supcapsular lenticular opacity. AD, Merlin defects

NF-Noonan overlap: AD, Neurofibromin defects

SPRED1 NF-1-like syndrome: Axillary freckling, CALM, macrocephaly, and Noonan-like appearance. AD, SPRED1 defects

TS: Angiofi bromas, angiomyolipomas, shagreen patch, Koenen tumors, ash leaf macules, CALM, lymphangioleiomyomatosis, dental pitting, cardiac rhabdomyomas, phalangeal cysts, retinal gliomas, szs, gingival fi bromas, brain calcifi cations, molluscum pendulum. AD, TSC-1 (Hamartin) and TSC-2 (Tuberin) defects

Craniofacial abnormalities

Apert: Craniosynostosis, craniofacial anomalies, severe syndactyly, acneiform lesions, hyperhidrosis, 10% cardiac defects, and 10% GU anomalies. Sporadic, FGFR2 defects

Beare–Stevenson cutis gyrata: Craniosynostosis, cutis gyrata, AN, ear anomalies, anogenital anomalies, acrochordons, and prominent umbilical stump. AD, FGFR2 defects

Cardio-facio-cutaneous: Sparse/absent eyelash, KP, low posterior hairline, ichthyosis, palmoplantar hyperkeratosis, sparse curly hair, short neck, pulmonary stenosis, AV septal defects, short stature, and similar to Noonan. AD, KRAS, BRAF, MEK1, MEK2 defects

Cornelia/Brachmann de Lange: Synophrys, hirsutism, low hairline, MR, heart defects, thin lips, small nose, low-set ears, livedo reticularis/cutis marmorata, small hands and feet, and cryptorchidism/hypospadias. Defects: NIPBL (AD), SMC1L1 (XL), or SMC3 (mild, AD) – all in cohesin complex

Costello: Cutis laxa-like skin, verruca-like papillomas (face, anus, and axillae), acrochordons, AN, PPK, coarse facies, macroglossia, hypertelorism, broad nasal root, thick lips, onychodystrophy, hyperextensible fi ngers, short stature, malignancies (bladder, neuroblastoma, rhabdomyosarcoma), nevi, must distinguish from Noonan and CFC. AR, HRAS or KRAS defects

Crouzon: Craniosynostosis, hypertelorism, parrot nose, and exophthalmos. AD, FGFR2 defects

Crouzon with Acanthosis Nigricans: AD, FGFR3 defects

Goldenhar/oculoauriculovertebral dysplasia/Hemifacial microsomia: Extraauricular appendage, choristoma, eyelid coloboma, cervical vertebral abnormalities, and cardiac defects

Fanconi anemia: Pancytopenia, diffuse hypo/hyperpigmentation, CALMs, absent thumbs and radius (~40%), retinal hemorrhage, strabismus, short stature, and GU anomalies. AR, defects in Fanconi anemia complementation group genes A–N

Nevus sebaceous syndrome: Linear NS, szs, CNS abnormalities, coloboma, and skeletal defects

Noonan: Mimics Turner syndrome in males, acral lymphedema, nevi, hypertelorism, low-set ears, coarse curly hair, low posterior hairline, broad/webbed neck, KP atrophicans, ulerythema ophryogenes, short stature, chest deformities, heart defects, and bleeding diathesis. AD, PTPN11/SHP2, KRAS, SOS1 defects

Treacher Collins: Mandibulofacial dysostosis, downward eyes, lid coloboma, ear anomalies, and NL intelligence. AD, TCOF1 defects

Trichorhinophalangeal: Sparse brittle hair, pear-shaped nose, long philtrum, brachyphalangia, cone-shaped digital epiphysis, crooked fingers, short, brittle nails, short, loose skin, and cartilaginous exostoses. AD, defects: Types 1 and 3 – TRPS1; Type 2: continuous TRPS1 and EXT1 deletion

Progerias

Acrogeria: May be a spectrum of Ehlers–Danlos IV, atrophic acral skin, mottled pigmentation, thin or thick nails, micrognathia, and atrophic tip of nose

Cockayne: Premature graying, cachetic dwarfism, retinal atrophy, deafness, sunken eyes, beak-shaped nose, large ears, photosensitivity, telangiectasia, dementia, premature aging, loss of subcutaneous fat, thin hair, flexion contractures, severe MR, and salt and pepper retina. AR, CSA – ERCC8 defects, CSB – ERCC6 defects

Progeria/Hutchinson–Gilford: Atrophic, sclerodermoid, poikilodermatous skin, prominent veins, alopecia, bird facies, failure to thrive, premature graying, short stature, coax valga, flexural contractures, abnormal dentition, and early death from atherosclerotic heart disease. AR, LMNA defects

Restrictive dermopathy: Taut, translucent skin, open mouth, joint contractures, arthrogryposis, and pulmonary insufficiency. AR, LMNA, or ZMPSTE24 defects

Rothmund–Thomson/hereditary congenital Poikiloderma: Photosensitivity, poikiloderma, dorsal hand keratoses (25% SCC transformation), sparse hair, loss of eyebrows/eyelashes, short, bone defects (radius and hands), cataracts (50% blind), MR, hypodontia, EPS, and osteosarcomas. AR, RECQL4 defects

Werner/adult progeria: Short, high-pitched voice, beak-shaped nose, cataracts, DM2, muscle atrophy, osteoporosis, sclerodermoid changes, painful callosities, severe atherosclerosis, progressive alopecia, canities, hyperkeratosis at elbows/knees/palms/soles, ischemic ulcers, reduced fertility, and sarcomas. AR, RECQL2 defects

Tumor syndromes

Birt–Hogg–Dube: Fibrofolliculomas, trichodiscomas, acrochordons, lipomas, collagenomas, RCC (50% chromophobe/oncocytic hybrid), PTX/lung cysts, hypercalcemia, and colon polyps. AD, FLCN defects

Brooke–Spiegler: Trichoepitheliomas, cylindromas, spiradenomas, and milia. AD, CYLD defects

Cowden: Tricholemmomas, oral mucosal papillomatosis/cobblestoning, acral keratoses, lipomas, sclerotic fibromas, thyroid gland lesions (2/3) (esp. a multiple adenomatous goiter or multiple follicular adenomas), fibrocystic breast lesions, breast cancer (3/4 of F), GI polyposis, GU lesions (1/2 of F) (esp. endometrial cancer), adenoid facies, high arched palate, lingua plicata, and acral papular neuromatosis. AD, PTEN defects

Gardner: Epidermal cysts (may be pilomatricoma-like), desmoid tumors, fibromas (esp. back/paraspinal/nuchal), osteomas, lipomas, leiomyomas, neurofibromas, supernumerary teeth, GI polyps – high rate of malignant transformation, CHRPE, dental anomalies, adrenal adenomas, hepatoblastoma, CNS tumors (Turcot), thyroid carcinoma. AD, APC defects

Li–Fraumeni – Diverse malignancies – breast cancer, acute leukemia, brain tumor, soft tissue/bone sarcomas, adrenal carcinoma, and melanoma

MEN I: Parathyroid, pituitary, pancreas, adrenal, thyroid tumors, lipomas, inclusion cysts, angiofibromas, collagenomas, CALMs, and gingival macules. AD, Menin defect

MEN IIa: Medullary thyroid CA, phaeochromocytoma, parathyroid adenomas, and macular and lichen amyloidosis. AD, RET defects

MEN IIb: Medullary thyroid CA, pheochromocytoma, mucosal neuromas, large lips, lordosis, genu valgum, kyphosis, CALMs, lentigines, marfanoid habitus, synophrys, and megacolon/ganglioneuromatosis. AD, RET defects

Multiple cutaneous and uterine leiomyomata (fibromas): 15–60% develop renal duct or papillary renal type II cancer, rarely cerebral cavernomas. AD, Fumarate Hydratase defects (homozygous mutations cause severe mitochondrial encephalopathy, and fumaric aciduria)

Multiple familial trichoepithelioma/epithelioma adenoides cysticum of Brooke: Trichoepitheliomas, milia. AD, maps to 9p21 (distinct from Brooke–Spiegler)

Schopf–Schulz–Passarge: Eyelid hydrocytomas, hypodontia, hypotrichosis, nail defects, PPK, eccrine syringofibroadenoma, and AR

Von Hippel–Lindau: Retinal angioma, cerebellar medullary angioblastic tumor, pancreatic cysts, RCC, pheochromocytoma, polycythemia, and AD

KA syndromes

Ferguson–Smith: Multiple self-healing KAs, onset: second decade, usually sun-exposed areas, scar, singly or in crops. AD, 9q31 (very close to PTCH1)

Grzybowski: Numerous small eruptive (2–3 mm), adult onset, oral mucosa and larynx may be involved, pruritus

Keratoacanthoma centrifugum marginatum: Large with peripheral growth and central healing, non-involuting dorsal hand or leg

Muir–Torre: KA, sebaceous carcinoma, sebaceous adenomas, colorectal cancer (50%), GU neoplasms (25%), and breast/lung neoplasms. AD, MSH2, MLH1, or MSH6 defects

Others: Subungual, KA dyskeratoticum and segregans, and KAs occurring post-UV, post-surgery, post-aldara, or post-laser resurfacing

Witten and Zak: Combo of Ferguson–Smith and Grzybowski

BCC sydromes

Bazex–Dupre–Christol: BCC, follicular atrophoderma, pili torti, milia, ulerythema ophryogenes, scrotal tongue, spiny hyperkeratoses, neuropsychiatric, and XLD

Gorlin/Basal cell nevus/nevoid BCC: BCC, palmoplantar pits, odontogenic jaw cysts, hypertelorism, frontal bossing, ovarian CA/fibroma, medulloblastomas, milia, lipomas, epidermal cysts, calcification of falx, fused/bifid ribs, eye anomalies, and hypogonadism. AD, PTCH1 defects

Rombo: BCC, trichoepitheliomas, hypotrichosis, atrophoderma vermiculata, milia, cyanosis of lips/hands/feet, telangiectasia, and AD

Disorders of vascularization

Alagille: Arteriohepatic dysplasia, nevus comedonicus, xanthomas, retinal pigment anomalies, peripheral arterial stenosis, pulmonic valvular stenosis, "butterfly" vertebrae, absent deep tendon reflexes, broad forehead, bulbous nasal tip, and foreshortened fingers. AD, JAG1, or NOTCH2 defects

Ataxia telangiectasia/Louis–Bar: Cerebellar ataxia starts first (at ~1 yo), wheelchair-bound by ~ 12 yo, oculocutaneous telangiectasias develop by 3–6 yo, sinopulm infxn, IgA and IgG are diminished, IgE and IgM may be diminished, premature aging, poikilodermatous and sclerodermatous skin, MR, insulin-resistant DM2, increased AFP (makes it difficult to screen for hepatic tumors) and CEA, radiosensitivity, lymphoid/solid (stomach, breast) malignancies, cutaneous granulomas. AR but cancer risk in heterozygotes, ATM defects

Beckwith–Wiedemann: Facial PWS, macroglossia, omphalocoele, hemihypertrophy, adrenocortical carcinomas, pancreatoblastomas, and hepatoblastomas. Defects: p57/KIP2/CDKN1C or NSD1

Blue rubber bleb nevus/Bean: Painful blue nodules with hyperhidrosis, GI bleeds.

Bloom: Short stature, telangiectatic facial erythema, malar hypoplasia, photosensitivity, hypogonadism/decreased fertility, high-pitched voice, leukemia, lymphoma, low IgM and IgA, recurrent pneumonia, CALM, crusted/blistered lips, narrow face, DM2 (and acanthosis nigricans), MR, loss of eyelashes. AR, RECQL3 = RECQ2 defects

Capillary malformation-ArterioVenous malformation/CM-AVM: Atypical capillary malformations + AVM, AV fistula, soft tissue overgrowth. AD, Germline RASA1 defects

CLOVES: Congenital lipomatous overgrowth, vascular malformation (may have spinal/paraspinal fast flow lesion), epidermal nevus, spinal/skeletal abnormalities, renal anomalies, inguinal hernia, undescended testicles, and increase risk of pulmonary embolism. Associated with Wilms tumor. Somatic mosaic, PIK3CA gene, activating mutation.

Cobb: Cutaneomeningospinal angiomatosis, hemangioma or vascular malformation of a spinal segment and its corresponding dermatome

Cutis marmorata telangiectatica congenita/Van Lohuizen: Persistant livedo, atrophy/ulceration, CNS defects, MR, craniofacial anomalies, glaucoma, syndromes with cutis marmorata: Adams–Oliver, Cornelia de Lange, Coffin–Siris (related condition: Macrocephaly-CMTC syndrome – macrocephaly + cutis marmorata + several additional features among the following: hypotonia, toe syndactyly, segmental overgrowth, hydrocephalus, midline facial nevus flammeus, frontal bossing)

Gorham–Stout/disappearing (aka Vanishing or Phantom) bone: Onset: childhood or young adulthood, progressive osteolysis of one or more bones, vascular malformations (bone and skin), pathologic fractures, limb tenderness and weakness, thoracic duct occlusion, and chylothorax, tx: radiation

Klippel–Trenaunay: Capillary malformation with limb hypertrophy, venous/lymphatic malformations, angiokeratomas, lymphangiomas, AV fistula, phlebitis, thrombosis, and ulcerations. PIK3CA.

Maffucci: Enchondromas, increased chondrosarcoma, venous malformation, ±spindle cell hemagioma, increased incidence of malignancies (brain, ovarian, and pancreatic). AD, IDH (isocitrate dehydrogenase). Ollier – no vascular malformations.

Multiple cutaneous and mucosal venous malformations/VMCM: AD, TIE2 defects

Osler–Weber–Rendu/Hereditary hemorrhagic telangiectasia: Telangiectasia of mucosa/ face/palms/soles, epistaxis, GI bleed, AVM in brain, lungs, and liver. AD.

HHT-1: Endoglin. Higher incidence of pulmonary AVMs

HHT-2: Activin receptor-like kinase-1

HHT-3: SMAD-replated protein 4

Parkes Weber: Capillary malformation, AVM, ±soft tissue overgrowth. Somatic RASA1.

PHACES: Posterior fossa abnormalities, Hemangiomas, Arterial anomalies (including intracranial aneurysms), Cardiac anomalies (often aortic coarctation), Eye anomalies, Sternal defects, usually females, most often left-sided hemangioma, Dandy–Walker malformation, and cleft palate

Proteus: Assymmetric progressive disproportionate partial gigiantism (hands and feet) and body hemihypertrophy, lipomas, cerebriform connective tissue nevus, macrocephaly, hyperostosis, vascular malformation (capillary, venous +/– lymphatic0, ocular anomalies, and scoliosis. Somatic mosaic, AKT1, activating mutation.

Roberts/SC phocomelia/SC pseudothalidomide: Facial PWS, hypomelia, hypotrichosis, growth retardation, cleft lip/palate, limb defects. AR, ESCO2 defects

Sturge–Weber: V1 PWS, V2, and V3 may be involved but must be in conjunction with V1, full V1 involvement has greater risk than partial V1 involvement, glaucoma, seizures, ipsilateral vascular malformation of meninges and train track calcifications, mental retardation, bone ± soft tissue overgrowth. Somatic mutation, QNAQ.

Thrombocytopenia-absent radius/TAR: Absent radius, decreased platelets, PWS

Von Hippel–Lindau: Capillary malformation of head/neck, retinal/cerebellar hemangioblastoma, renal cell CA, renal cysts, pheochromocytoma, adrenal CA, and pancreatic cysts. AD, VHL defects

Lymphedema

Meige/Lymphedema praecox: Most common form of primary lymphedema AD, FOXC2/MFH1 defects (also causes Yellow Nail, Lymphedema–Distichiasis, and Lymphedema and Ptosis syndromes)

Nonne–Milroy: Congenital lymphedema, unilateral or bilateral, pleural effusions, chylous ascites, scrotal swelling, protein-losing enteropathy, risk for lymphangiosarcoma and angiosarcoma, right > left leg. AD but F>M, FLT4/VEGFR3 defects

Yellow nail: Lymphedema, pleural effusions, bronchiectasis, and yellow nails. AD, FOXC2/MFH1 defects

Nonhereditary syndromic vascular disorders

APACHE: Acral Pseudolymphomatous Angiokeratoma of CHildrEn

Coats: Retinal telangiectasia, ipsilateral PWS

Hennekam: Congenital lymphedema, intestinal lymphangiectasia, MR

Kasabach–Merritt: Consumptive coagulopathy associated with large vascular lesion, especially kaposiform hemangioendothelioma or tufted angioma

Mondor: Thrombophlebitis of the veins in the thoracogastric area, often breast, sometimes strain/trauma

POEMS/Crow–Fukase: Glomeruloid hemangiomas, Polyneuropathy, Organomegaly (liver, lymph nodes, and spleen), Endocrinopathy, Monoclonal protein (IgA or G)/Myeloma (15% Castleman disease), Skin changes (hyperpigmentation, skin thickening, hypertrichosis, and sclerodermoid changes), sclerotic bone lesions, edema, and papilledema

Secretan: Acral factitial lymphedema

Stewart-Bluefarb: Pseudo-KS, leg AVM

Stewart–Treves: Mastectomy → angiosarcoma

Syndromes with photosensitivity: XP, Bloom, Rothmund-Thomson, Cockayne, Hartnup, porphyrias, TTD, Cockayne, Kindler, Prolidase deficiency, Hailey-Hailey, Darier

Wyburn-Mason: Facial PWS, ipsilateral AVM of retinal / optic pathway

Disorders of metabolism
Enzymatic deficiencies
Alkaptonuria: Dark urine/sweat, arthritis, discolored cartilage, kyphoscoliosis, joint destruction, tendon rupture, deafness, vs. exogenous ochronosis due to hydroxyquinone, phenol, or picric acid. AR, Homogentisic acid oxidase/Homogentisate 1,2-dioxygenase defects

Angiokeratoma	**Solitary papular**: usually extremity, preceding trauma
	Circumscriptum: large, single Blaschkonian plaque, extremity
	Corporis diffusum: Fabry, Fucosidosis
	Mibelli: fingers and toes, adolescence, cold-provoked
	Fordyce: scrotum, vulva, middle-aged
	Caviar spot: tongue

Fabry: Angiokeratoma corporis diffusum, whorl-like corneal opacities, "maltese cross" in urine, painful paresthesias, ceramide accumulates in heart, autonomic nervous system, and kidneys (main cause of mortality), CVA/MI (second most cause of mortality), autoantibodies (esp. LAC and antiphospholipid), and thrombosis. XLR, α-Galactosidase A

Fucosidosis: Angiokeratoma corporis diffusum, coarse thick skin, MR, szs, spasticity, dysostosis multiplex, visceromegaly, growth retardation, and respiratory infections. AR, α-L-Fucosidase

Gaucher: Glucosylceramide/GlcCer/glucosylcerebroside accumulates in the brain, liver, spleen, and marrow, Type 1: "nonneuronopathic," HSM, bronze skin, pinguecula of sclera, adults; Type 2: "acute neuronopathic," infant, may be preceded by ichthyosis; Type 3: "subacute neuronopathic," juvenile, chronic neuro sxs; Type 3C: with CV calcifications. AR, Acid β-Glucosidase defects (except Atypical Gaucher – PSAP/Saposin C defect)

Hartnup: Error in tryptophan secretion, pellagra-like rash, and psychiatric changes. AR, SLC6A19 defects

Homocystinuria: Marfanoid appearance, premature heart disease, low IQ, szs, osteoporosis, codfish vertebrae with collapse, livedo on legs, fine sparse hair, pigmentary dilution, and upward ectopia lentis. AR, Cystathione β-Synthase or MTHFR defects

Hurler: HSM, BM failure, thick lips, large tongue, MR, corneal opacities, broad hands with clawlike fingers, dried urine with toluidine blue turns purple, and dermatan sulfate and heparan sulfate in urine. AR, α-L-Iduronidase defects

Hunter: Like Hurler but milder, pebbly lesions over, XLR, iduronate sulfatase defects

Lesch–Nyhan: HGPRT deficiency, hyperuricemia, self-mutilation, MR, spastic CP, tophi. XLR, HPRT defects

Lipogranulomatosis/Farber: SQ masses over wrists/ankles, arthritis, hoarse, involves larynx, liver, spleen, kidneys, and CNS. AR, Acid ceramidase (also called N-acylsphingosine amidohydrolase – ASAH) defects

Niemann–Pick: Classical infantile form (A, Ashkenazi), visceral form (B, adults, nonneuropathic), subacute/juvenile form (C), Nova Scotia form (D), adult form (E), HSM, lymphadenopathy, MR, cherry red macula, yellow skin, and dark macules in mouth. AR, Sphingomyelinase or NPC1 defects

Oxalosis: Livedo, nephrocalcinosis, and cardiomyopathy. AR, Type 1 - Alanine–Glyoxylate Aminotransferase (AGXT) defects, Glyoxylate Reductase/Hydroxypyruvate Reductase (GRHPR) defects

PKU: MR, szs, pigmentary dilution, and atopic dermatitis. AR, Phenylalanine hydroxylase or Dihydropteridine reductase defects

Tangier: Alpha lipoprotein deficiency, orange yellow striations on large tonsils, splenomegaly, neuropathy, and decreased cholesterol. AR, ATP-Binding Cassette-1 (ABC1) defects

Lipomatosis

Dercum/Adiposa dolorosa: Psychiatric issues, obese women, multiple painful lipomas, asthenia, AD

Familial multiple lipomatosis: spares shoulders and neck, AD

Madelung/Launois–Bensaude/familial symmetrical lipomatosis: Alcoholism, liver disease, DM2, gout, hyperlipidemia, massive symmetrical lipomas around neck and upper trunk, and "body-builder" appearance

Total lipodystrophies

Bernadelli–Seip: Congenital total/generalized lipodystrophy, increased appetite, increased height velocity, AN, hyperpigmentation, thick curly hair, mild MR, DM2, CAD, hypertriglyceridemia, and hepatic steatosis. AR, Type 1 – 1-Acylglycerol-3-Phosphate O-Acyltransferase-2 (AGPAT2) defects, Type 2 – Seipin (BSCL2) defects

Seip–Lawrence: Acquired total lipodystrophy, begins before age 15, preceded by infxn or CTD, DM2, AN, liver involvement is worse and commonly fatal, muscle wasting, and growth retardation

Partial lipodystrophies

Barraquer–Simons: Acquired progressive lipodystrophy, first and second decade onset after viral illness, begins in face and progresses downwards to iliac crests/buttocks, increased C3 nephritic factor, GN, third trimester abortions, DM2, LMNB2 defects

Insulinopenic partial lipodystrophy w/ Rieger anomaly/SHORT: In infancy, loss of fat on face and buttocks, retarded growth, bone age, and dentition, DM2 with low insulin, NO AN, Rieger anomaly = eye and tooth anomalies, S = stature; H = hyperextensibility of joints or hernia; O = ocular depression; R = Rieger anomaly; T = teething delay

Kobberling–Dunnigan: At puberty, loss of SQ fat from extremities, buttocks, and lower trunk, gain fat on face, neck, back, and axilla, AN, hirsutism, PCOS, DM2, increased TG. AD or XLD, Type 1 – unknown genetic defect, Type 2 – LMNA defects, Type 3 – PPARG defects

Porphyrias
U: urine B: Blood

Pseudoporphyria	—	2/2 NSAIDS, tetracycline, hemodialysis, tanning booths, thiazide, and furosemide	Normal urine, blood, and feces
			PCT-like, photosensitive blistering and skin fragility; no hypertrichosis/hyperpigmentation/sclerodermoid changes
PCT	AD	Uroporphyrinogen decarboxylase	U/B: uroporphyrin 3× > coproporphyrin
			Stool: Isocoproporphyrin
			Photosensitive blistering, skin fragility, hypertrichosis, sclerodermoid changes
			Tx: phlebotomy, antimalarials. Check Fe, HCV, and hemochromatosis
Hepatoerythropoietic porphyria (Homozygous PCT)	AR	Uroporphyrinogen decarboxylase	Similar U/B/Stool as PCT, plus elevated protoporphyrins in RBCs
			Similar to CEP – photosensitive blistering in infancy, hypertrichosis, hyperpigmentation, neurologic changes, anemia, dark urine, and erythrodontia

continued p.192

Variegate porphyria	AD	Protoporphyrinogen oxidase	U: dALA, PBG (during attack); coproporphyrin > uroporphyrin (unlike PCT)
			B: 626 nm fluorescence
			Stool: elevated coproporphyrins > protoporphyrins
			Most often asx; may have PCT-like skin, AIP-like neurologic and GI sx
			Avoid precipitating factors
Acute intermittent porphyria	AD	Porphobilinogen deaminase	U: PBG, dALA B: dALA
			Abdominal pain, muscle weakness, psychiatric sx, no skin findings/photosensitivity, risk of liver cancer
Hereditary coproporphyria	AD	Coproporphyrinogen oxidase	U: coproporphyrin, dALA, PBG (during attack)
			Stool: coproporphyrin (always)
			PCT-like skin, AIP-like neurologic and GI sxneuron
Congenital erythropoietic porphyria (Gunther)	AR	Uroporphyrinogen-III synthase	U/Stool/RBC: uroporphyrin and coproporphyrin
			Severe photosensitivity, erythrodontia, mutilating scars, hypertrichosis, madarosis, scleromalacia perforans, red urine, anemia, and gallstones
			Tx: Transfuse to keep Hct 33% (turn off porphyrin production)
Erythropoietic protoporphyria	AD AR	Ferrochelatase	U: nl B/RBC/stool: protoporphyrin
			Severe photosensitivity (elevated protoporphyrin IX), purpura, erosions/scars, waxy/"weather beaten" thickening (nose, knuckles), gallstones, anemia, and liver dysfunction
			Tx: β-carotene, antihistamine, NBUVB to induce UV tolerance

Disorders of pigmentation

Albright hereditary osteodystrophy: Pseudo or pseudopseudo-hyper-parathyroidism, short fourth and fifth digits, osteoma cutis, short stature, dimpling over knuckles, and MR. Maternally inherited GNAS1 mutations

Acromelanosis progressiva: Rare, black pigment of hands/feet, spread by age ~5 years

Acropigmentation of dohi/dyschromatosis symmetrica hereditaria: Hypo- and hyperpigmented macules on extremeties in a reticulated pattern, especially dorsal hands/feets. AD, DSRAD defects

Bannayan–Riley–Revalcaba/Bannayan–Zonana: Macrocephaly, genital lentigines, MR, hamartomas (GI polyps), lipomas, trichilemmomas, vascular malformation, and thyroid disorder. High risk of malignancy (breast, thyroid, endometrium, Lhermitte–Duclos cerebrellar gangliocy-toma). AD, PTEN defects

Carney complex: NAME (Nevi, Atrial myxoma, Myxomatous neurofibromata, Ephelids), **LAMB** (Lentigines, Atrial myxoma, Myxoid tumors, Blue nevi), Sertoli cell tumors, melanotic schwannomas, mammary neoplasia, and CVA from cardiac emboli, pigmentary nodular adrenal tumors, pituitary adenomas. AD, PRKAR1A defects

Chediak–Higashi: Light cream skin, silvery hair, photophobia, nystagmus, usually present with recurrent infxn (lymphs and NK cells cannot secrete cytotoxic granules), giant lysosome granules in PMNs, giant melanosomes, bleeding diathesis, no neurologic defect. AR, LYST defects

Cross-McKusick/Oculocerebral syndrome with hypopigmentation: Albinism, MR, szs, spastic di/quadriplegia, silvery-gray hair

Dermatopathia pigmentosa reticularis: Generalized reticulate pigmentation, sweating disregulation, decreased dermatoglyphics, noncicatricial alopecia, onychodystrophy, and PPK. AD, KRT14 defects

De Sanctis–Cacchione: Type A XP, mental deficiency, dwarfism, hypogonadism. AR, ERCC6 defects

Dowling–Degos: Postpubertal, progressive, brown, reticulate hyperpigmentation of the flexures, no hypopigmented macules, soft fibromas, pitted perioral scars, rarely hidradenitis suppurativa, path = elongated pigmented rete ridges, thinned suprapapillary plates, dermal melanosis. AD, KRT5 defects (**Galli–Galli** – acantholytic Dowling–Degos; Dowling–Degos shares features with **Haber** – early rosacea, trunkal keratoses (esp. axillae SK/VV-like), pitted scars, PPK).

Familial GI stromal tumors (GISTs) with hyperpigmentation: GISTs, perineal hyperpigmentation, hyperpigmented macules (perioral, axillae, hands, perineal – not oral or lips), +/- urticaria pigmentosum. AD, C-KIT defects (activating mutations)

Familial progressive hyperpigmentation: Hyperpigmented patches at birth, spread, involve conjunctivae and buccal mucosa, AD

Hermansky–Pudlak: Tyrosinase +, hemorrhagic diathesis, absent dense bodies in platelets, nystagmus, blue eyes, granulomatous colitis, pulmonary involvement, progressive pigment recovery, Puerto Ricans, Jews, Muslims. AR, HPS1–8 defects (includes DTNBP1 and BLOC1S3)

IP acromians/hypomelanosis of Ito: Hypopigmented nevi (linear/whorled) + CNS anomalies, strabismus, szs, MR, mosaic chromosomal anomalies

IP/Bloch–Sulberger: Four stages: (i) Blistering, (ii) Verrucous, (iii) Hyperpigmented, (iv) Hypopigmented/Atrophic; Eosinophilia/leukocytosis, pegged teeth, szs, MR, strabismus, Scarring alopecia, onychodystrophy, ocular sxs. XLD, NEMO defects

Kindler–Weary: Acral, traumatic bullae during childhood, sclerotic poikiloderma, photosensitivity, periodontosis, pseudosyndactyly, scleroderma/XP-like facies, esophageal strictures, oral leukokeratoses, and SCC. AR, KIND1 defects

LEOPARD/Moynahan: Lentigines, EKG abnormalities, Ocular hypertelorism, Pulmonary stenosis, Abnormal genitalia, growth Retardation, Deafness. AD, PTPN11 defects

Linear and whorled/figurated nevoid hypo/hypermelanosis: No bullae, Blaschko distribution, often with MR, PDA, and ASD

McCune–Albright: "Coast of Maine" CALM, precocious puberty, polyostotic fibrous dysplasia (fractures, asymmetry, pseudocystic radiographic lesions), endocrinopathies (hyperthyroidism, Cushing, hypersomatotropism, hyperprolactinemia, hyperparathyroidism). Mosaic activating GNAS1 defects

OCA1A, 1B/tyrosine negative albinism (OCA = oculocutaneous albinism): 1A: No tyrosinase activity, strabismus, photophobia, reduced acuity, 1B: Slightly more tyrosinase activity. AR, Tyrosinase defects (if temperature sensitive mutation → "Siamese cat" pattern)

OCA2: Tyrosinase +, increased in Blacks/South Africa, 1% of Prader-Willi and Angelman patients have OCA2. AR, P gene defects

OCA3: Blacks, copper/ginger hair, light tan skin, ±eye involvement. AR, TYRP1 defects

OCA4: AR, MATP/SLC45A2 defect

Pallister–Killian: Hyperpigmentation in Blaschko lines, coarse facies, temporal hypotrichosis, CV anomalies, and MR. Mosaic tetrasomy 12p

Peutz–Jeghers: 90% small bowel involved, colic pain, bleeding, intussusception, rectal prolapse, 20–40% malignant transformation of GI polyps, cancer (breast, ovary, testes, uterus, pancreas, and lungs), sertoli cell tumors, oral lentigines (also facial, hands/soles, genital, and perianal), longitudinal melanonychia, presents before or in early puberty. AD, STK11 defects (vs. **Laugier–Hunziker.** Nonfamilial orolabial pigmented macules similar to P–J without GI involvement, Caucasians presenting between ages 20 and 40 years)

Piebaldism/Partial albinism: White forelock, depigmented patch ("diamond-patches"). AD, C-KIT defects (inactivating mutations)

Reticulate pigmentation of kitamura: Linear palmar pits, reticulate, hyperpigmented macules, 1–4mm on volar and dorsal hands, no hypopigmented macules. AD, KRT5 defects

Rufous oculocutaneous albinism/ROCA: Copper-red colored skin/hair, iris color diluted, South Africa. AR, TYRP1 defects

Russell–Silver: Growth retardation, feeding difficulties, triangular facies, downturned lips, blue sclerae, limb asymmetries, clinodactyly of fifth digit, CALM, urologic abnormalities, 10% demonstrate maternal uniparental disomy of chromosome 7

Waardenberg: Depigmented patches, sensorineural defects, white forelock, dystopia canthorum, iris heterochromia, broad nasal root, white eyelashes, cleft lip, scrotal tongue, megacolon (Type 4), limb defects (Type 3) AD>AR, Type 1: PAX3, Type 2A: MITF, Type 2D: SNAI2, Type 3: PAX3, Type 4: SOX10, Endothelin-B receptor, or Endothelin-3 defects

Xeroderma pigmentosa: Types A–G, Type A most severe, A is most common in Japan, Group C (30%) and D (20%) are most common overall defective UV damage repair, ectropion, blepharitis, keratitis, low intelligence, dementia, ataxia, lentigines, premature aging, NMSC, melanoma, KA, AR

Nonhereditary syndromic disorders of pigmentation

Alezzandrini: Unilateral degenerative pigmentary retinitis, ipsilateral vitiligo, and poliosis

Bronze baby syndrome: Complication of phototherapy for bilirubinemia, elevated direct bili, hepatic dysfunction, induced by photoproducts of bilirubin and biliverdin

Cronkhite-Canada: Melanotic macules on fingers, more diffuse hyperpigmentation than Peutz–Jeghers, alopecia, onychodystrophy, protein losing enteropathy, GI polyposis

Gray baby syndrome: Chloramphenicol

Riehl melanosis: Pigmented contact dermatitis on face, especially brown-gray discolored forehead/temples, often due to cosmetics, interface reaction on path

Vogt–Koyanagi–Harada: Depigmented skin/eyelashes, chronic granulomatous iridocyclitis, retinal detachment, and aseptic meningoenchalitis

Immunodeficiency syndromes

APECED: Autoimmune Polyendocrinopathy, (chronic mucocutaneous) Candidiasis, Ectodermal Dystrophy, frequent Addison and/or hypoparathyroidism, selective T cell anergy for candida, alopecia, vitiligo, and oral SCC. AR, AIRE defects

Chronic Granulomatous Disease/CGD: Recurrent purulent and granulomatous infxns of the long bones, lymphatic tissue, liver, skin, lungs, 2/3 in boys, eczema, defect in NADPH oxidase complex, autoimmunity, lupus-like sxs in XL carriers (rash, arthralgias, oral ulcers, fatigue, but usually ANA-), gene for XLR (60%): CYBB, AR forms: NCF1, NCF2, CYBA (p22-, p47-, p67-, and p91-phox)

CVID: Typical sx onset and diagnosis in late 20s, increased HLA-B8, DR3, recurrent sinopulmonary infxns, increased autoimmune dz, lymphoreticular and GI malignancies, arthritis, noncaseating granulomas (may be confused with sarcoidosis), some T cell dysfxn, reduced Ig levels (esp IgG and IgA, also IgM in ½ of patients), tx: IVIG

DiGeorge/thymic hypoplasia: Notched, low set ears, micrognathia, shortened philtrum, hypertelorism, absent parathyroids → neonatal hypocalcemia, thymic hypoplasia → T cell deficit, cardiac anomlies (truncus arteriosis, interrupted aortic arch), psychiatric sxs, cleft lip/palate, CHARGE overlap, 1/3 with Complete DiGeorge have eczematous dermatitis. AD, deletion in proximal long arm of chromosome 22 (TBX1 is especially important)

Hyper-IgM: Recurrent infxns, low IgG, E, A, respiratory infxn, diarrhea, otitis, oral ulcers, VV, recurrent neutropenia, tx with IVIG, BMT. XL (CD40L), AR (CD40, AICD, HIGM3)

Hyper-IgE: AD-like lesions, recurrent pyogenic infxns/cold abscesses, eosinophilia, may have PPK, asthma, chronic candidiasis, urticaria, coarse facies with wide nose, deep-set eyes, hyperextensible joints, fractures, lymphomas, pneumatoceles, retained primary teeth, scoliosis, and pathologic fractures. AD: STAT3 defects, AR: TYK2 defects (AR form has severe viral infections, HSV, extreme eosinophilia, neurologic complications, and no skeletal/dental defects), subset with **Job's**: Girls with red hair, freckles, blue eyes, hyperextensible joints

Isolated IgA deficiency: 50% with recurrent infxns, 25% with autoimmune dz, Celiac, UC, AD, asthma, IVIG infusion may cause allergic rxn 2/2 IgA Ab, hard to confirm dx before 4 yo because IgA is late to develop in children

Isolated IgM deficiency: 1/5 with eczematous dermatitis, VV, patients with MF and celiac disease may have secondary IgM deficiency, thyroiditis, splenomegaly, hemolytic anemia

Leukocyte Adhesion Molecule deficiency: Delayed umbilical separation, periodontitis, gingivitis, poor wound healing, Tx: BMT. AR, CD18 β2 integrin (can't bind CD11, C3b).

Myeloperoxidase deficiency: Most asymptomatic. AR, MPO defects
Omenn/Familial reticuloendotheliosis with eosinophilia: Exfoliative erythroderma, alopecia, eosinophilia, HSM, LAN, infections, diarrhea, hypogammaglobulinemia, hyper-IgE, decreased B cells, and increased T cells. AR, RAG1, RAG2 defects
SCID: Absent cellular and humoral immunity, monilithiasis, diarrhea, and pneumonia. AR, Adenosine deaminase, RAG1, RAG2 defects
Thymic dysplasia with normal immunoglobulins/Nezelof: T-cell deficit, severe candidiasis, varicella, diarrhea, pulm infxns, nl Ig, AR
Wiskott–Aldrich: Young boys, triad (atopic, recurrent infxn – esp. encapsulated organisms, thrombocytopenia), small platelets, lymphoid malignancies, cellular and humoral immunodeficiency, autoimmune disorders, often present with bleeding (from circumcision or diarrhea), defects in cellular and humoral immunity: IgM deficiency with IgA and IgE often elevated and IgM often normal, HSM, tx: BMT. XLR, WASP defects
X-linked agammaglobulinemia/Bruton: Males, onset: infancy, recurrent infxns (Gram+ sinopulmonary, meningoencephalitis, arthritis), reduced or undetectable Ig levels, atopy, vasculitis, urticaria, no germinal centers or plasma cells, RA-like sxs, neutropenia, chronic lung disease, defect in PreB to B cell differentiation, tx: IVIG. XL, BTK defects.

Silvery hair syndromes (Melanolysosomal neurocutaneous syndromes)

	Chediak–Higashi	Elejalde	Griscelli
Neurologic	Normal (rarely defects in adult form)	Severe defects, mental and motor, regressive	Defects in Type 1, normal in Types 2 and 3
Immunologic	PMN, NK, and lymph cell defects, fatal accelerated phase (uncontrolled macrophage and lymphocyte activation)	Normal	Normal in Types 1 and 3, Defects in Type 2 (lymphs and NK cells), no fatal accelerated phase
Hair	Silvery, regular melanin clumps in small granules (6X smaller than granules of Elejalde or Griscelli)	Silvery, irregular melanin clumps in large and small granules	Silvery, irregular melanin clumps in large and small granules
Skin	Pigment dilution	Pigment dilution	Pigment dilution
Platelet	Dense granule defects	Dense granule defects	Dense granule defects
Ophtho	Defects	Defects	Defects
Inheritance	AR, LYST	AR, MYO5A	AR, MYO5A (Type 1), RAB27A (Type 2), MLPH, or MYO5A (Type 3)

Hereditary periodic fever syndromes

Familial mediterranean fever/FMF: Recurrent fever (few hours to several days), recurrent polyserositis (peritoneum, synovium, and pleura), AA amyloidosis, renal failure, erysipelas-like erythema esp. BLE, rare associations: HSP and PAN. AR or AD, MEFV/Pyrin defects

Hyper-IgD with periodic fever/HIDS: Recurrent fever (3–7 days, 1–2 months apart), abdominal pain, diarrhea, headache, arthralgias, cervical lymphadenopathy, erythematous macules > papules and nodules, elevatated IgD and IgA, rare associations: HSP and EED, mevalonic aciduria. AR, MVK defects

TNF receptor-associated periodic/TRAPS/Hibernian fever: Recurrent fever (usu > 5 days, often 1–3 weeks), myalgia (w/ overlying migratory erythema), pleurisy, abdominal pain, conjunctivitis/periorbital edema, serpiginous, edematous, purpuric, or reticulated lesions esp. at extremities, AA amyloidosis, renal failure, leukocytosis, elevated ESR. AD, TNF-Receptor 1 defects

Cryopyrin-associated periodic syndromes

Histo: lots of PMNs, no Mast cells

Blau: Arthritis, uveitis, granulomatous dermatitis – early onset sarcoidosis. AD, NOD2/CARD15 defects

Familial cold autoinflammatory/Urticaria/FCAS: Urticaria-like eruption, limb pain, recurrent fever, flare with generalized cold exposure, normal hearing, AA amyloidosis. AD, CIAS1 defects

Majeed: Subacute or chronic multifocal osteomyelitis with neutrophilic dermatosis or Sweet syndrome. AR, LPIN2 defects

Muckle–Wells: Urticaria-like eruption, limb pain, recurrent fever, AA amyloidosis (more common than FCAS), deafness. AD, CIAS1 defects

Neonatal-onset multisystemic inflammatory disease/NOMID/CINCA: Triad of CNS disorder, arthropathy, and rash (edematous, urticarial-like papules and plaques, neutrophilic eccrine hidradenitis); also deafness and visual disturbance, recurrent fever, AA amyloidosis. AD, CIAS1 defects

Pyogenic sterile arthritis, Pyoderma gangrenosum, and Acne/PAPA: Periodic Fever with Aphthous Stomatitis, Pharyngitis, and Cervical Adenopathy (PFAPA), attacks last ~5 days. AD, PSTPIP1 defects (vs. SAPHO: synovitis, acne, pustulosis, hyperostosis, and osteitis)

Miscellaneous

Angelman: Happy puppet syndrome, MR, szs, pale blue eyes, tongue protrusion, unprovoked bouts of laughter, hypopigmentation, maternal chromosome 15 deletion or (1/4) Ubiquitin-protein Ligase E3A (UBE3A) defects

Barber–Say: Hypertrichosis, lax skin, abnormal fingerprints, ectropion, macrostomia, MR

Branchio-oculofacial/BOF: Laterocervical psoriasiform lesions, similar to aplasia cutis congenital, abnormal nasolacrimal ducts → infections, sebaceous scalp cysts, low pinnae, accessory tragus, broad nose, hypertelorism, loss of punctae, premature aging, AD

CADASIL: Cerebral Arteriopathy, Autosomal Dominant, with Subcortical Infarcts and Leukoencephalopathy, recurrent ischemic strokes, early dementia, granular osmiophilic deposits around vascular smooth muscles cells and under the basement membrane on EM. AD, NOTCH3 defects

CHIME: Migratory ichthyosiform dermatosis, Coloboma, Heart defects, migratory Ichthyosiform dermatitis, Mental retardation, Ear defects (deafness); also szs, abnormal gait.

Donahue: Leprechaunism, lipodystrophy, AN, and hypertrichosis. AR, INSR defects

Epidermodysplasia verruciformis: HPV types 3, 5, 8, SCC. AR, EVER1 or EVER2 defects

Heck/focal epithelial hyperplasia: Occurs in American Indians, Eskimos, Latin Americans, oral mucosa infections with HPV 13, 32

Iso-Kikuchi/COIF: Congenital onychodysplasia of the index fingers, inguinal hernia, radial or digital palmar artery stenosis, AD

Lafora: Onset: late adolescence with death within a decade, progressive myoclonic epilepsy, ataxia, cerebellar atrophy, PAS+_cytoplasmic eccrine duct inclusions. AR, EPM2A/Laforin defects

Lhermitte–Duclos: Dysplastic gangliocytoma, isolated or associated with Cowden. AD, PTEN defects

Fibrodysplasia Ossificans Progressiva: Malformed great toes, osteoma cutis (endochondral). AD, ACVR1 defects

Riley-Day/Familial dysautonomia: Feeding difficulties, lack of emotional tears, absent fungiform papillae (vs. absent filiform papillae in geographic tongue), diminished refl exes/pain/taste, no flare with intraepidermal histamine, drooling, labile BP, blotchy erythema while eating, pulmonary infxn, Ashkenazi. AR, IKBKAP defects

Melkersson–Rosenthal: Scrotal tongue, orofacial swelling, facial nerve palsy

Prader–Willi: Obesity after 12 months of age, MR, skin picking, chromosome 15 deletion in 60% (paternal imprinting), downslanting corners of mouth, almond-shaped eyes, and hypopigmentation

Van der Woude: Congenital lower lip pits, cleft palate, and hypodontia. AD, IRF6 defects

Setleis: Forcep mark-like, scar-like bitemporal lesions, leonine facies, low frontal hairline, periorbital swelling, flat nasal bridge, upslanting eyebrows, large lips, bulbous nose (Brauer syndrome – isolated temporal lesions), AD or AR

Miscellaneous nongenetic syndromes

Frey: Gustatory hyperhidrosis, usually following trauma/surgery to the parotid gland (auriculotemporal nerve)

Schnitzler: Urticarial vasculitis, bone pain, fever, hyperostosis, IgM monoclonal gammopathy, arthralgia, LAN, HSM, elev ESR

Dermatoses of pregnancy

Condition	Frequency	Synonyms	Onset	Course	Description	Path/labs	Treatment
Polymorphic eruption of pregnancy	1:160	PUPPP, Toxic erythema/rash of preg, Late-onset prurigo of pregnancy	Late third trimester or immediately postpartum	Often primiparous, no maternal/fetal risk, rarely recurs, resolves 1–2 wk postpartum	Urticarial papules/plaques in abdominal striae, spares umbilicus, spares face/palms/soles; rapid weight gain may be risk factor	Nonspecific path	Topical steroids, antihistamines
Pemphigoid gestationis	1:50 000	Herpes gestationis	Late pregnancy or immediately postpartum	Often recurs w/ subsequent preg, menstruation, and OCP, increased prematurity and SGA, ≤10% of neonates have skin lesions, BP2 Ag, assoc w/ Graves, resolves weeks–months postpartum	Intensely pruritic, vesiculobullous, trunk, 75% flare w/ delivery, spares face/palms/soles/oral, HLA-DR3/DR4 associated	Subepi vesicle, perivasc lymphs/eos, DIF: linear C3 ± IgG in along BMZ of perilesional skin	Systemic steroids
Atopic eruption of pregnancy	1:300	Prurigo of preg, Prurigo gestationis, Early-onset prurigo, Papular derm of preg, Pruritic folliculitis of preg	Usually first or second trimester	No fetal/maternal risk, may recur w/ subsequent preg, resolves weeks–months postpartum	2/3 eczematous, 1/3 papular or prurigo	Diagnosis of exclusion, nonspecific path	Emollients, urea, and topical steroids. If severe, systemic steroids, antihistamines, and UVB

Intrahepatic cholestasis of pregnancy	1:100–1,000, higher incidence with twins, + FH	Pruritus/prurigo gravidarum, Obstetric cholestasis, Jaundice of preg	Third trimester	Increased rates of prematurity, fetal distress/death, and meconium staining, pruritus resolves within days postpartum, malabsorption → Vit K def, 2/3 recur w/ subsequent preg, often recurs w/ OCP	Intensely pruritic, ± jaundice, no primary lesions, UTI in 50%, sxs worse at night and on trunk and palms/soles	Increased serum bile salts, Liver US nl, Biopsy: centrilobular cholestasis	Urodeoxycholic acid, UVB, Vit K
Impetigo herpetiformis	Rare	May represent acute generalized pustular psoriasis	Third trimester	Increased rates of placental insufficiency, stillbirth, fetal abnormality, hypocalcemia, vitamin D deficiency, often remits with delivery, recurs next preg	Sterile crusted pustules in flexures and inguinal, spreading centrifugally, fever, cardiac/renal failure possible	Pustular psoriasis-like path, DIF neg, hypocalcemia	Systemic steroids

DERMOSCOPY AND DERMATOPATHOLOGY

Dermoscopy

Polarized (PD) vs. Nonpolarized (NPD):

- NPD or contact immersion requires liquid interface, direct skin contact (using a gel rather than alcohol leads to less distortion from pressure)
- NPD better for milia-like cysts, comedo-like openings, peppering/regression, blue-white areas, lighter colors
- PD better for vessels, red areas, shiny-white streaks/fibrosis

Algorithms:
2-Step Algorithms

STEP 1) Determine if Melanocytic or Non-Melanocytic

Typical dermoscopic features of skin lesions	
Melanocytic	Pigment network, dots and globules, streaks, parallel patterns (acral skin), blue grey pigment, lack of specific features
Seb keratosis	Milia-like cysts – also seen in IDN
	Comedo-like openings – also seen in IDN
	Exophytic papillary structures
	Fat fingers
	Cerebriform surface – also seen in BCC
BCC	Absent pigment network
	(Maple) Leaf-like areas
	Arborizing vessels
	Blue-gray ovoid nests/globules
	Pink-white shiny areas
	Spoke wheels
Vascular lesions	Red-blue/black lacunas and homogenous areas
Dermatofibroma	Central star-like white area surrounded by peripheral delicate pigment network

STEP 2) If Melanocytic, differentiate benign from malignant using global features, patterns, and local features

	Features concerning for melanoma	Features suggestive of benign nevus
Global features	Asymmetry and multiple colors	Symmetry and uniform color
Patterns	Atypical reticular pattern: thick black, brown, or gray lines, irregular meshes, abrupt termination at the edges	Typical reticular pattern: brown, narrow, regular symmetric mesh, reticular pattern fades at periphery
Local features	Irregular dots/globules, streaks, atypical vessels, and blue-white veil	—

3-Point Checklist – 2 or more points = possible melanoma and needs bx

- Asymmetry in structure or color
- Atypical pigment network
- Blue-white structure

7-Point Checklist – 3 or more points = possible melanoma and needs bx

Major criteria = 2 points each
- Atypical pigment network
- Blue-white veil
- Atypical vascular pattern

Minor criteria = 1 point each
- Irregular pigment
- Irregular dots/globules
- Irregular streaks
- Regression

Patterns of Pigment Network:

- **Reticular pattern:** pigmented "lines" = rete ridges; hypopigmented "holes" = dermal papillae
  - Benign = Typical reticular pattern: brown, narrow, regular symmetric mesh, reticular pattern fades at periphery
  - Melanoma = Atypical reticular pattern: thick black, brown, or gray lines, irregular meshes, abrupt termination at the edges

- **Globular pattern:** varying sizes of round/ovid structures. Typical in acquired melanocytic nevi in young patients.
- **Cobblestone pattern:** large aggregates of blobules or dermal nests arranged in a square or angulated shape-like cobblestones. Typical in dermal nevi.
- **Homogeneous pattern:** diffuse area of color without any pigmented network or structures. Common in blue nevi, SK, and benign nevi.
- **Parallel pattern:** seen on acral surface. Benign lesions have pigment in "furrow" or sulci of the dermal papilla. Melanoma has pigment along the "ridge" or base of the papilla (99% specificity).
- **Starburst pattern:** pigmented streaks in a radial arrangement. Found in spitzoid melanoma and pigmented spindle cell nevus of Reed.
- **Pseudopigmented network** – on face
- **Pigment network but not melanocytic** – SK, DF, accessory nipple

Features Suggestive of Melanoma:

Streaks – melanoma

Blue-white veil – melanoma, Spitz, angiokeratoma

Black blotches – if irregular, suggestive of melanoma (if uniform, consider Reed)

Regression structures – melanoma (especially with melanin peppering)

Radial streaming/pseudopods/branched streaks/broken network – melanoma

Milky-Red areas – early melanoma

Dots/globules – if irregular, suggestive of melanoma

Acral Melanocytic Lesions:

- Parallel-Furrow, Fibrillar, Lattice-like or Homogeneous patterns – acral melanocytic nevi
- Parallel-Ridge pattern – acral melanoma (acrosyringia open onto ridges, ridges are wider than furrows)

Features Suggestive of Other Lesions:

Moth-Eaten Border and Fingerprint pattern – solar lentigo

Steel Blue areas – blue nevi

EB Nevi – often demonstrate certain specific features associated with melanoma (atypical pigment network, irregular dots/globules, atypical vascular pattern), but not other features (blue-white veil, regression structures/blue-white areas, irregular streaks, black dots)

LPLK – depends on involution stage, localized (early) or diffuse (late) pigmented granular pattern, regressive features (blue-white scar-like depigmented or vascular structures)

Facial Lentigo Maligna – asymmetric pigmented follicular openings, dark rhomboidal structures, slate-gray dots and globules

Dermoscopic Vessels:
Comma-Like vessels – benign melanocytic lesion
Arborizing vessels – BCC
Hairpin vessels – SK, melanoma (if irregular), KA, SCC
Dotted/Irregular vessels – melanoma
Polymorphous vessels – melanoma
Corkscrew vessels – amelanotic melanoma metastases
Corona/Wreath/Crown vessels – surround sebaceous hyperplasia (central yellow globular structure)
Glomerular vessels – SCC, SCCIS
Point vessels – melanocytic neoplasms, superficial epithelial neoplasms (AK, SCCIS)

Histopathologic Correlates of Dermoscopic Features:
Color according to melanin location:

Black	Melanin in upper epidermis
Brown	Melanin in DEJ
Grey Blue	Melanin in papillary dermis
Blue	Melanin in reticular dermis (blue nevus)
Brown	Symmetry and uniform color
White	Evidence of fibrosis or regression
Red	Presence of hemoglobin inside vessels

Pigment network – lines = rete ridges; spaces = superpapillary plates
Pseudopigmented network on face – adnexal structures = holes (face has minimal rete ridges)
Dots and globules – nests of melanocytic cells at different depths
Black blotches – pigment everywhere (radially, epidermal, dermal)
Cerebriform surface – gyrus = fat fingers; sulcus = pigmented keratin
Leaf-like areas – islands of pigmented BCC (large islands = blue-gray ovoid nests)
Blue-white veil – white = orthokeratotic hyperkeratosis; blue = dermal melanin

Dermatopathology

Histochemical staining

Stain	Purpose
Hematoxylin-Eosin	Routine
Masson trichrome	Collagen (green), Muscle (red), Nuclei (black). Helps to distinguishing leiomyoma (red) from dermatofibroma (green)
Verhoeff von Gieson	Elastic fibers
Pinkus acid orcein	Elastic fibers
Gomori's aldehyde fuchsin	Elastic fibers (blue); collagen (red)
Movat's Pentachrome	Connective tissue
Silver nitrate	Melanin, reticulin fibers
Fontana Masson	Melanin
Schmorl's	Melanin
DOPA-oxidase	Melanin
Gram	Gram +:blue-purple; Gram −:red
Methenamine silver (Gomori, GMS)	Fungi, Donovan bodies, Frisch bacilli, BM, sodium urate
Grocott	Fungi
Periodic Acid-Schiff (PAS)	Glycogen, fungi, neutral MPS (diastase removes glycogen)
Alcian blue pH 0.5	Sulfated MPS
Alcian blue pH 2.5	Acid MPS
Toluidine blue	Acid MPS
Colloidal iron	Acid MPS
Hyaluronidase	Hyaluronic acid
Mucicarmine	Epithelial mucin
Leder	Mast cells (chloroacetate esterase)
Giemsa	Mast cell granules, acid MPS, myeloid granules, leishmania
Fite	Acid-fast bacilli
Ziehl–Neelson	Acid-fast bacilli
Kinyoun's	Acid-fast bacilli
Auramine O	Acid-fast bacilli (fluorescence)
Perls potassium ferrocyanide	Hemosiderin/Iron
Prussian blue	Hemosiderin/Iron
Turnbull blue	Hemosiderin/Iron
Alkaline Congo red	Amyloid (the Congo red variant pagoda red No. 9/Dylon is more specific for amyloid)
Thioflavin T	Amyloid
Acid orcein Giemsa	Amyloid
Cresyl violet	Amyloid, ochronosis

Nerve blocks for the face

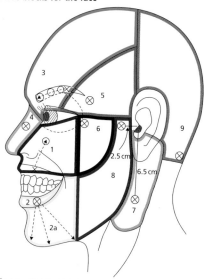

1. <u>Infraorbital</u> (30 g, 1", 2 cc): Nose, cheek, upper lip, lower eyelid
   Intraoral: Enter above first premolar (third lateral) in gingival-labial sulcus, aim toward foramen in mid-pupillary line 1 cm below orbital rim.
2. <u>Mental</u> (30 g, 1", 2 cc): Lower lip
   Intraoral: Enter gingival-labial sulcus at base of second lower bicuspid
2a. <u>Mental plus</u> (30 g, 1.5", 2–4 cc): Chin
   After the mental nerve is blocked, pass 1 cm beyond in all directions toward inferior mandibular border
3. <u>Supraorbital</u>: Med/lat forehead, anterior scalp (30 g, 1.5", 3 cc)
   <u>Supratrochlear</u>: Mid-forehead
   <u>Infratrochlear</u>: Medial upper eyelids, upper side of nose
   Enter along the orbital rim at the lateral 1/3 of the eyebrow aiming toward the supraorbital notch. Inject 1 cc lateral to the notch, 1 cc medial to the notch, and 1 cc when the needle advances to the nasal bone.
4. <u>Dorsal nasal</u> (30 g, 1", 1–2 cc): Cartilaginous nasal dorsum and tip.
   Inject ~1 cc lateral to the distal tip of the nasal bone.
5. <u>Zygomaticotemporal</u> (30 g, 1.5", 1–2 cc): Lateral orbital rim/temple.
   Inject inferior to the zygomaticofrontal suture, 1 cm lateral to the orbital rim. Inject 1 cc over the lacrimal gland for upper lateral eyelid (lacrimal nerve).
6. <u>Zygomaticofacial</u> (30 g, 1.5",1–2 cc): Superior/lateral cheek.
   Inject just lateral to the lateral/inferior border of the orbital rim.
7. <u>Great auricular</u> (30 g, 1", 1–2 cc): Lower 1/3 ear, lower postauricular
   Inject over mid-SCM, 6.5 cm below the external auditory meatus.
8. <u>V3-mandib</u> (22–23 g spinal needle, 3–4 cc): Most of cheek, upper preauric.
   Insert 90° at the sigmoid notch (b/n condyle and coronoid process) 2.5 cm anterior to the tragus. Advance to the ptyergoid plate, mark needle, retract to skin, redirect 1 cm posterior, insert to mark, then aspirate and inject.
9. <u>Occipital</u> (30 g, 1", 5 cc): Posterior scalp
   Inject medial to the occipital artery (palpate at the superior nuchal line) OR inject along superior medial line b/n occipital protuberance and mastoid.

Plate 1. Nerve block for the face. (Courtesy of Dr. Stacey Tull.)

Handbook of Dermatology: A Practical Manual, Second Edition.
Margaret W. Mann and Daniel L. Popkin.
© 2020 John Wiley & Sons Ltd. Published 2020 by John Wiley & Sons Ltd.

Blocks for the digits, hands, and feet

Digital block

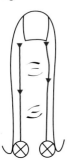

- Two dorsal and two volar nerves
- Inject 1–2 cc of 2% plain lido on each side of digit distal to the MCP (or MTP) joint
- Maximum of 6–8 cc to avoid circulatory compromise

Plate 2. Digital nerve block (Courtesy of Dr. Stacey Tull.)

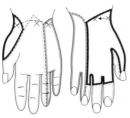

Wrist

■ <u>Radial</u>: Inject lateral to the radial artery at the proximal wrist crease to the midpoint of the dorsal wrist

■ <u>Ulnar</u>: Inject at the proximal wrist crease medial to the flexor carpi ulnaris (ring finger)

■ <u>Median</u>: Inject at the proximal wrist crease b/n palmaris longus and flexor carpi radialis (long finger)

Plate 3. Nerve block of the hand (Courtesy of Dr. Stacey Tull.)

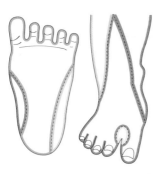

Ankle

■ <u>Sural</u>: Inject 5 cc midway between Achilles and lateral malleolus

■ <u>Post tibial</u>: Inject 3–5 cc posterior to PT artery below the medial malleolus

■ <u>Saphenous</u>: Inject 5 cc along the long saphenous vein 1 cm above the medial malleolus

■ <u>Sup. peroneal</u>: Inject 5 cc from 5 cm above lateral malleolus to the anterior tib

□ <u>Deep peroneal</u>: Skip it (mostly for deep structures) – use local for skin here.

Plate 4. Nerve block of the feet (Courtesy of Dr. Stacey Tull.)

Stain	Purpose
Von Kossa	Calcium
Alizarin red	Calcium
Pentahydroxy flavanol	Calcium
Scarlet red	Lipids
Oil red O	Lipids
Sudan black	Lipids, lipofuscin
Osmium tetroxide	Lipids
Dopa	Tyrosinase
Warthin Starry	Spirochetes, Donovan bodies
Dieterle silver	Spirochetes
Steiner	Spirochetes
Bodian	Nerve fibers
PGP 9.5	Nerve fibers
GFAP	Glial, astrocytes, Schwann cells
Feulgen	DNA
Methyl-green Pyronin	DNA
Foote's, Snook's	Reticulin fibers
PTAH	Fibrin, infantile digital fibromatosis
	Inclusions (also stained by Trichrome), granules of granular cell tumor, amoeba
Methylene blue	Ochronosis
Brown–Hopps	Bacteria
Brown–Brenn	Bacteria
McCallum–Goodpasture	Bacteria
DeGalantha	Urate crystals (20% silver nitrate also stains Gout; Gout preserved with etoh)
Ulex europaeus lectin	Endothelial cells
Peanut agglutinin	Histiocytes
Neuron-specific enolase	Neural, neuroendocrine, Merkel, granular cell tumor
Gross Cystic Dz Fluid Protein	Apocrine, Paget's, met breast CA

Immunohistochemical staining

Epidermal

Cytokeratin 20	Merkel cell (perinuclear dot)
Cytokeratin 7	Paget's
EMA	Eccrine, apocrine, sebaceous (also plasma cells, LyP, anaplastic CTCL – primary systemic not primary cutaneous)

continued p.208

| CEA | Met adenoca, Paget's, eccrine, apocrine |
| BerEP4 | BCC+, Merkel cell+, SCC- |

Mesenchymal

Desmin	Muscle
Vimentin	Mesenchymal cells (AFX, melanoma, and sarcomas)
Actin	Muscle, glomus cell tumors
Factor VIII-related Ag (VWF)	Endothelial cells, megakaryocytes, platelets
Ulex europasus agglutinin I	Endothelial cells, angiosarcoma, Kaposi, keratinocytes
CD31	Endothelial cells, vascular tumor, angiosarcoma, NSF, scleromyxedema
CD34	DFSP^1: CD34+, Factor XIIIa-
	DF: CD34-, Factor XIIIa+
	Endothelial cells, NSF, scleromyxedema
	Morphea: CD34+ spindle cells selectively depleted
	Focal CD34+ spindle cells around trichoepithelioma but not BCC
Procollagen I	Scleromyxedema > NFD/NSF
GLUT1	Positive in infantile hemangiomas and placenta. Negative in vascular malformations, RICH, NICH, PG, tufted angiomas, kaposiform hemangioendotheliomas (reduced or negative in subglottic infantile hemangiomas)
WT1 and LeY	Positive in infantile hemangiomas, negative in vascular malformations
D2-40* and LYVE-1	Lymphatics and kaposiform hemangioendothelioma

Neuroectodermal

S100	Melanocytes, nerve, Langerhans, eccrine, apocrine, chondrocytes, and sebocytes
HMB-45	Melanocytes
MART-1	Melanocytes
Mel-5	Melanocytes
CD1A	Langerhans cells
Synatophysin	Merkel cells
Chromogranin	Merkel cells

Hematopoeitic

Factor XIIIa	PLTs, macrophages, megakaryocytes, dendritics (NSF**, scleromyxedema), DF but not DFSP
HAM-56	Macrophages
Alpha-1-Antitrypsin	Macrophages
κ and λ	Mature B cells and plasma cells
BCL1	Mantle cell lymphoma

BCL2	Follicular center lymphoma (except primary cutaneous follicle center lymphoma), BCC, trichoepithelioma (bcl2- except outer layer)
BCL6	Follicular center lymphoma
CD2	T cell
CD3	Pan T cell marker, NK cells
CD4	T helper cell, Langerhans
CD5	T cells, some B calls in mantle zone, depleted in MF†
CD7	T cells, depleted in MF
CD8	T cytotoxic cells
CD10	B cell in BL, follicular center lymphoma, lymphoblastic lymphoma, AFX
CD14	Monocytes
CD15	Granulocytes, Hodgkin's
CD16	NK cells
CD20	B cells
CD22	B cells
CD23	B cells, marginal zone lymphoma, CLL
CD25 (IL-2R)	Activated B/T/Macs, evaluate before denileukin diftitox
CD30 (Ki-1)	Anaplastic CTCL, LyP, anaplastic large cell lymphoma, activated T and B cells, RS cells (Hodgkin's)
CD43 (Leu-22)	Pan T cell marker, mast cells, myeloid cells
CD45 (LCA)	CD45RO: memory T cells
	CD45RA: B cells, naive T cells
CD56	NK cells, angiocentric T cell lymphoma, Merkel cell
CD68	Histiocytes, AFX, NSF, scleromyxedema, mast cells, myeloid cells
CD75	Follicular center cells
CD79a	B cells, plasma cells (plasmacytoma)
CD99	Precursor B-lymphoblastic leukemia/lymphoma, Ewing's, PNET
CD117 (c-kit)	Mast cells
CD138	Plasma cells

---

‡DFSP: CD34+ XIIIa- Stromelysin-3- CD68- CD163- HMGA1/2- vs. DF: CD34- XIIIa+ Stromelysin-3+ CD68+ CD163+ HMGA1/2+; Increased hyaluronate in the stroma of DFSP vs. DF; Tenascin positivity at DEJ overlying DF but not DFSP

*D2-40 – Often negative, but may have focal positivity in congenital hemangioma and tufted angioma

**"circulating fibrocyte" – procollagen I+ C11b+ CD13+ CD34+ CD45RO+ MHCII+ CD68+

†MF – usually CD3+ CD4+ CD5- CD7- CD8- Leu-8- CD45RO+ with $\alpha\beta$ TCR; MF is also usually CD30- but not all CD30+ cases undergo anaplastic large cell transformation (anaplastic large cell transformation from MF, Hodgkin's, or LyP is usually ALK- and EMA- similar to primary systemic anaplastic large T-cell lymphoma but unlike primary cutaneous anaplastic large T-cell lymphoma)

Pathologic bodies

Body/sign/clue	Features	Diagnosis
Antoni A tissue	Densely cellular areas with palisaded nuclei, fasicles, and Verocay bodies	Schwannoma
Antoni B tissue	Loose, gelatinous stroma, fewer cells, microcystic changes	Schwannoma
Arao–Perkins bodies	Elastin bodies in connective tissue streamers below vellus follicles	Androgenic alopecia
Asteroid bodies	Star-like cytoplasmic inclusions in giant cells	Sarcoidosis and other granulomatous diseases (TB, botryomycosis, sporotrichosis, actinomycosis, leprosy, foreign body granuloma, and berylliosis)
Azzopardi effect	Basophilic vascular streaking (encrusted nuclear material/DNA around vessels)	Tumor necrosis, crush
Banana bodies	1) Curvilinear, membrane-bound bodies in Schwann Cells on EM 2) Crescentic, ocher bodies in the dermis	1) Farber disease 2) Ochronosis
Beanbag cells	Large macrophages demonstrating cytophagocytosis	Subcutaneous panniculitis-like T-cell lymphoma/Cytophagic histiocytic panniculitis
Birbeck granules	Tennis racket structures on EM	Langerhans cells
Busy dermis	—	GA, interstitial granulomatous dermatitis, resolving vasculitis, folliculitis, early KS, desmoplastic MM, chronic photodermatosis, breast CA mets
Caspary–Joseph spaces	Clefts at DEJ associated with basal layer injury, aka Max Joseph Cleft	LP, lichen nitidus
Caterpillar bodies	Eosinophilic, segmented, elongated (epidermal) bodies on roof of blisters (Col IV)	Porphyrias

Body/sign/clue	Features	Diagnosis
Cholesterol clefts	Needle-like crystals	Sclerema neonatorum, subcutaneous fat necrosis of the newborn, post-steroid panniculitis, NXG, cholesterol emboli, NLD, trichilemmal cysts
Chunks of coal	Large atypical lymphoid cells with hyperchromatic nuclei	Lymphomatoid papulosis
Cigar bodies	Oval, elongated yeast cells	Sporotrichosis
Colloid/Civatte bodies	Apoptotic bodies in epidermis (Civatte) or extruded into papillary dermis (Colloid)	Lichen planus and variants
Comma-shaped bodies	Cytoplasmic worm-like bodies on EM	Benign cephalic histiocytosis
Conchoidal bodies (Schaumann bodies)	Shell-like, lamellated, basophilic, calcified protein complexes in giant cells	Sarcoidosis and other granulomatous diseases
Corps grains	Small, dyskeratotic, acantholytic keratinocytes with elongated grain-shaped nuclei seen in stratum corneum	Darier, Grover, warty dyskeratoma, Hailey–Hailey (rare)
Corps ronds	Enlarged, dyskeratotic, acantholytic keratinocytes with round nuclei and perinuclear halo seen in Malpighian layer and surrounding basophilic dyskeratotic material	Darier, Grover, warty dyskeratoma, Hailey–Hailey (rare)
Councilman bodies	Cytoplasmic inclusion	BCC
Cowdry Type A and B	Eosinophilic, intranuclear inclusions surrounded by clear halo	A – HSV, CMV (+ "owl's eye cells" – viral inclusions in endothelial cells), VZV; B – Polio
Cytoid bodies	Heterogeneous round, oval, or polygonal deposits, usually in dermis	Collective term for colloid bodies, Russell bodies, amyloid, elastic globes
Donovan bodies	Single or clustered rod safety pin-like bacteria in macrophages	Granuloma inguinale
Dutcher bodies	Intranuclear pseudoinclusions in malignant plasma cells, Ig	B-cell lymphoma, multiple myeloma
Farber bodies	Comma-shaped tubular structures in cytoplasm of fibroblasts and endothelial cells on EM	Farber disease

continued p.212

Body/sign/clue	Features	Diagnosis
Flame figures	Poorly circumscribed, small areas of amorphous eosinophilic material adherent to dermal collagen	Eosinophilic cellulitis + flame figures = Well's syndrome > arthropod bites, parasites, BP, DH, eosinophilic panniculitis
Floret cells	Multinucleated giant cells with marginally placed nuclei	Pleomorphic (spindle cell) lipoma
Flower cells	Atypical CD4+ T-cells, prominent nuclear lobation	HTLV-1, ATL
Ghost cells	Calcified necrotic anucleate adipocytes with thickened membrane	Pancreatic panniculitis (+saponification) (vs. shadow/ghost cells in pilomatricomas)
Giant granules in neutrophils	Large granules	Chédiak–Higashi
Globi	Globular clumps of AFB in macrophages (Foam/Lepra/ Virchow cells)	Lepromatous leprosy
Guarnieri bodies	Cytoplasmic, eosinophilic inclusions in epidermal cells	Smallpox, caccinia
Henderson–Patterson bodies	Large, cytoplasmic, eosinophilic inclusions in keratinocytes	Molluscum contagiosum
Homer–Wright rosettes	Central nerve fibrils, peripheral small tumor cells	Cutaneous neuroblastoma
Jordans' anomaly	Vacuolated leukocytes on peripheral smear	Dorfman–Chanarin
Kamino bodies	Eosinophilic globules at DEJ made of BMZ components	Spitz nevus
Lafora bodies	Concentric amyloid deposits (=polyglucosan bodies)	Lafora disease
Lipofuscin-like granules	Yellow-brown granules in dermal macrophages	Amiodarone hyperpigmentation
Macromelanosomes	Large melanosomes	Café au lait macules, Chédiak–Higashi, XP macules, Hermansky–Pudlak
Marquee sign	Organisms at the periphery of macrophages	Leishmania
Medlar/Sclerotic bodies	Muriform cells, "copper pennies," round thick-walled brown fungi	Chromoblastomycosis
Michaelis–Gutman bodies	Calcified, degraded bacteria in macrophages, lamellated	Malakoplakia

Body/sign/clue	Features	Diagnosis
Mikulicz cells	Large macrophages containing Klebsiella rhinoscleromatis	Rhinoscleroma
Morulae	Leukocyte intracytoplasmic inclusions, Ehrlichia multiplying in cell vacuoles	Ehrlichiosis
Mulberry bodies	Dermal mulberry-like endosporulation/sporangia	Protothecosis (vs. "mulberry-like figures" on EM in Fabry eccrine glands)
Mulberry cells	Moruloid, granular, eosinophilic adipocytes – "ping pong balls"	Hibernoma
Negri bodies	Eosinophilic, cytoplasmic inclusions in neurons	Rabies
Odland bodies	Small, lamellated granules rich in lipids in granular layer, membrane-coating granules on EM	Important for permeability barrier, absent in harlequin fetus
Onion skinning	Perivascular, hyaline material	Lipoid proteinosis (onion skin fibrosis in GF, angiofibroma)
Papillary mesenchymal bodies	Germinal hair bulb	Trichoblastoma, trichoepithelioma
Pautrier microabscesses	Three or more atypical lymphocytes within epidermis	Mycosis fungoides
Pericapillary fibrin caps	—	Venous leg ulcers, venous stasis, venous hypertension, non-venous leg ulcers
Pohl–Pinkus marks	Isolated hair shaft narrowing (severe = bayonet hair)	Surgery, trauma
Psammoma bodies	Concentrically laminated, round, calcified bodies	Cutaneous meningioma, ovarian and thyroid neoplasms, papillary kidney carcinoma, mesothelioma
Pustulo-ovoid bodies of milian	Large eosinophilic granules with clear halo	Granular cell tumor
Russell bodies	Immunoglobulin deposits in plasma cells	Rhinoscleroma, plasmacystosis
Spiderweb cells	Globular, striated, vacuolated cells	Adult rhabdomyoma
Splendore–Hoeppli deposits	Flame figure-like eosinophilic deposits around organisms	Parasites, fungus, bacteria

continued p.214

Body/sign/clue	Features	Diagnosis
Verocay bodies	Palisading nuclei in rows around eosinophilic cytoplasm	Schwannoma
Weibel–Palade bodies	Dense rod or oval organelles on EM	Endothelial cells

Source: Adapted from Benjamin A. Solky, MD, Jennifer L. Jones, MD, Claire A. Pipkin, MD. Boards' Fodder – Histologic Bodies.

Cysts

Cysts	Lining, contents	Clinical, hints
Keratinous, infundibular type (epidermoid)	Epidermis-like, includes granular layer, loose orthokeratin	Punctum, foreign body giant cell reaction
Milia	Like KCIT but thin wall and small	—
Keratinous, trichilemmal type (pilar)	Stratified squamous, no granular layer, cholesterol clefts, compact keratin	Scalp, may calcify
Steatocystoma	Ruggated, thin stratified squamous, glassy pink surface, sebaceous glands	Pachyonychia congenital type II, KCIT-like keratin, trunk
Vellus hair cyst	Thin epidermal-like lining, laminated keratin, vellus hairs	Small, trunk, AD, numerous, ±pigment
Pigmented follicular	Stratified squamous, many pigmented hairs	M>F, pigmented, face
Apocrine hidrocystoma	Apocrine cells	Solitary, small, H/N, Schopf–Schulz–Passarge, focal dermal hypoplasia
Dermoid	Stratified squamous, adnexal structures	Lateral eyebrow, periocular, midline, newborn/infant
HPV-related	Epideral-like + inclusions, vacuolar changes, hypergranulosis, verrucous lining	HPV-60-related version on soles
Thyroglossal duct	Stratified squamous, may have cilia, columnar/cuboidal elements	Thyroid follicles, midline neck
Branchial cleft	Stratified squamous, may have cilia, pseudostatified columnar elements	Lymph tissue, lateral neck, jaw, preauricular

Bronchogenic	Goblet cells, cilia, respiratory epithelial lining	Suprasternal, precordial, smooth muscle, cartilage, often neck
Cutaneous ciliated	Cilia, columnar/cuboidal	F>M, thighs/buttocks
Median raphe	Pseudostratified columnar, mucinous cells	Ventral penis/scrotum
Thymic	Stratified squamous or cuboidal, ± cilia	Thymic tissue, neck, mediastinum
Pseudocyst of auricle	Within cartilage, no lining	Often asx, upper pinna
Digital mucous	No true lining, stellate fibroblasts, myxoid, thin overlying epidermis	Dorsal digit
Mucocele	No true lining, mucin, fibrous tissue, macs	Lower lip, buccal, salivary glands
Pilonidal	Sinus tract, inflammation, hair shafts	Sacrococcygeal

Other derm path buzzwords, patterns, DDx

Findings	Association(s)
Buzzwords	
"Sawtoothing"	Lichen planus
"Ball and claw"	Lichen nitidus (also see histiocytes)
"Swarm of bees"	Alopecia areata
"Toy soldiers," "strings of pearls," "fettucine collagen"	Mycosis fungoides
"Coat-sleeve" perivascular lymphocytosis	Gyrate erythema (consider lymphocytic vasculitis)
"Tea cup" scale/Tea cup sign (oblique, upwardly angulated parakeratosis)	Pityriasis rosea
"Dirty feet"	Solar lentigo (vs. "dirty fingers" – lentigo simplex), Becker's nevus
"Bubblegum stroma"	Neurofibroma
"Glassy collagen"	Keloid
"Tadpoles/sperm in the dermis"	Syringoma (if clear cell variant think diabetes)
"Corn flakes"	Keratin granuloma
"Red crayons" (blood vessels)	Atrophie blanche

continued p.216

Findings	Association(s)
Eyeliner sign ("the thin brown line" – basal layer preventing invasion), "windblown"	Bowen
"Caput medusa" (radially streaming follicles/sebaceous glands)	Trichofolliculoma
"Crazy pavement"	Colloid milium > nodular amyloidosis
Collagen trapping	DF, DFSP (+ fat entrapment)
Squamous eddies	Irritated seborrheic keratosis, inverted follicular keratosis, incontinentia pigmenti
Checkerboard alternating para/ortho-keratosis	Pityriasis rubra pilaris
Mounding parakeratosis	Pityriasis rosea, (+ spongiosis, RBC extravasation), guttate psoriasis (+ PMNs), PL (interface, lymphocytic vasculitis) nummular eczema
Layered dermal infiltrate	Necrobiosis lipoidica diabeticorum (+ necrobiosis, plasma cells)
Sandwich sign (PMNs between ortho and parakeratosis)	Tinea
Cysts with arabesques lining	Lipodermatosclerosis
Nuclear molding	Merkel cell carcinoma, ('bunch of grapes') metastatic neuroendocrine carcinoma
Comedonecrosis ("comedo" pattern with central necrosis)	Sebaceous carcinoma
Wiry collagen (fibroplasias of papillary dermis)	Mycosis fungoides
Growth patterns	
Storiform/Cartwheel pattern	Storiform/sclerotic/plywood collagenoma, DF, DFSP, fibromyxoid sarcoma, schwannoma, solitary fibrous tumor, perineurioma, primary cutaneous meningioma
Herringbone pattern	Fibrosarcoma
Jigsaw puzzle pattern (+ "pink cuticle")	Cylindroma
Tissue culture pattern (+ microcysts)	Nodular fasciitis ("myxoid scar")
Chicken-wire vascular pattern	Myxoid liposarcoma (collapsed linear blood vessels)

Findings	Association(s)
Swiss cheese pattern ("oil cysts")	Sclerosing lipogranuloma
Reticulated pattern	Fibroepithelioma of pinkus, reticulated seborrheic keratosis, tumor of the follicular infundibulum
Peripheral palisading	Tumors: BCC, trichoepithelioma (thick BM), basaloid follicular hamartoma, trichilemmoma, tumor of the follicular infundibulum, sebaceoma, pilar tumor, schwannoma, epitheliod sarcoma (necrobiosis); Rashes: GA (mucin), RA/RF nodule (fibrinoid necrosis), gout urate (crystals), NLD (necrobiosis), NXG (degenerated collagen), palisaded neutrophilic and granulomatous dermatitis, eruptive xanthoma

Differential diagnoses

Eosinophilic spongiosis	Arthropod bite, incontinentia pigmenti (first stage – look for necrotic keratinocytes), pemphigus (esp. vegetans), BP, CP, herpes gestationis, PUPPP, ACD, eosinophilic folliculitis, id, drug
Grenz zone	GF, EED, leprosy, lymphocytoma cutis, B cell lymphoma/leukemia, acrodermatitis chronica atrophicans, DFSP/DF
Bland dermal spindle cell proliferations	DF, DFSP, neurofibroma, dermatomyofibroma, leiomyoma (perinuclear halo), solitary fibrous tumor
Atypical dermal spindle cell proliferations	AFX, melanoma, SCC, leiomyosarcoma, angiosarcoma ("falling apart" appearance), Kaposi (+ eosinophilic globules, promontory sign, plasma cells)
Small blue cell tumors dermal proliferations	Glomus tumor, Merkel cell carcinoma, lymphoma, eccrine spiradenoma, metastatic carcinoma
Small red deep well-circumscribed tumor	Angioleiomyoma
Busy dermis	GA, interstitial granulomatous dermatitis, resolving vasculitis, folliculitis, early KS, desmoplastic MM, chronic photodermatosis, breast CA recurrence
Boxcar/Square biopsy	Scleroderma, scleredema, scleromyxedema, NLD, nl back skin, radiation (prominent telangiectasia)
~Normal appearance	TMEP, amyloidosis (lichen/macular – look for pigment incontinence), connective tissue nevus, myxedema, ichthyosis, cutis laxa, anetoderma, tinea versicolor, GVHD, argyria
Single filing of cells	Leukemia, (pseudo)lymphoma, metastatic carcinoma (breast), glomus cell tumor, GA, congenital melanocytic nevus, microcystic adnexal carcinoma
Pseudobullae (massive superficial dermal edema)	PMLE, Sweet, erysipelas, erysipeloid, arthropod bite reaction
Pale epidermis	Pellagra, acrodermatitis enteropathica, necrolytic migratory erythema, Hartnup, clear cell acanthoma/papulosis

continued p.218

Basement membrane thickening (with rash)	Lupus, lichen sclerosis, dermatomyososits
Accessory polypoid lesion	Accessory tragus (vellus hairs), accessory nipple (smooth muscle, traumatic/amputation neuroma), accessory digit (nerves – vs. prominent often vertical collagen in acquired digital fibrokeratoma)
Pagetoid spread	Paget's (spares basal layer), melanoma, SCC, Bowen, sebaceous carcinoma, MF, neuroendocrine tumor, rectal carcinoma
Wedge-shaped	Lymphomatoid papulosis (infiltrate), tick bite reaction (infiltrate), Degos (infarct), PLEVA (infiltrate: EM-like with parakeratosis), lichen planus (wedge-shape hypergranulosis), melanocytic nevi (esp. with halo)
Peripheral collarette	Lobulated capillary hemangioma, cherry angioma, myxoid cyst, angiokeratoma, AFX, sebaceous adenoma, clear cell acanthoma
Lymphoid follicles	ALHE, pseudolymphoma (top heavy, well-formed, tingible body macs), B-cell lymphoma (bottom heavy, poorly-formed)

Artifacts

Vacuolated keratinocytes	Freeze artifact
Ribbon-like blue material	Gel foam artifact
"Chafs of wheat" (spindled epidermal cells)	Electrodessication artifact
Minocycline pigmentation	
Type I: Facial, blue-black, scars	Iron stains +, melanin stains – (unlike types II and III, type I is not related to prolonged exposure to MCN)
Type II: Extremities, blue-gray	Iron stains +, Fontana reaction + but not melanin
Type III: Photodistributed or generalized, muddy brown	Epidermal hypermelanosis, melanin stains +, iron stains -

Giant cells

Touton	Circumferential arrangement of nuclei ("wreath"), central glassy and foamy peripheral cytoplasm
Langhans	Horseshoe arrangement of nuclei
Foreign body	Haphazard nuclei

Part 2
Surgical and Cosmetic Dermatology

Handbook of Dermatology: A Practical Manual, Second Edition.
Margaret W. Mann and Daniel L. Popkin.
© 2020 John Wiley & Sons Ltd. Published 2020 by John Wiley & Sons Ltd.

SURGICAL DERMATOLOGY

Skin cancer
Surgical margin guidelines

Tumor Type	Tumor characteristics	Excision Margin
Melanoma (see melanoma guide pg.) consider SLN Bx for > 0.8 mm or ulceration	In-situ	0.5–1 cm or Slow Mohs
	≤1 mm	1 cm
	1.01–2 mm	1–2 cm
	>2 mm	2 cm
Basal Cell Carcinoma (BCC)	**Low risk BCC**	3–4 mm
	Well-defined borders	
	Small size	
	Area L < 20 mm	
	Area M < 10 mm	
	Area H < 6 mm	
	Nodular or superficial subtype	
	Primary tumor	
	High Risk BCC	Mohs or 5–10 mm
	Poorly defined margins	
	Larger Size	
	Area L > 20 mm	
	Area M > 10 mm	
	Area H > 6 mm	
	High risk tumor or patient features *(see indication for mohs below)*	
Squamous Cell Carcinoma (SCC)	**Low risk SCC**	4–6 mm
	Well-defined borders	
	Small size	
	Area L < 20 mm	
	Area M < 10 mm	
	Area H < 6 mm	
	Well differentiated histology	
	Primary tumor	
	High Risk SCC	Mohs or 6–10 mm
	Poorly defined margins	
	Larger Size	
	Area L > 20 mm	
	Area M > 10 mm	
	Area H > 6 mm	
	High risk tumor location (ear, lip)	
	High risk tumor or patient features *(see indication for mohs below)*	

continued p.222

Tumor Type	Tumor characteristics	Excision Margin
Dermatofibrosarcoma protuberans (DFSP)	NCCN favors Mohs over WLE	2–4 cm to level of deep fascia
Merkel Cell Carcinoma	NCCN favors WLE. Can do Mohs if it does not interfere with SNLBx	1–2 cm to investing fascia layer Advised SLNBx.

Indication for Mohs micrographic surgery

Adapted from Ad Hoc Task Force, et al. AAD/ACMS/ASDSA/ASMS 2012 appropriate use criteria for Mohs micrographic surgery. *J Am Acad Dermatol* 2012; 67:531.

Location
- High risk/area "H": "mask" areas of face (central aspect of face, eyelids [including inner/outer canthi], eyebrows, nose, lips [cutaneous/mucosal/vermillion], chin, ear and periauricular skin/sulci, temple), genitalia (including perineal and perianal), hands, feet, nail units, ankles, and nipples/areola.
- Moderate risk/area "M": cheeks, forehead, scalp, neck, jawline, and pretibial surface.
- Low risk/area "L": trunk and extremities (excluding pretibial surface, hands, feet, nail units, and ankles).

High-risk tumor features
- *Recurrence/incomplete* prior excision
- *Aggressive features (high risk of recurrence):*
  - BCC: with morpheaform, fibrosing, sclerosing, infiltrating, micronodular, or metatypical/keratotic type.
    - Size: Area L > 20 mm; Area M > 10 mm; Area H > 6 mm
  - SCC with sclerosing, basosquamous, small cell, poorly/undifferentiated, spindle cell, pageotid, infiltrating, keratoacanthoma on the face, single cell, clear cell, lymphoepithelial, sarcomatoid, Breslow depth 2 mm or greater, and Clark's level IV or greater
  - Perivascular/perineural invasion
  - Other tumors: adenocystic carcinoma, adnexal carcinoma, apocrine/eccrine carcinoma, atypical fibroxanthoma, DFSP, extramammary paget disease, leiomyosarcoma, merkel cell carcinoma, and malignant fibrous histiocytoma

High-risk patient features
- Immunocompromised (IC): transplant recipient, HIV, hematologic malignancy, or immunosuppressive medications
- Genetic syndromes: basal cell nevus, XP, and bazex syndromes
- Prior radiated skin: tumor arising in site of prior radiation treatment
- Patient with history of aggressive skin cancer with no known risk factors

Melanoma - AJCC TNM classification
Major changes in AJCC eighth edition
- Round to 0.1 mm decimal for tumor depth
- Changes to T1a and T1b to 0.8 mm threshold
- Removal of mitotic rate for T category (recorded but not impacting T category)
- N category – "microscopic" vs. "macroscopic" redefined as "clinically occult" and "clinically apparent".
- Pregnostic stage III subgroup changed (increased to IIIA–IIID)
- N subcategories revised based on number of tumor involved lymph nodes
- M1 categories changed – LDH no longer upstage to M1c, additional of CNS metastases to M1d.

Tips:
- 0.8–1.0 mm = T1b or Stage IB
- Nodal involvement → at least stage III
- Distant mets → stage IV

T classification

Tx	1° tumor cannot be assessed	
T0	No evidence of 1° tumor	
Tis	Melanoma *in situ*	
T1	≤1.0 mm	a: <0.8 mm with no ulceration
		b: 0.8–1.0 mm with no ulceration
		or <1.0 mm with ulceration
T2	1.0–2.0 mm	a: no ulceration
		b: + ulceration
T3	2.0–4.0 mm	a: no ulceration
		b: + ulceration
T4	>4.0 mm	a: no ulceration
		b: + ulceration

N classification

			Survival %	
			5 yr	10 yr
Nx	Nodes cannot be assessed/not performed			
N0	No regional lymphadenopathy/metastases detected			
N1	1 node	a: no MSI, node clinically occult	84	75
		b: no MSI, node clinically detected	76	71
	0 node	c: MSI present	81	75
N2	2–3 nodes	a: no MSI, node clinically occult	79	71
		b: no MSI, node clinically detected	71	71
	1 node	c: MSI present, node detectable or occult	69	59
N3	4+ nodes	a: no MSI, node all clinically occult	60	46
		b: no MSI, >1 node clinically detected or matted	64	57
	2+ more nodes	c: MSI present, node clinically detectable or occult	52	43

Microsatellite instability (MSI) = any in-transit, satellite, locally recurrent, or microsatellite metastases

M classification

M	Site	Serum LDH
Mx	Distant mets cannot be assessed	N/A
M0	No distant mets	N/A
M1a	Distant skin, soft tissue including muscle, and/or nonregional lymph node	(0) Normal
		(1) Elevated
M1b	Lung mets	(0) Normal
		(1) Elevated
M1c	Non-CNS visceral mets	(0) Normal
		(1) Elevated
M1d	CNS mets	(0) Normal
		(1) Elevated

Adapted from AJCC Cancer Staging manual, Eighth Edition (2017). Balch CM et al. Final version of 2009 AJCC melanoma staging and classification. *J Clin Oncol* 2009; 27:6199–6206. Gershenwald JE et al. Melanoma staging: evidence-based changes in the American Joint Committee on cancer eighth edition cancer staging manual. *CA Cancer J Clin* 2017;67:472–492.

Clark level

Level I	Confined to the epidermis (MIS)
Level II	Invasion past basement membrane into the papillary dermis
Level III	Tumor filling papillary dermis to the junction of the superficial reticular dermis
Level IV	Invasion into the reticular dermis
Level V	Invasion into the subcutaneous tissue

Clark level is no longer recommended as a staging criterion and is used for staging tumors ≤1 mm^2 only if mitotic rate cannot be determined.

Breslow depth

Breslow tumor thickness is measured in mm from the top of the granular layer of the epidermis (or the base of an ulcer) to the deepest point of tumor invasion using an ocular micrometer.

Melanoma - AJCC TNM staging and survival

	Clinical staging			Pathologic staging			Survival (%)	
	T	N	M	T	N	M	5 yr	10 yr
IA	T1a	0	0	T1a	0	0	99	98
IB	T1b	0	0	T1b	0	0	99	96
				T2a			96	92
IIA	T2b	0	0	T2b	0	0	93	88
				T3a			94	88
IIB	T3b	0	0	T3b	0	0	86	81
	T4a			T4a			90	83
IIC	T4b	0	0	T4b	0	0	82	75
IIIA	Any T*	N1–3	0	T1–2a	N1a	0	93	88
				T1–2a	N2a			
IIIB				T0	N1b–c	0	83	77
				T1–2a	N1b–c			
				T1–2a	N2b			
				T2b–3a	N1a–2b			
IIIC				T0	N2b–c	0	69	60
				T0	N3b–c			
				T1a–3a	N2c–3c			
				T3b–4a	Any N			
				T4b	N1a–2c			
IIID				T4b	N3a–c	0	32	24
IV	Any T	Any N	M1	AnyT	Any N	M1a	9–27	16
						M1b		3
						M1c		6
						M1d		

Gershenwald JE et al. Melanoma staging: evidence-based changes in the American Joint Committee on Cancer Eighth Edition cancer staging manual. *CA Cancer J Clin* 2017;67:472–492.
*There are no Stage III subgroups in clinical staging.

Melanoma: treatment guidelines

Breslow depth (mm)	Margin (cm)	SNL*	Physical exam**	Workup***	Adjuvant treatment
In situ	0.5–1	No	q6 mo × 1 yr then yearly	• Symptom specific (CT, PET, MRI)	—
<1	1	No*	q6–12 mo × 5 yr then yearly	• Symptom specific (CT, PET, MRI)	—
1.01–2.00	1–2	Yes		• Symptom specific (CT, PET, MRI)	• Clinical trial • Observe
2.01–4.00	2	Yes	q3–6 mo × 2 yr, q3–12 mo × 3 yr, then yearly		• Clinical trial • Observe • IFN α
>4	2	Yes			
Stage III SLN +, micromet	WLE (as above)	LND or clinical trial	q3–6 mo × 2 yr, q3–12 mo × 3 yr, then yearly	• CXR, CT, brain MRI, and/or PET/CT scans q3–12 mo (optional) • Baseline imaging for staging and symptom-specific evaluation (CT, PET, MRI)	• Clinical trial • Observe • IFN α • High-dose ipilimumab
Stage III Clinical + nodes, macromet	WLE	FNA or bx of + LN, then LND			• Clinical trial • Observe • IFN α • High-dose ipilimumab • Biochemotherapy† • ±RT to nodal basin if Stage IIIC

Stage III in-transit	WLE / FNA or Bx of in-transit lesions	...?	...CT, CT, brain MRI, and/or PET/ CT scans q3–12 mo (optional) • Baseline imaging for staging and symptom-specific evaluation (CT, PET, MRI)	...intralesional BCG, IL-2, IFN, talimogene laherparepvec (T-VEC) • IFN α • Limb perfusion with melphalan • Clinical trial (preferred) • Radiation tx • Systemic tx
			q3–6 mo × 2 yr, q3–12 mo × 3 yr, then yearly	

Stage IV	FNA or bx	Yes	q3–6 mo × 3 yr, q4–12 mo × 2 yr, then yearly	• Chest/abd/pelvic CT, MRI brain and/or PET CT for baseline staging and symptom-specific evaluation, LDH
				BRAF testing (metastatic disease)
					• Systemic therapy preferred
					• See NCCN Guidelines
					• Clinical trial
					• Anti-PD1 monotherapy
					• BRAF mutated: Targeted therapy (combination therapy with dabrafenib/trametinib or vemurafenib/cobimetinib)
					• Second line:
					  o Dacarbazine
					  o Temozolomide
					  o High-dose IL2

Source: Adapted from NCCN Practice Guideline in Oncology- v.2 2016 Melanoma.

*Sentinel lymph node should be performed at the time of the Wide Local Excision. Consider in tumor <1 mm if initial bx with mitotic rate ≥1 mm², ulceration, positive deep margin, angiolymphatic invasion, or young age. The yield and clinical significance of SLNBx in Stage IA is unknown and is generally not recommended.

**Followup: At least annual skin exam for life, educate patient in monthly self-skin and lymph node exam. (Bichakjian et al. Guidelines of care for the management of primary cutaneous melanoma. *JAAD* 2011; 65:1032–1047).

***Evaluation: Routine imaging/lab tests not recommended in Stage 0/IA disease. In Stage IB, may consider nodal basin ultrasound prior to SLNB for patients with equivocal regional lymph node physical exam (NCCN guidelines 2.2016). CT, PET, and MRI may be performed to evaluate specific sxs.

†Regimens include dacarbazine, temozolomide, paclitaxel, vinblastine, IL-2, IFNα-2b, and combinations thereof (see NCCN guidelines).

Squamous cell carcinoma (SCC)
NCCN stratification of low versus high risk cutaneous SCC

Parameters	Low risk	High risk
Clinical H&P		
Location/size (including peripheral rim of erythema)	Area L < 20 mm Area M < 10 mm	Area L ≥ 20 mm Area M ≥ 10 mm Area H
Borders	Well defined	Poorly defined
Primary vs. recurrent	Primary	Recurrent
Immunosuppression	–	+
Site of prior radiation or chronic inflammatory process	–	+
Rapidly growing tumor	–	+
Neurological symptoms	–	+
Pathology		
Degree of differentiation	Well or moderately differentiated	Poorly differentiated
High-risk histological subtype	–	+
Depth (thickness or Clark's level)	<2 mm or I, II, III	≥2 mm or IV, V
Perineural, lymphatic, or vascular involvement	–	+
Recommended TX	• EDC in nonterminal hair-bearing area • Standard excision with 4–6 mm margin to subq • RT for nonsurgical cases	• Mohs surgery • Standard excision may be considered with 6 mm margins • RT for nonsurgical cases

Source: Adapted from National Comprehensive Cancer Network stratification of low versus high-risk cSCC. National Comprehensive Cancer Center. NCCN Clinical Practice Guidelines in Oncology; Squamous Cell Carcinoma (V2.2018). 2018; www.nccn.org, 1 February 2018.
Area H = "mask areas" of face (central face, eyelids, eyebrows, periorbital, nose, lips [cutaneous and vermilion], chin, mandible, preauricular and postauricular skin/sulci, temple, and ear), genitalia, hands, and feet.
Area M = cheeks, forehead, scalp, neck, and pretibia.
Area L = trunk and extremities (excluding pretibia, hands, feet, nail units, and ankles).
High-risk histologic subtype: Acantholytic (adenoid), adenosquamous (showing mucin production), desmoplastic, or metaplastic (carcinosarcomatous) subtypes.

SCC TNM classification: tumor classification AJCC vs BWH

BWH classification provides better prognostication in patients with localized disease (stratifies T2 into a and b)

	AJCC eighth ed	Brigham and Women's Hospital
Tx	1° tumor cannot be assessed	1° tumor cannot be assessed
Tis/T0	SCC *in situ*	SCC *in situ*
T1	<2 cm in greatest diameter with fewer than two "high-risk" features	0 risk factors
T2	2–4 cm, or with two or more "high-risk" features	T2a: 1 risk factor T2b: 2–3 risk factors
T3	• >4 cm • minor bone erosion • perineural invasion (tumor cells within nerve sheath >0.1 mm or clinical/radiographic involvement of names nerves) • or deep invasion (beyond subq fat or >6 mm to the base of tumor)	4 risk factors or bone invasion
T4a	Tumor with gross cortical bone/marrow invasion	
T4b	Tumor with skull base invasion and/or skull base foramen involvement	
	AJCC high-risk factors: • >2 mm thickness • Clark level ≤IV • perineural invasion • primary site ear, non-hair-bearing lip • Poorly differentiated histology	BWH risk factors: • tumor diameter ≥2 cm • poorly differentiated histology • perineural invasion • tumor invasion beyond the subcutaneous fat

SCC AJCC TNM staging

	T	N	M
0	Tis	0	0
I	T1	0	0
II	T2	0	0
III	T3	0	0
	T1–3	1	0
VI	T1–3	2	0
	Any T	3	1
	T4	Any N	
	Any T	Any N	

continued p.234

SURGICAL DERMATOLOGY

T	N	M
	N1 = 1 LN+ ≤3 cm ENE−	M0 = no distant mets
	N2 = 1 LN+ ≤3 cm ipsilateral ENE+	M1 = distant mets
	1 LN+, >3 and ≤6 cm ipsilateral ENE− or	
	1 LN+ ≤3 cm ipsilateral ENE+	
	≥2 LN+ all ≤6 cm ipsilateral ENE−	
	N3 = ≥1 LN+ >6 cm ENE+	
	1 LN+ ≤3 cm ENE+ contralateral or	
	≥1 LN+ >3 cm ipsilateral ENE+ or ≥2	
	LN+, any ENE+	
	ENE+, with extranodal extension; ENE−,	
	without extranodal extension	

SCC - Treatment of advanced disease

- **Regional disease** (in-transit and regional LN mets) – LN dissection, adjuvant radiation ± concurrent systemic therapy
- **Distal mets** – Multidisciplinary approach (NCCN)
  - First line: Cisplatin ± 5-Fluorouracil
  - Second line: Epidermal Growth Factor Receptor (EGFR) inhibitors
    - Monoclonal antibodies: Cetuximab, Panitumumab
    - Tyrosine kinase inhibitors: Erlotinib, Gefitinib
  - Emerging: Checkpoint inhibitors – Anti-PD-1 inhibitors: Nivolumab, Pembrolizumab

Prophylactic antibiotics and antivirals

Guideline for Prophylactic antibiotics

Use of antibiotic prophylaxis for endocarditis indicated for surgical procedure on infected tissue in patients with high-risk cardiac lesion or as detailed below

Antibiotic (trade size)	Adults	Children
All sites except oral and groin/lower extremity:		
Cephalexin (500 mg, 250 mg/5 ml)	2 g	50 mg/kg
Dicloxacillin (500 mg, 250 mg/5 ml)	2 g	50 mg/kg
If penicillin allergic		
Azithromycin (250, 500 mg)	500 mg	15 mg/kg
Clarithromycin (500 mg, 250 mg/5 ml)	500 mg	15 mg/kg
Clindamycin (300 mg)	600 mg	20 mg/kg
Oral site:		
Amoxicillin (500 mg, 250 mg/5 ml)	2 g	50 mg/kg
If penicillin allergic		
Azithromycin (250, 500 mg)	500 mg	15 mg/kg
Clarithromycin (500 mg, 250 mg/5 ml)	500 mg	15 mg/kg
Clindamycin (300 mg)	600 mg	20 mg/kg

Antibiotic (trade size)	Adults	Children
Groin and lower extremity site		
Cephalexin (500 mg, 250 mg/5 ml)	2 g	50 mg/kg
If penicillin allergic		
Trimethoprim-Sulfamethoxazole, double strength	1 tab	
Levofloxacin	500 mg	

One hour prior to surgery: (all p.o. doses).

Algorithm for antibiotic prophylaxis

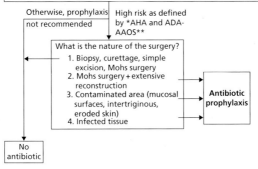

High-risk cardiac conditions:*
• Prosthetic cardiac valve or prosthetic material used for valve repair
• Prior infective endocarditis
• Cardiac transplant recipients who develop valvulopathy
• Congenital heart disease (CHD), specifically, unrepaired cyanotic CHD, first 6 months after completely repaired CHD with prosthetic material or device, repaired CHD with residual defects which inhibit endothelialization (at or adjacent to prosthetic patch or device)

High risk for prosthetic joint infection:**
• First 2 years post joint replacement
• History of joint infections
• Immunocompromised/immunosuppressed patients
• Patients with malignancy, malnourish, hemophilia, or Type I diabetes

Otherwise, prophylaxis not recommended | High risk as defined by *AHA and ADA-AAOS**

What is the nature of the surgery?
1. Biopsy, curettage, simple excision, Mohs surgery
2. Mohs surgery + extensive reconstruction
3. Contaminated area (mucosal surfaces, intertriginous, eroded skin)
4. Infected tissue

→ **Antibiotic prophylaxis**

No antibiotic

Adapted from *Wilson W. et al. Prevention of Infective Endocarditis, *Circulation* 2007; 116: 1736–54; Messingham MJ and Arpey CJ. Update on the Use of Antibiotics in Cutaneous Surgery. *Derm Surg* 2005; 31: 1068–78; **Wright TI, et al. Antibiotic prophylaxis in dermatologic surgery: advisory statement 2008. *J Am Acad Dermatol* 2008; 59:464–73.

Guideline for prophylactic antivirals

History of HSV infection of the orofacial area is an indication for prophylaxis for facial resurfacing, chemical peels, dermabrasion, PDT, and orofacial surgery. Treat for 7–14 days with acyclovir, valacyclovir, or famciclovir to suppress viral reactivation during reepithelialization.

Acyclovir (Zovirax)	400 mg tid × 7–14 d
Valacyclovir (Valtrex)	500 mg bid × 7–14 d
Famciclovir (Famvir)	250 mg bid × 7–14 d

SURGICAL DERMATOLOGY

Antiseptic scrubs

Agent	Mechanism of action	Gram +	Gram −	Mycobacteria	Viruses	Fungi	Spores	Speed of action	Residual activity	Other
Alcohol 60–95%	Denature proteins (bacterial cell wall)	+++	+++	+++	+++	+++	−	Fast	None	Flammable with laser/cautery Allow to dry on surface
Chlorhexidine 2–4% (Hibiclens)	Impairs cell membrane	+++	++	+	+++	+	−	Intermed	Excellent	Ototoxicity, keratitis, skin irritant
Iodine 3% (Lugol)	Oxidation	+++	+++	+++	+++	++	+	Intermed	Minimal	Skin irritant Inactivated by blood/sputum
Iodophors– (Betadine) Povidone-iodine 7.5–10%	Oxidation/substitution by free iodine: disrupts S–H and N–H bonds, C=C bonds in fatty acids	+++	+++	+	++	++	−	Intermed (needs to dry)	Minimal	Skin irritant (less than iodine) Inactivated by blood/sputum May cross-react with radiopaque iodine Surfactant + iodine = iodophor
TechniCare PCMX Chloroxylenol	Disrupts cell membrane	+++	+	+	+	+	Unknown	Slow	Good	Addition of EDTA increases its activity against pseudomonas

	Mechanism									Comments
Triclosan 0.2–2%	Disrupts cell wall, inhibits fatty acid synthesis, binds bacterial enoyl–acyl carrier protein reductase (ENR, *fabI*)	+++	++	+	+++	–	Unknown	Intermed	Good	Forms chloroform and dioxins when combined with chlorine in tap water
Benzalkonium (Quaternary ammonium)	Dissociation of cell membranes; disrupts intermolecular interactions	++	+	+/–	+ Lipophilic	+/–	Unknown	Slow	Good	Use only in combination with alcohols. Eyedrop preservative. Easily inactivated by cotton gauze/organic materials

Source: Adapted from CDC. *MMWR Recomm Rep.* 2002 Oct 25;51(RR-16):1–48.

Anesthetics

Mechanism of action
Reversibly inhibit nerve conduction by blocking sodium ion influx into peripheral nerve cells = prevent depolarization of nerves.

Practical tips to decrease pain with injections:
The patient
- Distract, pinch the skin
- Consider topical anesthesia (i.e. LMX) prior to infiltration

The anesthetic agent
- Warming to 37–42 °C
- Buffered lidocaine with bicarb (increase the pH 3.3 → 7.4)
  Add 1 cc 8.4% $NaHCO_3$ to 10 cc Lidocaine 1% with epi

The injection technique
- Fine needle (27, 30, or 32 gauge)
- Inject slowly
- If possible, through a dilated pore or wound edge
- Deeper injections into SQ area hurts less (go from deep subdermal to tight dermal)
- Minimize needle punctures by moving in a fan shape
- Consider nerve blocks or ring blocks

Dose calculation	1% = 1 g/100 ml = 10 mg/cc
	0.1% = 0.1 g/100 ml = 1 mg/cc

Standard formula for buffered Lidocaine
1% Lidocaine with epinephrine 1:100 000

Ingredient	Quantity
Lidocaine 1%	50 ml
Sodium bicarbonate 8.4%	5 ml
Epinephrine 1:1000	0.5 ml

Tumescent anesthesia
Lidocaine 0.05–0.1% + Epinephrine 1:1 000 000
Max Tumescent is 35–50 mg/kg
Peak Lidocaine level at 12–14 hours

Ingredient	Quantity
Normal saline 0.9%	1000 ml
Lidocaine 1%	50–100 ml
Sodium bicarbonate 8.4%	10 ml
Epinephrine 1:1000	1 ml

SURGICAL DERMATOLOGY

Topical anesthetic (see drug section pg 197)

EMLA cream*	lidocaine 2.5% and prilocaine 2.5%
LMX	lidocaine 4 and 5% in liposomal delivery cream
Lida-Mantle	lidocaine 3% cream
Topicaine	lidocaine 4% and 5% gel
Pliaglis	lidocaine 7% and tetracaine 7% cream

Source: Cavef et al. *Arch Derm* 2007;143:1074–1076.
*Risk of methemoglobinemia. Also, may create artefactual vacuolization/swelling of the upper epidermis and basal layer damage/clefting.

Pharmaceutically compounded topical anesthetic

BLT	20% benzocaine, 6% lidocaine, 4% tetracaine
TAC	0.5% tetracaine, 1:2000 epineprine, 11.8% cocaine
LET	4% lidocaine, 1:2000 epineprine, 0.5% tetracaine
Lasergel	10% lidocaine, 10% tetracaine
23/7	23% lidocaine, 7% tetracaine

Adverse reaction to local anesthetics

Condition	Pulse	BP	Signs and symptoms	Management
Vasovagal Rxn	▼	▼	Diaphoresis, hyperventilation, nausea	Trendelenburg, cool compress
Epinephrine Rxn	▲	▲	Sweating, tachypnea, HA, palpitation	Reassurance, beta-blocker
Anaphylaxis	▲	▼	Tachycardia, bronchospasm	Epinephrine 1:1000 × 0.3 ml SQ. Antihistamine, airway maintenance
Lidocaine toxicity				
1–6 µg/ml	NI	NI	Tongue and circumoral paresthesia, metallic taste, tinnitus, lightheadedness	Observe
6–9 µg/ml	NI	NI	Tremors, nausea, vomiting, hallucination, muscle fasciculations	Diazepam, airway maintenance
9–12 µg/ml	▼	▼	Seizures, cardiopulmonary depression	Respiratory support
>12 µg/ml	—	—	Coma, cardiopulmonary arrest	CPR/ACLS

Source: Adapted from Snow SN and Mikhail GR. *Mohs Micrographic Surgery* Second Edition. Chapter 14. Table 14–3.

SURGICAL DERMATOLOGY

Local anesthetic

Generic name	Trade name	Pregnancy category[†]	Potency	Onset (min)	Without epinephrine		With epinephrine[†]	
					Duration (min)	Max dose (mg/kg) for adults	Duration (min)	Max dose (mg/kg) for adults
Amide ("i" before – caine = amide)								
Lidocaine	Xylocaine	B	Intermed	<2	30–120	4.5 (30 cc for 70 kg)	60–400	7 (50 cc for 70 kg)
Bupivacaine	Marcaine, Sensorcaine	C*	High	2–10	120–240	2.5	240–480	3
Mepivacaine	Carbocaine	C*	Intermed	3–20	30–120	6	60–400	8
Prilocaine	Citanest	B	Intermed	5–6	30–120	7	60–400	10
Etidocaine	Duranest	B	High	3–5	200	4.5	240–360	6.5
Ester								
Procaine	Novocain	C	Low	5	15–30	10	30–90	14
Chloroprocaine	Nesacaine	C	Low	5–6	30–60	10	—	—
Tetracaine	Pontocaine	C	High	7	120–240	2	240–480	2
Other – in patients who might be allergic to above								
Diphenhydramine hydrochloride1% solution		B	—	5	15–180	Sedation with >25 mg (2.5 cc of 1%)	—	—
Normal saline with benzoyl alcohol preservative		—	—	—	—	—	—	—

†Epinephrine is pregnancy category C. Low doses (diluted 1:300,000 can be used during pregnancy)
*Pregnancy category C

236

	Metabolized by	Excretion	Allergic reaction
Amide	Liver p450 enzyme (caution in patients with liver disease)	Kidney	Rare, due to preservative methylparaben (if allergic: switch to preservative-free lidocaine)
Ester	Tissue pseudocholinesterase	Kidney	More common Due to metabolite to PABA (p-aminobenzoic acid) (if allergic: switch to amides)

Nerve blocks*

See Plates 1–4.

Surgical Anatomy

Anatomy of the face
Cosmetic unit of the central face

SURGICAL DERMATOLOGY

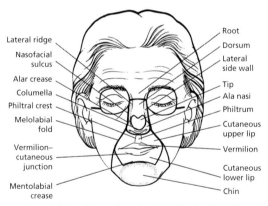

Lateral ridge
Nasofacial sulcus
Alar crease
Columella
Philtral crest
Melolabial fold
Vermilion–cutaneous junction
Mentolabial crease

Root
Dorsum
Lateral side wall
Tip
Ala nasi
Philtrum
Cutaneous upper lip
Vermilion
Cutaneous lower lip
Chin

From Robinson JK (ed.). *Atlas of Cutaneous Surgery*, first edition. WB Saunders: 1996, p. 2, figure 1.2, with permission.

Cosmetic units of the cheek

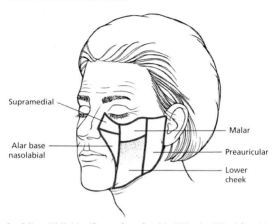

Supramedial

Alar base
nasolabial

Malar

Preauricular

Lower
cheek

From Robinson JK (ed.). *Atlas of Cutaneous Surgery*, first edition. WB Saunders: 1996, p. 2, figure 1.4, with permission.

Cosmetic units of the forehead

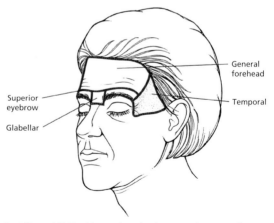

General
forehead

Superior
eyebrow

Glabellar

Temporal

From Robinson JK (ed.). *Atlas of Cutaneous Surgery*, first edition. WB Saunders: 1996, p. 2, figure 1.3, with permission.

Cosmetic units of the nose

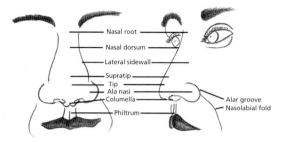

- Nasal root
- Nasal dorsum
- Lateral sidewall
- Supratip
- Tip
- Ala nasi
- Columella
- Philtrum
- Alar groove
- Nasolabial fold

Courtesy of Dr. Quan Vu

Anatomy of the nasal cartilage

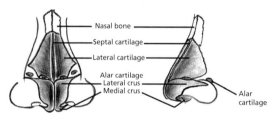

- Nasal bone
- Septal cartilage
- Lateral cartilage
- Alar cartilage
- Lateral crus
- Medial crus
- Alar cartilage

Courtesy of Dr. Quan Vu

Anatomy of the ear

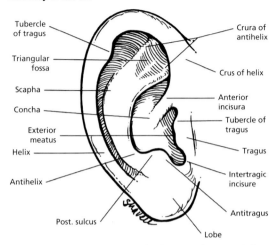

From Robinson JK (ed). *Atlas of Cutaneous Surgery*, first edition. WB Saunders: 1996, p. 186, figure 3.1, with permission.

Cosmetic units of the eye

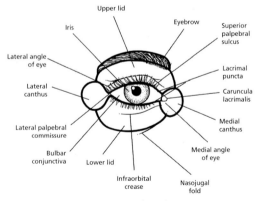

From Robinson JK (ed). *Atlas of Cutaneous Surgery*, first edition. WB Saunders: 1996, p. 3, figure 1.5, with permission.

Anatomy of the eye

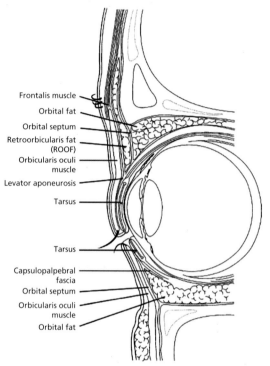

Frontalis muscle
Orbital fat
Orbital septum
Retroorbicularis fat (ROOF)
Orbicularis oculi muscle
Levator aponeurosis
Tarsus

Tarsus
Capsulopalpebral fascia
Orbital septum
Orbicularis oculi muscle
Orbital fat

From Robinson JK (ed.). *Atlas of Cutaneous Surgery*, first edition. WB Saunders: 1996, p. 3, figure 1.5, with permission.

Danger zones in surgery

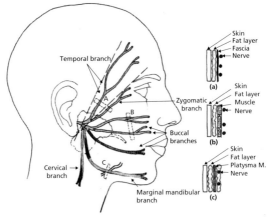

From G Bernstein. *J Dermatol Surg Oncol*, 1986; 12(7):725, figure 6, with permission.

1. *Temporal branch of CN VII:*
   Most vulnerable location: mid-zygomatic arch.
   Nerve course: Nerve exits the superior–anterior portion of the parotid gland, then courses 0.5 cm below the tragus to 1.5 cm above the lateral eyebrow. Nerve lies just beneath the skin, subcutaneous fat, and SMAS.
   Motor innervation: frontalis, upper portion of the orbicularis oculi and corrugator supercilii
   Damage: inability to raise eyebrow and wrinkle forehead. Results in a flat forehead and droopy eyebrow.

2. *Marginal mandibular branch of CN VII:*
   Most vulnerable location: mid-mandible 2 cm lateral to the oral commissure.
   Nerve course: Nerve exits the inferior–anterior portion of the parotid gland, then courses along the angle of the mandible across the facial artery and vein. May be 2 cm or more below the inferior edge of the mandible if the head is rotated or hyperextended. Lies beneath the skin, subcutaneous fat, and SMAS.
   Motor innervation: orbicularis oris, risorius, mentalis, and depressor muscles of the mouth.
   Damage: drooping of the mouth, inability to pull the lip laterally and inferiorly with smiling.

3. *Great auricular nerve (C$_2$ and C$_3$):*

　Most vulnerable location: 6.5 cm below the external auditory canal along the posterior border of the sternocleidomastoid muscle.

　Nerve course: Nerve courses toward the lobule posterior to the external jugular vein.

　Damage: Sensory innervation, results in numbness of the inferior 2/3 of the ear and adjacent cheek and neck

4. *Spinal accessory nerve (CN XI):*

　Most vulnerable location: Erb's point.

　Nerve course: Nerve exits from behind the SCM at Erb's point and courses diagonally and inferiorly across the posterior triangle. Draw a line from the angle of the jaw to the mastoid process – Erb's point is located 6 cm vertically below the midpoint of this line at the posterior border of the sternocleidomastoid (within a 2 cm area). Also may define area by drawing a line horizontally across the neck from the thyroid notch to the posterior border of the sternocleido-mastoid (1 cm above and 1 cm below).

　Innervation: location of the great auricular, less occipital, and spinal accessory nerve. The spinal accessory nerve innerves the trapezius muscle.Damage: winged scapula – inability to shrug the shoulder and abduct the arm.

Danger zone of the neck: Erb's point

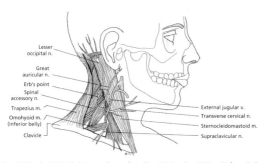

From RG Wheeland RG (ed.). *Cutaneous Surgery*, first edition. WB Saunders: 1994, p. 61, figure 5.13, with permission.

Dermatomal distribution of sensory nerves

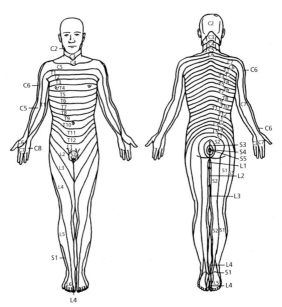

From Leventha: Fractures, dislocations, and fracture-dislocations of the spine. In Canale et al (eds.) *Campbell's Operative Orthopaedics*, tenth edition. Mosby: 2003, Figure 35.1, with permission.

Anatomy of the lower extremity venous system

Modified from Min RJ, et al. Duplex ultrasound evaluation of lower extremity venous insufficiency. *J Vasc Interv Radiol* 2003 14: 1233–1241, with permission.

Anatomy of the great saphenous vein

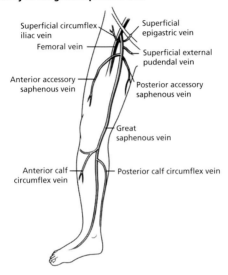

Anatomy of the perforator veins

Anatomy of the short saphenous vein

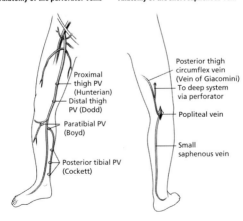

Anatomy of the nail

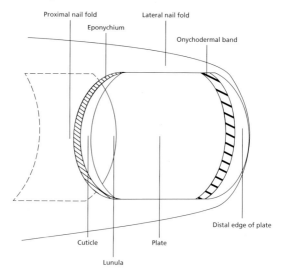

From RK Scher and CR Daniel. Nails: Therapy, Diagnosis, Surgery, second edition. WB Saunders: 1997, p. 13–14, figures 2.1, 2.2a, 2.2b, with permission.

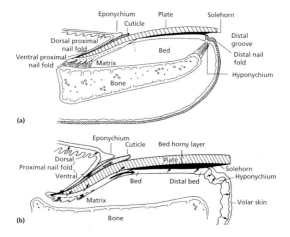

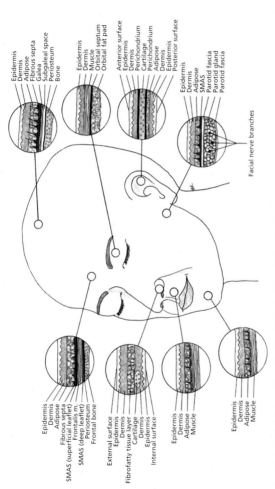

Epidermis
Dermis
Adipose
Fibrous septa
Galea
Subgaleal space
Periosteum
Bone

Epidermis
Dermis
Muscle
Orbital septum
Orbital fat pad

Anterior surface
Epidermis
Dermis
Perichondrium
Cartilage
Perichondrium
Adipose
Dermis
Epidermis
Posterior surface

Epidermis
Dermis
Adipose
SMAS
Parotid fascia
Parotid gland
Parotid fascia

Facial nerve branches

Epidermis
Dermis
Adipose
Fibrous septa
Frontalis m.
SMAS (superficial leaflet)
SMAS (deep leaflet)
Periosteum
Frontal bone

External surface
Epidermis
Dermis
Fibrofatty tissue layer
Cartilage
Dermis
Epidermis
Internal surface

Epidermis
Dermis
Adipose
Muscle

Epidermis
Dermis
Adipose
Muscle

From Wheeland RG (ed.). *Cutaneous Surgery*, first edition. WB Saunders; 1994, p. 51, figure 5.6, with permission.

Undermining depths in reconstruction

Scalp	Subgaleal (relatively avascular)
Forehead	Subgaleal (for large defects) or subcutaneous fat above frontalis fascia
Temple/zygomatic arch	Superficial subcutaneous fat above temporal branch of facial nerve
Mandible	Superficial subcutaneous fat above marginal mandibular branch of facial nerve
Ear	Above perichondrium
Lip	Above orbicularis oris
Nose	Above perichondrium/periosteum
Rest of face	Superficial subcutaneous fat, above the parotid duct
Terminal hair-bearing area	Deep to hair papillae
Lateral neck	Superficial subcutaneous fat above spinal accessory nerve
Trunk/extremities	Above muscular fascia
Hands and feet	Subdermal

Reconstruction algorithm: STAIRS

Reconstruction algorithm: STAIRS

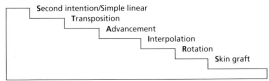

Second intention/Simple linear
Transposition
Advancement
Interpolation
Rotation
Skin graft

Second intention
Cosmetic result of wound healing by second intention according to anatomical site

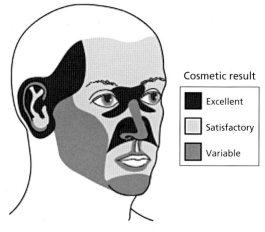

Cosmetic result

- ⬛ Excellent
- ⬜ Satisfactory
- ▧ Variable

- Ideal for

   1. Concave areas: Periorbital (medial canthus), temple, conchal bowl, and alar crease
   2. Shallow defects: i.e. shins
   3. Fair-skinned patient (wound tends to heal with whiten scar)
   4. Poor operative candidates

- May take weeks/months to heal, so patient must be able to perform wound care
- May heal with atrophic, hypertrophic, white scar
- Can perform delayed repair/graft at 2–4 weeks

Cosmetic result of wound healing by secondary intention according to anatomical site. From Zitelli JA. Wound healing by secondary intention. *JAAD* 1983;9(3) 407–415; with permission

Simple linear closure
- 3–4:1 Length:width ratio
- Orient along relaxed skin tension lines (RSTLs) at junction of cosmetic subunits

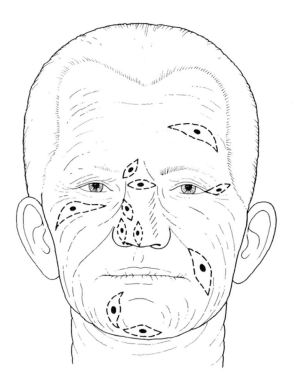

RSTL on the face showing orientation of simple linear closure.

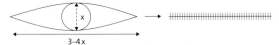

From S Burge, R Rayment. *Simple Skin Surgery*. Blackwell Scientific Publications: 1986; with permission.

M-plasty

- Modification of the linear closure
- GOAL: Shortens the length of a scar

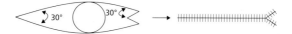

Transposition flap

- GOAL: Redistribute tension vectors
- Flap rotates about a pivotal point at the base of the pedicle and is transposed over an island of normal skin
- Pivotal restraints may limit its movement
- Wide undermining necessary to prevent pincushioning
- Common flaps: rhombic, bilobe, z-plasty, banner, and nasolabial (melolabial)

Rhombic

- Used for small defects where adjacent tissue is available to rotate onto defect.
- Changes the tension vector along the secondary defect (perpendicular to tension across primary defect).
- Classic rhombic (Limberg) consists of parallelogram with 60° and 120°.
- Common locations: medial canthus, upper 2/3 of nose, lower eyelid, temple, and peripheral cheek.

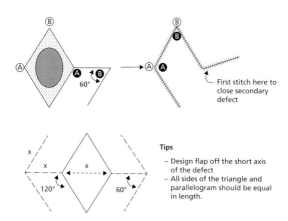

First stitch here to close secondary defect

Tips
- Design flap off the short axis of the defect
- All sides of the triangle and parallelogram should be equal in length.

SURGICAL DERMATOLOGY

Modifications of rhombic flaps

<u>Webster 30°</u>

Narrower flap, easier to close secondary defect

Less reorientation of tension vectors

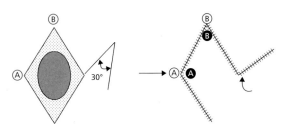

<u>Dufourmentel</u>

Compromise between Limberg and Webster flap

Extend dotted lines then bisect them

Second incision parallel to defect midline

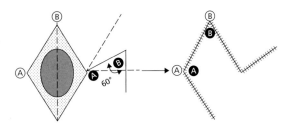

<u>Bi-rhombic flap</u>

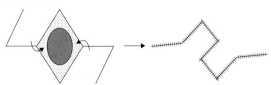

Bilobe

- Used for small defects 1–1.5 cm in size. Common location: lower 1/3 of nose
- Tension is shared between the secondary and tertiary defects

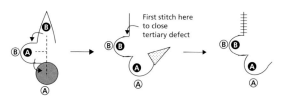

Zitelli modified bilobe flap

- Determine the location of standing cone, then draw ~90° (Zitelli modification) line
- First lobe is at 45° – equal or slightly smaller than defect
- Second lobe is at 90° to the standing cone
- Wide undermining in the submuscular plane to prevent trapdoor effect

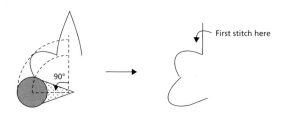

Z-plasty

- GOAL: changing the direction of a scar or to elongate a scar.
- Limbs of the Z should be equal lengths.

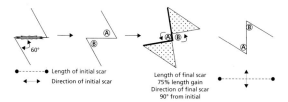

- The degree of the limbs determines both the direction and length of final scar.

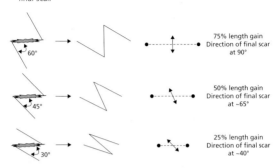

75% length gain
Direction of final scar at 90°

50% length gain
Direction of final scar at ~65°

25% length gain
Direction of final scar at ~40°

Advancement flap
- GOAL: modification of the linear closure, with standing cones (burow triangle) displaced to a more desirable position (i.e. away from free margin).
- Tension vector remains parallel to the motion of the flap.
- Types of advancement flaps: U-plasty, H-plasty, burow advancement, modified crescentic advancement, O → T, and island pedicle.

U-plasty/O → U: unilateral advancement
- Burow triangles created away from defect in one direction.
- Useful along eyebrow and helical rim.

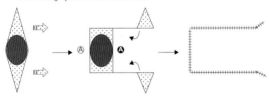

H-plasty/O → H: bilateral advancement
- Burow triangles created away from defect bilaterally.
- Useful if tissue reservoir is available bilaterally.

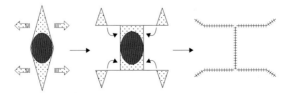

Burow's advancement flap: unilateral advancement

- Displaces one of the standing cone to a more desirable location.
- Useful if defect is along lateral upper cutaneous lip → may displace one of the standing cone to the nasolabial folds.

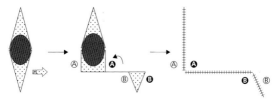

Modified crescentic advancement flap: unilateral advancement

- Modification of the burow triangle.
- Crescentic standing cone removed along the flap to lengthen it.
- Eliminates the need for excision of a standing cone.

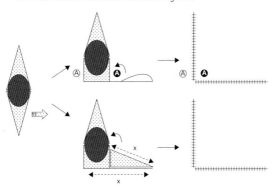

O→ T/T-plasty/A → T: bilateral advancement

- Displaces one of the standing cone bilaterally.
- Useful adjacent to a free margin or along the junction between two cosmetic units (brow, eyelid, forehead, and lip).

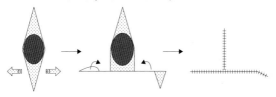

V→Y advancement/Island pedicle/Kite flap

- Island of tissue detached from periphery but with underlying subcutaneous and muscular pedicle.
- Caution: no undermining to base of island – must keep flap attached to underlying pedicle to ensure good blood supply.

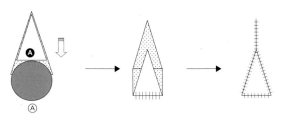

Interpolation flap

- GOAL: coverage of large defects requiring flap with robust blood supply.
- Commonly axial pattern flap – based on named direct cutaneous artery.
- Robust blood supply allow greater length:width ratio.
- Two-staged procedure.
- Base is usually located at some distance from defect. Pedicle must pass over or under an intervening bridge of intact skin.
- Types of flaps: paramedian, nasolabial, and abbe.

Flap	Arterial supply	Defect location	Pedicle division
Paramedian forehead	Supratrochear artery	Large distal nasal defect	2–3 wk
Retroauricular helical	Random flap: rich vascular supply from posterior auricular, superficial temporal, and occipital branches	Large helical rim defect	3 wk
Nasolabial	Angular artery	Large ala defects	2–3 wk
Abbe	Superior or inferior labial artery	Large lip defect	3 wk

Rotation flap

- GOAL: covering a defect when there is an abundant surrounding tissue reservoir.
- Pivotal flap with a curvilinear incision – the flap and defect form a semicircle.
- Rotates in an arc about a pivotal point near the defect.

- Distributes the tension vector along the curvilinear line.
- Common locations: scalp, lateral cheek, infraorbital, and temple.
- Types of rotation flaps: unilateral rotation, bilateral rotation (O → Z), pinwheel, dorsal nasal flap, and Tenzel/ Mustarde flaps.

Unilateral rotation flap
- Usually flap is inferiorly/laterally based to improve lymphatic drainage and decrease flap edema.
- Consider backcut to improve mobility.

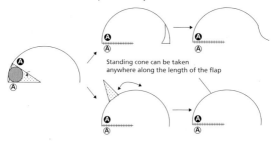

Standing cone can be taken anywhere along the length of the flap

O–Z plasty/bilateral rotation flap
- Useful when there is insufficient tissue reservoir for unilateral flap.
- Common location: scalp.

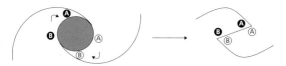

Dorsal nasal rotation/Reiger/Hatchet flap
- Useful for nasal defect <2.5 cm on the lower 2/3 of the nose, best if midline.
- Flap along the entire nasal dorsal.
- Undermine at the level of the perichondrium/periosteum
- Backcut in the glabella.

Mustarde/Tenzel rotation flap
- Laterally based cheek rotation flap.
- Useful for defect along supramedial cheek/lower eyelid.
- Mustarde flap mobilizes entire cheek for defect >½ of eyelid.
- Tenzel flaps mobilizes partial cheek for defect <½ eyelid.

SURGICAL DERMATOLOGY

Skin graft

- GOAL: surgical defect which cannot be closed with adjacent local skin or allowed to heal by second intention; useful for larger wounds, especially in areas that require tumor surveillance.
- Stages of skin graft

Stage	Events	Graft	Timeline
Imbibition	"Ischemic period" – nutrient through osmosis (bolster improves osmosis)	Dark color, edematous	24–48 h
Inosculation	Anastomosis of existing blood vessels	Pink	48–72 h (up to 10 d)
Neovascularization	New capillary ingrowth to graft from wound bed	Hypopigment, less edema	6–7 d

- Three major types:
  1. Full thickness skin graft (FTSG) = epidermis + full dermis
  2. Split thickness skin graft (STSG) = epidermis + partial dermis
  3. Composite graft = skin (epidermis and dermis) + additional component (cartilage or fat)

FTSG

- Minimal contraction ~15%.
- Better cosmesis than STSG – good color, texture, and thickness match.
- Must have intact perichondrium/periosteum for survival – higher metabolic demand than STSG = higher rates of graft failure.
- Most useful for defects less than 3 cm.
- Common sites: eyelids, medial canthus, helical rim, conchal bowl, nasal tip, and digits.
- Good donor sites: preauricular/postauricular area, supraclavicular, standing cones (burow graft), conchal bowl, upper eyelid, and forehead.

STSG

- Higher risk for contraction, poor cosmesis.
- Useful for very large defects: can use fenestration/meshing to enlarge size.
- Donor site heal by second intention can be painful.
- Large grafts need to be harvested with special equipment.

- Better survival than FTSG due to low nutritional requirements
  - Thin: 0.005–0.012 in.
  - Medium: 0.012–0.018 in.
  - Thick: 0.018–0.028 in.

Composite graft
- Less likely to contract, better cosmesis.
- Highest risks for necrosis due to avascular tissue (cartilage) and thicker graft.
- Useful when bulk and structural support is needed – i.e. nasal alar defects.

Type of graft	Nutritional needs	Risk of graft failure	Cosmesis and tissue match	Contraction risk	Durability/ strength	Sensation
FTSG	High	Higher	Good	Low	Good	Good
STSG	Low	Lower	Poor	High	Poor	Fair
Composite	High	Highest	Good	Low	Excellent	Fair

Causes of graft failure
- *Poor blood and nutritional supply*: nicotine use, nutritional deficiency, and collagen vascular disease.
- *Poor graft bed contact*: graft movement (activity, trauma, and poor immobilization), hematoma, seroma.
- *Infection*: immunosuppression, diabetes, systemic disease, and poor wound care.
- *Physician technique*: incomplete defatting, high tension due to inadequate size, rough tissue handling, and excessive cautery.

SURGICAL DERMATOLOGY

Sutures

Absorbable

Material	Origin	Filament	Tensile strength 50%	Absorption	Reactivity	Degradation
Plain gut	Animal collagen*	Twisted	1 wk	14–80 d	High	Proteolysis
Fast absorbing gut	Animal collagen*	Twisted	3–7 d	21–42 d	High	Proteolysis
Vicryl rapide	Polyglactin	Braided	5 d	42 d	Moderate	Hydrolysis
Monocryl	Poliglecaprone	Monofil	1 wk	90–120 d	Low	Hydrolysis
Chromic gut	Plain gut tanned with chromium salts	Twisted	2–3 wk	30–80 d	High, less than plain gut	Proteolysis
Dexon	Polyglycolic acid	Braided	2–3 wk	90 d	Low	Hydrolysis
Vicryl	Polyglactin	Braided	3 wk	80–90 d	Moderate	Hydrolysis
PDS	Polydioxanone	Monofil	4 wk	180 d	Low	Hydrolysis
Maxon	Polyglyconate	Monofil	4 wk	180 d	Very low	Hydrolysis

*Gut made from mucosa/submucosa of sheep or beef intestine.

Nonabsorbable

Material	Origin	Filament	Tensile strength	Reactivity	Elasticity	Handling
Silk	Silk	Braided or twisted	Low, 3–6 mo	High	Inelastic Soft suture	Best
Prolene/Surgilene	Polypropylene	Monofil	High, 2 yr	Least	Very elastic Stiff suture	Fair–good
Ethilon/Monosol/Dermalon	Nylon	Monofil	High, losing 10–20%/yr	Low	Mild elasticity Stiff suture	Fair
Surgilon/Nurolon/Mersilene	Nylon	Braided	High, Losing 10–20%/yr	Moderate	Mild elasticity	Good
Ethibond/Dacron/Novafil	Polyester	Monofil or braided	High, Permanent	Low	Mild elasticity	Very good
	Polybutester	Monofil	High	Low	Very elastic	Very good

Suture removal time

Area	Removal time (days)
Face	4–5
Neck	5–7
Scalp	7
Trunk	7–12
Extremities	10–14

Electrosurgery*

Modality	Terminals	Gap output	Voltage	Amperage	Capability
Electrodessication	1	Markedly damped	High	Low	Superficial destruction
Electrofulguration	1	Markedly damped	High	Low	Superficial destruction (Spark gap)
Electrocoagulation	2	Moderately damped	Mod	Mod	Deep penetration and destruction, Good hemostasis
Electrosection	2	Undamped	Low	High	Cutting

*Electrocautery = not electrosurgery, no electric current, uses heat conduction.

Wound healing

Time	Tensile strength vs. baseline
1 wk	5%
1 mo	40%
1 yr	80%

- Three phases of wound healing: Inflammatory (days) → Proliferation (weeks) → Remodeling (months)
- Platelets are the first cells to appear
- Collagen: Early in wound healing, Collagen III predominates, then later replaced by Collagen I.

Wound dressing

Type	Brand name	Composition	Absorptive	Others	Indications
Adhesive dressing					
Hydrocolloids	Duoderm Hydrocol	Hydrophilic base and adhesive with polyurethane	Good, absorbs water and forms gel with exudates	May leave in place 1–7 d depending on exudate	Pressure ulcers, second intention wounds Wound with low-to-moderate exudates
Film dressing	Tegederm Op-site Bioocclusive	Polyurethane file	None (may cause fluid collection) Gas permeable	Impermeable to bacteria	Best used in conjunction with alginate/hydrogen. Good for monitoring wounds. Lacerations/abrasions/STSG donor site
Nonadhesive dressing					
Alginates	Sorbsan Algiderm	Cellulose like polysaccharide Alginic acid	Highly	Hemostatic agent: releases Ca++	Highly exudative wounds Contraindicated for dry wounds
Hydrogels	Tegagel Flexigel Curagel	Cross-linked polymers with up to 80–90% water Semitransparent gel	Limited, not suitable for exudative wounds	Cooling/pain relief Useful for dry wounds by rehydrating the area	Abrasion wounds (post laser, peels)
Foam dressing	Flexzan Allevyn Aquacel Kendall	Hydrophilic foam, polyurethane, silicone	Highly, gas and water permeable	Compresses chronic leg wounds, conforms to body contours	Pressure ulcer, exudative wound
Gauze dressing	Telfa pad Vaseline gauze, Xeroform		Excellent	Cheap, readily available	Use to cover nonocclusive, nonadherent dressing

Cosmetic Dermatology

Laser

Laser fundamentals: type, wavelength, depth, target and usage

Laser	Wavelength (nm)	Type	Depth (μm)	Target	Usage
CO_2	10 600	IR	20	Water	Resurface, destruction, coagulation, cut
Erbium: YAG	2 940	IR	1	Water	Superficial resurface, destruction
Thulium	1 927	IR	400	Water	Nonablative fractional resurfacing
Erbium:glass	1 550	IR	400–1500	Water	Nonablative fractional resurfacing
Nd:YAG	1 440, 1 450	IR	400–2000	Water	Nonablative resurfacing, nonablative fractional resurfacing
Long pulsed Nd:YAG	1 320	IR	400–2000	Water	Nonablative resurfacing
Nd:YAG	1 064	IR	1600–3000	Mel, Hb	Deep dermal pigment, black/ blue tattoo, hair removal, non-ablative resurface, leg veins, telangiectasia
Diode	800, 810, 930	R	1400	Mel	Dermal pigment, hair removal, leg veins, vascular
Q-Switched Alexandrite	755	R	1300	Mel	Tattoo (black, blue, and green), epilation, pigmentation
Q-Switched Ruby	694	R	1200	Mel	Epidermal/dermal pigment, tattoo (black, blue, and green), hair removal
Argon-pumped dye	630, 514, 488	O, G, B	600	Hb, mel	Vascular, epidermal pigment
Pulsed dye laser (PDL)	585–595	Y	600	Hb, mel	Vascular, hypertrophic scar

Laser	Wavelength (nm)	Type	Depth (μm)	Target	Usage
Copper (Bromide) vapor	578, 511	Y, G	400, 300	Hb, mel	Vascular, epidermal pigment
Krypton	568 531	Y G	400	Hb, mel	Vascular, epidermal pigment
Frequency-doubled Q-switched Nd:YAG/ KTP	532	G	400	Mel, Hb	Vascular, epidermal pigment, red tattoo
Flash lamp pumped PDL	510	G	300	Mel, Hb	Vascular, hypertrophic scar
Argon	488, 514	B	200, 300	Mel, Hb	Vascular, epidermal pigment
Excimer	351, 308, 193	UV	0.5	Protein	Psoriasis, vitiligo, LASIK
Intense pulsed light (IPL)	515–1,200		Up to 3000	Hb, mel	Epidermal/dermal pigment, vascular, hair removal

IR: infrared; R: red; O: orange; Y: yellow; G: green; B: blue; UV: ultraviolet; Mel: melanin; Hb: hemoglobin; KTP: Potassium-titanyl-phosphate.

Laser definitions

	Unit	Definition
Wavelength	nm	—
Energy	J	—
Power	W	Rate of energy delivery, laser output
Fluence	J/cm²	Amount of energy delivered per area
Pulse width	sec	Duration of laser exposure
Spot size	mm	Diameter of laser beam
Thermal relaxation time	sec	Time needed for the heated target to cool by 50% of its peak temperature through diffusion
Chromophore		Target of laser

Laser principles (LASER = Light Amplification by Stimulated Emission of Radiation)

1. monochromatic (single wavelength)
2. coherent (in phase with time and space)
3. collimated (parallel waves)

Selective photothermolysis: selective heating of a target chromophore occurs:

1. selected wavelength is preferentially absorbed by the target chromophore
2. energy is high enough to damage the chromophore
3. pulse duration of the laser is shorter than the thermal relaxation of the target

$$\text{Laser output} = \text{Power(W)} = \frac{\text{Fluence(J/cm}^2) \times \text{Spot Size(mm}^2)}{\text{Pulse Width(s)}}$$

To increase laser output → increase fluence
→ increase spot size
→ decrease pulse width

Thermal relaxation time of major skin chromophores

Chromophore target	Size (μm)	Thermal relaxation time
Melanosome	0.5–1.0	20–40 ns
Tattoo pigment particles	0.5–100	20 ns–3 ms
Epidermis	50	1 ms
Telangiectasias	30–50	1 ms
Blood vessel	100–300	5–30 ms
Melanin in hair follicle	200	20–100 ms

Laser treatment of tattoo pigment

Tattoo	Pigment	Wavelength absorbed (nm)	Laser
Black	Carbon (India ink),	1064	Picosecond Nd:YAG
	Iron oxide, Logwood	1064	Q-switched Nd:YAG
		755	Picosecond Alexandrite
		755	Q-switched Alexandrite
		694	Q-switched Ruby
Blue	Cobalt aluminate	1064	Picosecond Nd:YAG
		1064	Q-switched Nd:YAG
		755	Picosecond Alexandrite
		755	Q-switched Alexandrite
		694	Q-switched Ruby

Tattoo	Pigment	Wavelength absorbed (nm)	Laser
Green	Chromic oxide, Lead chromate,	755	Picosecond Alexandrite
		755	Q-switched Alexandrite
	Malachite, Ferro- and ferricyanides, Phthalocyanine dyes, Curcuma	694	Q-switched Ruby
Yellow	Cadmium sulfide	1064/532	Picosecond Nd:YAG
Red	Mercury sulfide (cinnabar),	1064/532	Picosecond Nd:YAG
	Cadmium selenide,	532, 510	Q-switched Nd:YAG
	Iron oxide (may turn black with laser tx)		

Photoinduced eye injury

	Wavelength (nm)	Exposure risk	Ocular target	Eye effect
UVB/UVC	200–320	Sunburn	Cornea	Photokeratitis (Snow blindness)
UVA	320–400	PUVA, Excimer	Lens	Photochemical UV cataract, delayed (yr)
Visible	400–760	Ruby, PDL, Argon	Retina (melanin, photoreceptors)	Photochemical and thermal retinal injury (Flash blindness)
Infrared A	760–1400	Nd:YAG	Retina	Same as above
Infrared B	>1400	CO_2, Erb:YAG	Cornea (water)	Corneal burn

Laser wavelength, depth of penetration and the electromagnetic spectrum

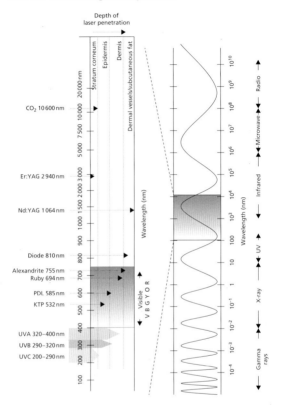

Absorption spectra of major skin chromophores

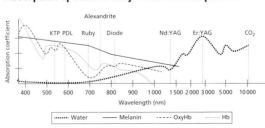

Photodynamic therapy

Basic principles
- Components: (i) Photosensitizer, (ii) Light source, (iii) Tissue oxygenation
- Two steps: (i) administration of photosensitizer (topical or systemic), (ii) irradiation with visible light
- Effects:
  - Through type 2 photooxidative reactions, PDT produces cytotoxic-reactive oxygen species (singlet oxygen, superoxide anion, hydroxyl radical, hydrogen peroxide) → oxidation of amino acids, proteins, lipids → necrosis, apoptosis
  - Modifies immune responses, i.e. cytokine expression
  - For acne, targets sebaceous glands and decreases P. acnes (P. acnes accumulates porphyrins)

Applications
AKs, acne, BCC, Bowen, photoaging, verruca vulgaris, hidradenitis suppurativa, sebaceous hyperplasia

Photosensitizer properties and options

Methyl aminolevulinic acid (MAL)	Aminolevulinic acid (ALA)
METVIX® cream 160 mg/g	Levulan® Kerastick® topical solution 20%
	Ameluz® 78 mg/g nanoemulsion gel 10%
More lipophilic (some passive transmembrane diffuse)	More hydrophilic (needs active transport)
Deeper penetration	Poorer penetration*
Intracellularly, MAL is demethylated to ALA	Not a photosensitizer but converted to protoporphyrin IX (through heme biosynthesis pathway)
Red light (Aktilite)	Blue light (Blu-U) – Levulan® Kerastick®
	Red Light (BF-RhodoLED) – Ameluz®
FDA approved for treatment of AK. Approved in Europe for treatment of BCC.	FDA approved for treatment of AK.

*Can increase ALA penetration by increasing the application time, occluding, scrubbing with acetone, or using iontophoresis or electroporation.

- Selectivity: MAL and ALA (i) concentrate in tumor cells and newly formed endothelium and (ii) require specific wavelengths to become activated.
- Heme pathway:
  - In the cytoplasm, ALA → porphobilinogen → uroporphyrinogen III → coproporphyrinogen III.
  - In the mitochondria, coproporphyrinogen III → protoporphyrinogen IX → protoporphyrin IX → iron incorporated by ferrochelatase.
- Systemic photosensitizers – have tetrapyrrolic structure and are given intravenously due to their low cutaneous penetration; examples: HpD and porfimer sodium (Photofrin®).

Light source
- ALA and MAL converts to protoporphyrin IX, which has an absorption peak at the Soret band (~405 nm, within blue light) as well as peaks at higher wavelengths (Q-bands – at 510, 545, 580, and 630 nm).
- Q-band peaks are ~15× smaller than the Soret band peak.
- Red light (Aktilite 630 nm) penetrates deeper into skin than blue light (Blu-U – 405–420 nm).

Adverse effects:
- Topical: mild, transient burning pain, pruritus, erythema, edema, crusting, and scaling.
- Systemic: longer-lasting generalized phototoxicity and sensitivity (sometimes months), photophobia, ocular pain, pigmentary changes, N/V, liver toxicity, metallic taste, SLE exacerbation.

Precautions/contraindications:
- Contraindicated in patients with porphyria, cutaneous sensitivity to the light source's wavelength(s), and allergies to porphyrins or any part of the ALA solution/MAL cream (MAL cream contains peanut/almond oils).
- Contraindicated in patients who are pregnant or breast-feeding.
- Patients should reveal all medications (OTC, herbal, rx – TCNs, thiazides, griseofulvin, sulfonamides, sulfonylureas, phenothiazines) which may impact (i) photosensitivity and (ii) ALA/MAL penetration (retinoids).
- Deep recurrence can occur with partial (superficial only) tx of malignancies.

PDT Protocol
Levulan® ALA PDT:

- Wash the treatment area with non-soap cleanser. Consider acetone scrub prior to applying ALA.
- Per package instructions: crush Levulan® Kerastick at two points, then sequentially down the stick. Shake stick vertically for two mintues. Must be used within two hours of resuspension.
- Avoid applying ALA to ocular/mucosal surfaces.
- For large areas, wait 30 minutes to 2 hours after applying ALA (~15 hours ok for small isolated lesion)
- For anesthetic effect, may apply topical lidocaine immediately following ALA application.
- Avoid bright artificial light and sunlight during incubation period.
- Use protective glasses.
- If situated 2–4 in. from Blu-U light, tx time ~ 16 minutes 40 seconds ($10 \, J/cm^2$).
- After tx, avoid sunlight (or intense light) for two days (sunscreen would not block visible light).
- Re-tx in two months prn.

Ameluz® ALA PDT:

- Degrease area with alcohol.
- Remove hyperkeratotic areas with curette but avoid bleeding.
- Apply gel to cover the lesions and approximately 5 mm surrounding area with a film of 1-mm thickness.
- Should not exceed area of 20 cm^2 and no more than 2 g (one tube) of Ameluz.
- Avoid applying to ocular/mucosal surfaces.
- Cover the area with light impermeable occlusive dressing and incubate for three hours.
- Avoid bright artificial light and sunlight during incubation period.
- Remove residual gel after incubation.
- Use protective glasses.
- Illuminate entire treatment areas with BF-RhodoLED® at 635 nm for 10 minutes at a distance of 2–3 in. from the skin surface (approximately 37 J/cm^2).
- After tx, avoid sunlight (or intense light) for two days (sunscreen would not block visible light).
- Re-tx in three months prn.

MAL PDT:

- Curette treatment area to remove scale.
- Apply MAL cream (nitrile gloves and spatula) under occlusion.
- Avoid sunlight, bright artificial lights, or cold during three hours incubation period.
- Use protective glasses.
- Tx time: 8–10 minutes at 5–8 cm from red light (37 J/cm^2).
- Re-tx in one week prn.

UV spectrum

UV spectrum and wavelengths

Infrared	>760 nm	
Visible	400–760 nm	
UV	<400 nm	
UVAI	340–400	Soret band (400–410 nm)
UVAII	320–340	Wood lamp (320–400, peak at 365 nm)
UVB	290–320	NBUVB (311 nm)
UVC	200–290	

UVB protection vs SPF

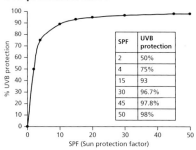

SPF	UVB protection
2	50%
4	75%
15	93
30	96.7%
45	97.8%
50	98%

UV protection measurements

- SPF = Sun Protection Factor = sunscreen protected:unprotected ratio of duration of UVB exposure to produce 1 MED.
- Water-resistant product maintains SPF level after 40 minutes of water immersion.
- Waterproof (very water-resistant) maintains SPF level after 80 minutes of water immersion.
- Measures of UVA protection: persistent pigment darkening, immediate pigment darkening, protection factor UVA.
- Critical wavelength (CW) = wavelength at which the integral of the spectral absorbance curves equals 90% of the integral from 290 to 400 nm (CW of at least 370 nm for broad-spectrum sunscreen).

Sunscreen	Max % conc.*	UVB	UVA II	UVA I
Anthranilates – meradimate, menthyl anthranilate	5	▨	■	
Avobenzone (Parsol 1789)	3		▨	■
Benzophenones – oxybenzone	6	■	■	▨
dioxybenzone	3			
Cinnamates – octinoxate	7.5	■		
cinoxate	3			
Mexoryl SX (Ecamsule)	3	▨	■	▨
PABA derivatives – padimate O	8	■		
benzoic acid	15	■		
Octocrylene	10	■	▨	
Salicylates – homosalate	15	■		
trolamine salicylate	12	■		
Titanium dioxide	25	■	■	▨
Zinc oxide	25	■	■	■

* % Maximum FDA-approved concentration

■ Maximum protection   ▨ Partial protection

UV associations/specificities

UVA	UVB	UVA and UVB
Immediate tanning	Delayed tanning	AKs
Photoaging (UVA > UVB)	Photocarcinogenesis (UVB > UVA)	Fine wrinkles
Hydroa vacciniforme	Persistent light reaction	Solar urticaria
Phytophotodermatitis	Sunburn	(or visible light)
Photoallergic drug reaction	Xeroderma pigmentosa	
PMLE (UVA > UVB, UVC, or visible)	Cockayne syndrome	
	Lupus erythematosus photosensitivity (UVB > UVA)	

Glogau Wrinkle scale

Glogau type	1	2	3	4
	No wrinkles	Wrinkles in motion	Wrinkles at rest	Only wrinkles
Age (years)	~20–30 s	~30–40 s	~50–60 s	~60–70 s and older
Photoaging	Early photoaging	Early–moderate photoaging	Advanced photoaging	Severe photoaging
Pigmentary changes	Mild/early pigmentary changes	Early lentigines	Dyschromia, telangectasia	Yellow-gray discoloration
Keratoses/ skin cancers	No keratoses	Palpable keratoses	Visible keratoses	Skin cancers
Wrinkles	Minimal wrinkles	Dynamic wrinkles – parallel smile lines	Wrinkles without motion	Wrinkles throughout

Fitzpatrick skin type

Skin type	Color	Tanning response
Type I	White	Always burns, never tans
Type II	White	Usually burns, sometimes tans
Type III	White	Sometimes burns mildly, always tans
Type IV	Olive	Rarely burns, always tans
Type V	Dark brown	Never burns, tans very easily
Type VI	Black	Never burns, tans very easily

Chemical peels

Pre-peel consideration:
- HSV prophylaxis (i.e. Acyclovir 400 TID × 4–7 days) for all medium and deep peels.
- Consider preconditioning skin with topical retinoids for an even peel. Stop two to four days prior to peel and resume two to four days after reepithelization
- Wash hair morning of procedure. No makeup, jewelry, and contact lens.

Peel prep:
- Informed consent signed.
- Ensure preop med taken.
- Cleanse with Septisol to remove oils. Rinse thoroughly.
- Wipe area with alcohol.
- Degrease area with 100% acetone to further debride oil and strateum corneum.
- Apply peel to area with 2 × 2 gauze or Q-tips.
- Neutralize (for Glycolic peels) or cool water compress for non-neutralizing peels.
- Review postop instructions.

Post-peel wound care (for medium/deep peels)
- Vinegar soak 3–4× per day with 0.25% acetic acid compress (1 tbsp white vinegar in 1 pint cool water).
- White petrolatum or emollient to face and neck (for deeper peels) or Eucerin cream (for superficial/medium depth peels). May cover neck with saran wrap.
- Hydroquinone posttreatment for PIH.

Peeling agents

Depth of peel	Layer	Peel	Amount	Component
Very superficial	Strateum corneum/ ganulosum	Retinoids		Retinoic acid
		TCA 10–25%	1 coat	Trichloroacetic acid (TCA)
		Resorcin 20–30%	5–10 min	Resorcinol
		Gycolic 30–50%	1–2 min	Alpha hydroxy acid
		Salicylic acid 20–35%		Beta hydroxy acid
		Jessner	1–3 coats	Resorcinol/ Salicylic acid/Lactic acid/ETOH
Superficial	Basal layer/ papillary dermis	TCA 35%	1 coat	TCA
		Gycolic 50–70%	5–20 min	Alpha hydroxyl acid
		Resorcin 50%	30–60 min	Resorcinol
Medium	Upper reticular dermis	Combination peels		Jessner + 35% TCA
				CO_2 + 35% TCA
				Glycolic 70% + 35% TCA
				50% TCA
Deep	Mid-reticular dermis	Baker-Gordon		Phenol/Septisol/ Croton oil
		Phenol 88%		Carbolic acid
		TCA 70–100%		Cross technique for ice-pick scars with toothpicks

Salicylic acid peels

For acne and melasma. 20–30% SA. White pseudofrost precipitate forms immediately. Use two to three coats. Solution can be left on for more drying effect.

Glycolic acid peels

Endpoint is pink edema (mild), perifollicular edema (moderate), and vesiculation (max). **Must be neutralized** with 10% sodium bicarbonate.

TCA peel

End point is frosting (self-neutralizing). Depth based on the number/amount of application (wait three to four minutes after each application to access the amount of frost). May use cold compress after appearance of light frost to reduce discomfort.

Level	Frosting	Depth of peel	Healing time
0	No frost, minimal erythema	Removes stratum corneum	—
1	Partial light frost, some erythema	Superficial peel	2–4 d
2	White frost with erythema show through	Full thickness epidermal peel	5 d
3	Solid white frost, no pink	Papillary dermis	5–7 d

Jessner solution

Resorcinol (14 g); Salicyclic acid (14 g); Lactic acid (14 g); Ethanol 95% (100 ml)
- Combination Jessner's/TCA produces a more even peel than TCA only
- Salicylate toxicity: tinnitus, headache, and nausea
- Recorcinol toxicity: methemoglobinemia, syncope, and thyroid suppression

Baker-Gordon phenol

88% Phenol (3 ml); Distilled water (2 ml); Septisol (8 drops); Croton oil (3 drops)

Rapidly absorbed through skin, metabolized by the liver, excreted by renal system

Risk of renal failure, hepatotoxicity, and cardiac arrthymias

Cook total body peel

70% glycolic acid gel followed immediately by 35–40% TCA

Neutralize with 10% sodium bicarbonate solution once scattered frosting is noted

Hetter Peel formulas with 35% Phenol/Croton oil

(Adapted from International Peel Society Workshop, Harold Brody, Peter Rullan, Richard Bensimon)

Hetter Peel strength based on % of croton oil – Can be made with volume or drops

Endpoint: Papillary dermis: transparent frost with pinkish background

Upper/mid-reticular dermis: Solid thick frost

Mid-dermis: Thick, gray white frost with eventual red-brown overtones

Recommended croton oil concentration based on location

Perioral	0.4–1.1%/medium light–heavy
Cheeks	0.4–0.7%/medium light–medium heavy
Forehead	0.2–0.4%/medium light
Eyelids	0.1%/very light
Neck	0.1%/very light feathering

Hetter formulation using volume

Croton oil/ phenol	0.1%/ 35%	0.2%/ 35%	0.4%/ 35%	0.8%/ 35%	1.2%/ 35%	1.6%/ 0%
Stock solution*	—	0.5 ml	1.0 ml	2.0 ml	3.0 ml	4.0 ml
USP Phenol 88%	1.2 ml	3.5 ml	3.0 ml	2.0 ml	1.0 ml	0 ml
Water	1.8 ml	5.5 ml	5.5 ml	5.5 ml	5.5 ml	5.5 ml
Septisol	—	0.5 ml	0.5 ml	0.5 ml	0.5 ml	0.5 ml
0.4% Hetter	1 ml	—	—	—	0.5 ml	0.5 ml
Total	4 ml	10 ml	10 ml	10 ml	10 ml	10 ml

*Stock solution: 24 ml phenol 88% + 1 ml Croton oil (=0.04%CO/ml)

Hetter formulation using drops

Croton oil/phenol	Very light peel 0.1%/28%	Medium light 0.35%/35%	Medium heavy 0.7%/35%	Heavy 1.1%/35%
Drops of croton oil*	—	1 drop	2 drops	3 drops
USP phenol 88%	2 ml	4 ml	4 ml	1.0 ml
Water	5 ml	6 ml	6 ml	6 ml
Septisol	—	16 drops	16 drops	16 drops
Medium light formula	3 ml	—	—	—
Total	10 ml	10 ml	10 ml	10 ml

*Stock solution: 24 ml phenol 88% + 1 ml Croton oil (=0.04% CO/ml)

Botulinum toxin

- Produced by Clostridium botulinum (gram negative anaerobic bacterium)
  Mechanism of action
  - Block Ach release from presynaptic nerve terminal of the motor end plate. Heavy chain irreversibly binds to the botulinum toxin receptor for endocytosis. Light chain then cleaves specific SNARE protein complex
    - BTX-A: cleaves SNAP-25
    - BTX-B: cleaves synaptobrevin/VAMP

Comparison of botulinum toxins

	OnabotuliumtoxinA	AbobotulinumtoxinA	IncobotuliumtoxinA
Manufacturer	Allergan	Ipsen/Medicis	Merz
Brand name US	Botox Cosmetic®	Dysport®	Xeomin®
Brand name Europe	Vistabex	Azzalure	Bocouture
FDA approval	2002 for moderate-to-severe glabella lines	2009 for moderate-to-severe glabella lines	2011 for moderate-to-severe glabella lines
	2013 for moderate-to-severe lateral canthal lines		
	2004 for axillary hyperhidrosis		
Serotype	A	A	A
Clostridium strain	HALL A	NCTC 2916	HALL A
Molecular weight + Protein complex (kDa)	~900	500–900	150 (free from complexing proteins)
Stabilization	Vacuum-drying	Lyophilized	Lyophilized
Storage (before and after reconstitution)	2–8 °C/2–8 °C	2–8 °C/2–8 °C	25 °C/2–8 °C
Shelf life	24 mo	15 mo	36 mo
Units/package	50 and 100	300 and 500	100
Approximate equivalency	1	2.5	1

- Reconstitution
  - Potency can be maintained for up to six weeks.
  - Reconstitution with sterile saline *with* preservative (0.9% benzyl alcohol) provides local anesthetic effect

Diluent added (0.9% NaCl) to 100 unit vial	1.0 ml	2.0 ml	2.5 ml	4.0 ml	8.0 ml
Resulting dose/units per 0.1 ml	10.0 U	5.0 U	4.0 U	2.5 U	1.25 U

- Response
  - Clinical effect one to three days following injection with maximal effect by two weeks
  - Benefits last three to six months
- Adverse effects/complications
  - Common: redness, ecchymosis, headache, bruising, edema, inflammation, and erythema

- Ptosis: minimize by careful selection of injection site. (1–1.5 cm away from the orbital rim at the midpupillary line)
  - If ptosis, use Iopidine (apraclonidine) drops. α2-adrenergic agonist which stimulates Muller's muscles to provide an elevation of 1–3 mm.
- Contraindications: infection at site of injection, known hypersensitivity to formulation.
- Caution:
  - Peripheral motor neuropathic disease, neuromuscular disorder (myasthenia gravis, Eaton-Lambert have increased risk of systemic side effects)
  - Aminoglycosides, penicillamine, and Ca+ channel blockers may potentiate BOTOX
  - Pregnancy category C
  - Lactation: not known whether toxin is excreted in human milk

Location	Muscles	Recommended Botox units	Comments
❶ Glabella frown lines	Corrugator, procerus, orbicularis oculi, depressor supercilii	10–30 U women 20–40 U men	Keep >1 cm superior to orbital rim
❷ Horizontal forehead lines	Frontalis	10–20 U women 20–30 U men ~ 2–8 sites at 1 cm apart	Avoid treating lower 1/3 of lateral forehead to avoid brow ptosis
❸ Crow's feet	Lateral fibers of orbicularis oculi	6–15 U per side subdermal plane	keep >1–1.5 cm lateral to orbital rim
❹ Bunny lines	Upper nasalis Procerus	2–4 U per side	1 U midline if needed to procerus
❺ Marionette lines and Mouth frown	Depressor anguli oris	5–10 U	Inject 1 cm lateral and 1–2 cm inferior to angle of mouth
❻ Mental crease	Mentalis	4–10 U	Deep injection
❼ Perioral rhytides	Orbicularis oris	1–2 U per quadrant	Superficially over vermillion
❽ Platysmal bands	Platysma	10–30 U women 10–40 U men	Grasp band and inject into belly of muscle

Botox injection sites

● Recommended sites ○ Optional sites

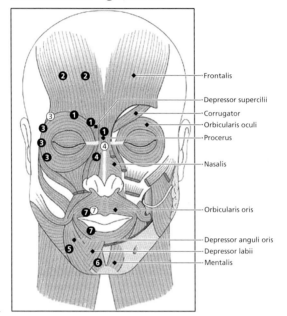

- Frontalis
- Depressor supercilii
- Corrugator
- Orbicularis oculi
- Procerus
- Nasalis
- Orbicularis oris
- Depressor anguli oris
- Depressor labii
- Mentalis

(Modified from Sommer B, Sattler G (eds.). *Botulinum Toxin in Aesthetic Medicine*. Boston: Blackwell Science, Ltd.; 2001, with permission.)

Injectable for adipolysis

- Deoxycholic acid (Kybella®) – FDA approved in 2015 for submental fat adipolysis
- Causes focal adipocyte lysis.
- Clear, colorless sterile solution, 10 g/ml, 2 ml vials. Store at room temperature.
- Injected 0.2 ml spaced 1 cm apart in the subcutis. Consider pinching preplaysmal fat between fingers to isolate fat.
- Risk of marginal mandibular injury, avoid injecting 1.0–1.5 cm from the inferior border of mandible.
- Side effects: common = swelling (87%), bruising/hematoma (72%), pain (70%), numbness (66%), erythema (27%), induration (23%); rare = marginal mandibular nerve injury with asymmetric smile/facial muscle weakness (4%), dysphagia (2%), alopecia, ulceration, necrosis.

Fillers

Brand name (Company)	Composition	How supplied	Duration of effect	FDA approval/CE mark	Location of injection	Side effects/adverse effects
COLLAGEN						
Zyderm I (Inamed, division of Allergan)	Bovine collagen 35 mg/ml Contains 0.3% lidocaine	0.5, 1.0, 1.5 ml	3–4 mo	FDA 1981 CE mark 1995	Superficial dermis – superficial rhytids, scars	Hypersensitivity to bovine collagen. Need two skin testing (2–4 wk apart). Wait 4 wk before treatment
Zyderm II (Inamed)	Bovine collagen 65 mg/ml Contains 0.3% lidocaine	0.5, 1.0 ml	3–4 mo	FDA 1983 CE mark 1995	Mid-dermis – moderate rhytids	Lidocaine sensitivity
Zyplast (Inamed)	Bovine collagen 35 mg/ml Cross-linked with glutaraldehyde Contains 0.3% lidocaine	1.0, 1.5, 2.0, 2.5 ml	3–5 mo	FDA 1985 CE mark 1995	Mid to deep dermis – deep rhytids, lip augmentation	
Cosmoderm I (Inamed)	Human collagen 35 mg/ml Contains 0.3% lidocaine	1.0 ml	3–4 mo	FDA 2003	Superficial dermis – superficial rhytids, scars	Lidocaine sensitivity
Cosmoderm II (Inamed)	Human collagen 65 mg/ml Contains 0.3% lidocaine	1.0 ml	3–4 mo	FDA 2003	Mid-dermis – moderate rhytids	
Cosmoplast (Inamed)	Human collagen 35 mg/ml cross-linked with glutaraldehyde Contains 0.3% lidocaine	1.0, 1.5 ml	3–4 mo	FDA 2003	Deep dermis – deep rhytids, lip augmentation	

continued p.282

Brand name (Company)	Composition	How supplied	Duration of effect	FDA approval/CE mark	Location of injection	Side effects/adverse effects
EVOLENCE 30 (ColBar LifeScience)	Porcine collagen 30 mg/ml. Glymatrix technology cross-link collagen to ribose – mimic human collagen. Dispersed in phosphate-buffered saline solution.	1.0 ml	Up to 12 mo	FDA 2008, voluntarily removed from US market in 2009. CE 2004. Approved in Canada	Upper to mid dermis	Nonhuman collagen with potential for allergic reaction, though pretesting is not required
HYALURONIC ACID – correction possible with hyaluronidase (not FDA approved)						
Belotero Balance (Merz)	Hyaluronic acid 22.5 mg/ml Varying degree of cross-link density By bacterial fermentation from *Streptococcus equi*	0.4 ml	6–12 mo	FDA 2011. CE mark.	Superficial to mid dermis – superficial rhytids, scars	—
Restylane Silk (Galderma)	Hyaluronic acid 20 mg/ml By bacterial fermentation from *Streptococcus equi*	1.0 ml	3–6 mo	FDA 2014.a CE mark.	Submucosal and dermis – Lip augmentation and perioral rhytids	—
Restylane ±L (Galderma)	Hyaluronic acid 20 mg/ml ± 0.1% lidocaine Average particle size 300 μm By bacterial fermentation from *Streptococcus equi*	0.4, 1.0 ml	4–6 mo	FDA 2003. CE mark.	Mid/deep dermis – moderate/severe rhytids, folds, lip	Rare allergic/ hypersensitivity reactions, granulomas

Restylane Refyne (Galderma)	Hyaluronic acid 20 mg/ml ± 0.1% lidocaine XpresHAn Technology By bacterial fermentation from *Streptococcus equi*	1.0 ml	12 mo	FDA 2016. CE mark	Mid/deep dermis – moderate/severe rhytids, folds, lip	Rare allergic/ hypersensitivity reactions, granulomas
Restylane Defyne (Galderma)	Hyaluronic acid 20 mg/ml ± 0.1% lidocaine XpresHAn Technology By bacterial fermentation from *Streptococcus equi*	1.0 ml	12 mo	FDA 2016 CE mark	Mid/deep dermis – moderate/severe rhytids, folds, lip	Rare allergic/ hypersensitivity reactions, granulomas
Restylane Lyft formerly Perlane ±L (Galderma)	Hyaluronic acid 20 mg/ml ± 0.1% lidocaine Average particle size 650 μm By bacterial fermentation from *Streptococcus equi*	1.0 ml	3–9 mo	FDA 2007	Deep dermis and subcutaneous to supraeriosteal – moderate/severe rhytids and cheek augmentation	Rare allergic/ hypersensitivity reactions, granulomas
Juvederm Ultra ±XC (Allergan)	Hyaluronic acid 24 mg/ml ± 0.3% lidocaine (9% cross-linked) produced by *Streptococcus equi*	1.0 ml	6–12 mo	FDA 2006	Mid/deep dermis – mod/severe rhytids, folds, lip	—
Juvederm Ultra Plus ±XC (Allergan)	Hyaluronic acid 24 mg/ml ± 0.3% lidocaine (11% cross-linked) produced by *Streptococcus equi*	1.0 ml	9–12 mo	FDA 2006	Deep dermis – severe rhytids, folds	—

COSMETIC DERMATOLOGY

continued p.284

Brand name (Company)	Composition	How supplied	Duration of effect	FDA approval/CE mark	Location of injection	Side effects/adverse effects
Juvederm Voluma ±XC (Allergan)	Hyaluronic acid 20 mg/ml ± 0.3% lidocaine (Vycross™ technology) produced by *Streptococcus equi*	1.0 ml	Up to 24 mo	FDA 2013 CE 2009	Subcutaneous to supraeriosteal – cheek augmentation	—
Juvederm Vollure ±XC (Allergan)	Hyaluronic acid 17.5 mg/ml ± 0.3% lidocaine (Vycross™ technology) produced by *Streptococcus equi*	1.0 ml	Up to 18 mo	FDA 2017 CE 2013 (Volift)	Submucosal and dermal – lip augmentation and perioral rhytids	—
Juvederm Volbella ±XC (Allergan)	Hyaluronic acid 15 mg/ml ± 0.3% lidocaine (Vycross™ technology) produced by *Streptococcus equi*	1.0 ml	Up to 12 mo	FDA 2016 CE 2013	Submucosal and dermal – lip augmentation and perioral rhytids	
Prevelle Silk (Mentor)	Hyaluronic acid 5.5 mg/ml (hylan B gel) + 0.3% lidocaine	0.75 ml	3–5 mo	FDA 2008	Mid/deep dermis – mod/severe rhytids, folds, lip	
Hylaform (Inamed/ Allergen)	Hyaluronic acid 5.5 mg/ml 20% cross-linking Derived from rooster comb	0.4, 0.75 ml	3–6 mo	FDA 2004 CE 1995	Mid/deep dermis – moderate/severe rhytids, lips	Contraindicated if allergic to avian product. Rare allergic/ hypersensitivity reactions, granulomas
Hylaform Plus (Inamed/ Allergen)	Hyaluronic acid 5.5 mg/ml 20% cross-linking Larger particle size Derived from rooster comb	0.4, 0.75 ml	3–6 mo	FDA 2004 CE 1995	Deep dermis – severe rhytids	

Captique (Allergan)	Hyaluronic acid 5.5 mg/ml 98% highly cross-linked By bacterial fermentation from *Streptococcus equi*	0.75 ml	3–5 mo	FDA 2004	Mid/deep dermis – mod/severe rhytids, folds, lip

Synthetic fillers

Radiesse formerly Radiance (Merz)	Calcium hydroxylapatite (25–45 µm) microspheres suspended in carboxymethylcellulose gel	0.8, 1.5 ml	1 mo +	FDA 2006	Subdermis – deep rhytids, folds, lipoatrophy, volume loss for dorsal hands	Rare allergic reactions. Reports of granulomas and nodules (not indicated for lips). Detectable on X-ray and CT scans
Radiesse Plus (Merz)	Same as above but with 0.3% lidocaine	0.8, 1.5 ml	12 mo +	FDA 2015	Subdermis – deep rhytids, folds, lipoatrophy volume loss for dorsal hands	Rare allergic reactions. Reports of granulomas and nodules (not indicated for lips). Detectable on X-ray and CT scans

continued p.286

COSMETIC DERMATOLOGY

Brand name (Company)	Composition	How supplied	Duration of effect	FDA approval/CE mark	Location of injection	Side effects/adverse effects
Sculptra (Galderma)	Poly-L-lactic acid (150 mg) suspended in mannitol (127.5 mg) and sodium carboxymethylcellulose (90 mg). Rehydrate with sterile water + 1% Lidocaine (last least 3 h prior to injection)	1 vial (150 µg)	Up to 2 yr after first tx. Need 3–6 tx spaced 2–4 wk apart	FDA 2004	Deep dermis/Subcutaneous plane – Restoration and correction of facial fat loss (HIV lipoatrophy)	Potential for lumpiness – need to massage area posttreatment
Bellafill Formerly Artefill and Artecoll (Suneva)	20% polymethylmethacrylate microspheres (32–40 µm) suspended in 3.5% bovine collagen with 0.3% lidocaine	0.4, 0.8 ml	Permanent filler up to 5 yr +	FDA 2006 CE 1994	Deep dermis – deep rhytids, folds, moderate-to-severe acne scars	Lidocaine sensitivity Potential for sensitivity to bovine collagen, need skin test 4 wk prior Reports of allergic reactions, foreign body granulomas 0.01%
Silikon (Alcon) AdatoSil (Bausch & Lomb)	Silicone, pure polymers from siloxane	1 vial 8.5 ml (2 ml max per tx)	Permanent	Off-label use. FDA approved for retinal tamponade	Subcutaneous plane – deep rhytids, folds	Granuloma formation, migration, inflammatory reactions

Homologous material

	Material	Status	Duration	Location	Notes
Autologen (Collagenesis)	Autologous human collagen, elastin, glycosaminoglycans, and fibronectic. Prepared from patient tissue	No longer available	4 mo–2 yr	No longer available	Mid dermis – mod/severe rhytids, lip, folds
Dermalogen (Collagenesis)	Pooled human cadaveric proteins, primarily type I and III collagens	No longer available	3–6 mo	No longer available	Mid and deep dermal filler for rhytids and folds
Fascian (Fascia Biosystems)	Freeze-dried irradiated cadaveric fascia lata reconstituted with saline and 0.5% lidocaine	No longer available	3–8 mo	No longer available	Superficial, mid, deep dermis based on particle size
Azficel-T/ laViv (Fibrocell Science)	Autologous fibroblasts culture from biopsy of the patient's skin	1.2 ml = ~18 million fibroblast	6 mo +	FDA	Mid/deep dermis
					Potential for hypersensitivity to polymyxin B sulfate, bacitracin, and gentamicin
					Requires patient biopsy then manufacturing takes 11–22 wk. Recommended series of three intradermal injection
Autologous fat	Autologous fat	20–50 cc based on harvest	6–24 mo	Subdermal	Need donor sites – thighs, buttocks, and abdomen

Source: Adapted from Injectables at Glance. The American society for aesthetic plastic surgery. http://www.surgery.org/download/injectablechart.pdf, 11/25/07. RD Sengelmann et al. Soft-tissue augmentation. In JK Robinson et al (eds.). *Surgery of the Skin*, first edition. Philadelphia: Mosby; 2005. Robert, B et al. Dermal Fillers: Overview, Collagen, Hyaluronic Acid. Emedicine.medscape.com. Retrieved 29 January 2017, from http://emedicine.medscape.com/article/1125066-overview#showall

COSMETIC DERMATOLOGY

Protocol for vascular occlusion from fillers

Adapted from Beer K, et al. *J Clin Aesthet Dermatol*. 2012 May; 5(5): 44–47. Dayan S et al. Management of impending necrosis associated with soft tissue filler injections. *J Drugs Dermatol*. 2011;10:1007–1012. Beleznay et al. *J Clin Aesthet Dermatol*. 2014 Sep; 7(9): 37–43.

- If suspecting vascular occlusion (blanching, mottled purplish discoloration, and severe pain), stop injection immediately.
- **Hyaluronidase** high-dose (at least 200u) injection into area. Reinject if no improvement within 60 minutes. Can be used even if non-HA filler. While skin testing is recommended prior to treatment due to risk of hypersensitivity (1/2000), in case of vascular compromise and impending necrosis, it is not necessary to do skin testing.
- Massage treatment area vigorous.
- Apply warm compress – apply for 5–10 minutes every 1–2 hours to promote vascular dilation.
- **Nitroglycerin 2% paste** – ?? efficacy. Apply immediately to area, then five minutes for every one to two hours. Sent home to apply up to three times a day. Monitor of dizziness and hypotension.
- **Aspirin 325 mg** under tongue immediately, then 650 mg daily for one week. Consider antacid to prevent aspirin associated gastritis.
- **Prednisone 20–40 mg** daily for three to five days to decrease inflammation.
- **Sildenafil citrate 50 mg** daily for three to five days to increase blood flow.
- Consider hyperbaric oxygen.

Venous disease treatment

Vein treatment algorithm

1. Superficial venous system is interconnected – treat the most proximal point of reflux first prior to sclerotherapy.
2. Recognize PATTERNS (see vein anatomy diagram pg 145–146)
   a. Great saphenous vein – courses from medial ankle → inner thigh. May have the presence of corona phlebectasia at medial ankle.
   b. Small saphenous vein – course from lateral ankle → popliteal fossa.
   c. Lateral subdermis system – all by itself. Can do sclerotherapy here.
3. Order a VENOUS REFLUX study NOT duplex ultrasound as duplex ultrasound only reports DVT and not superficial venous reflux.
4. Treatment algorithm (top down)
   a. Truncal disease – GSV or SSV reflux: Endovenous ablation, nonthermal ablation
   b. Varicose veins – microphlebectomy, US-guided sclerotherapy
   c. Reticular veins – foam sclerotherapy
   d. Spider veins – sclerotherapy, laser therapy

Sclerotherapy

Mechanism of action	Brand name	Sclerosing agent	FDA approval	Maximum dosage	Pain	Necrosis	Pigmentation	Other
Detergent/ emulsifier	Sotradecol	Sodium tetradecyl sulfate STS1%,3%	Yes, 2004	10cc of 3% solution	Mild/ Minimal	Occasional, at conc >1%	+++	0.1–0.3% anaphylaxis
	Asclera	Polidocanol POL 0.5%, 1%	Yes, 2010	2 mg/kg 10cc of 1%	Minimal	Rare	++ at high concentrations	0.2% anaphylaxis
	Scleromate	Sodium morrhuate	Yes, 1930	10cc	Moderate	Frequent	+++	3–10% cases of anaphylaxis (highest risk)
	Etholamin	Ethanolamine oleate	Off-Label use; for esophageal varices only	10cc	Mild	Occasional	+++	Risk of RBC hemolysis and renal failure Allergic rxn
Hyperosmotic agent	Hypertonic saline	Hypertonic saline 23.4% (NaCl)	Off-label use	10–20cc	Painful, muscle cramps	Significant if extravasated	++	No allergic rxn
	Sclerodex	10% Saline + 5% dextrose	No	10–20cc	Painful	Significant if extravasated	+	Low risk of allergic rxn
Chemical irritant	Chromex Scleremo	Glycerin 72%	No	5–10 cc	Moderate	Rare	Least likely	Viscous solution, rare allergic rxn
	Varigloban, Variglobin, Sclerodine	Polyiodine iodine	No	3 cc of 6%	Painful	Occasional	++	Viscous solution, rare allergic rxn- to iodine Renal insufficiency

Source: Adapted from Sadick N and Li C. Small Vessel Sclerotherapy. *Dermatologic Clinics.* 2001;19(3): 475–481 and Duffy DM. Cutaneous Necrosis Following Sclerotherapy. *J Aesth Dermatol Cosmetic Surg.* 1999;1(2): 157–168

COSMETIC DERMATOLOGY

Use needle gauge to determine vessel size

Needle Gauge	Vessel Size
30 gauge	0.32 mm
25 gauge	0.50 mm
18 gauge	1.25 mm

Recommended sclerotherapy concentration for varying vessel sizes

Vessel size (mm)	Recommended maximum effective concentration (%)					
	Liquid sclerosant				Foam sclerosant	
	Sotradecol (STS)	Polidocanol (POL)	Hypertonic saline	Glycerin	Foam STS	Foam POL
Matting	—	—	—	40–50	—	—
<1 mm	0.1	0.25	11.7	50–72	—	—
1–2 mm	0.2	0.5	11.7–23.4	—	—	—
2–4 mm	0.2–0.5	0.5–2.0	23.4	—	0.2–0.5	0.5–1
>4 mm	0.5–1.0	2.0–5.0	—	—	0.5–1.0	0.75–2.5

Preparing dilution of sclerosants
Sodium tetradecyl sulfate/STS

Stock concentration 3% solution, 2 cc per vial

Final solution	3% STS	Normal saline	Final amount
0.1%	1 cc	29 cc	30 cc
0.2%	2 cc	28 cc	30 cc

Polidocanol/POL

Stock concentration 0.5% and 1% solution, 2 cc per vial

Final solution	1% POL	Normal saline	Final amount
0.25%	2 cc	6 cc	8 cc
0.5%	2 cc	2 cc	4 cc

STS (Sodium tetradecyl sulfate) is 2–3× stronger than POL (polidocanol)
Foam sclerosant is 2–3× stronger than liquid sclerosant

- Foam concentration is always the concentration of initial liquid sclerosant prior to mixing (i.e. STS 0.2% foam means STS 0.2% liquid × 1 cc mixed with 4 cc of air).

- Tessari method = 1 cc of liquid to 4 cc of room air.
- Can use either two-way connector or three-way stopcock.
- Can aspirate before injecting to see flashback to ensure you are in the vein.

Tips to optimize sclerotherapy results and minimize complications

- Treat an entire vein cluster – reticular veins then spider veins
  Use lowest concentration necessary
  o Spider veins: STS 0.1%; POL 0.25%
  o Reticular veins: STS 0.2% Foam; POL 0.5% Foam
- Bend needle 45°, inject very superficially and parallel to the skin "like landing a plane".
  Low injection pressure, inject slowly
  o For spider vein, should see clearance of the veins immediately.
  o For reticular veins, might be difficult, so consider aspirating to see flashback.
- Stop immediately when extravasation occurs (bleb, white blanching).

Compression
- Increase the direct apposition of the treated vein walls → enhance the effectiveness of sclerosant.
- Decrease the incidence of recanalization and coagulum formation.
- Reduce the risk of hyperpigmentation.
- 20–30 mm Hg for one to three weeks

Minimizing hyperpigmentation
- Use the lowest conc/volume
- Use compression stockings
- Extract coagulum promptly
- Ask about minocycline use

Minimizing telangiectatic matting
- Use gentle sclerotherapy – low concentration, glycerin
- Avoid treating multiple times, sometimes these will resolve
- May consider ultrasound to rule out reflux disease
- Ask about estrogen/progesterone
- Consider treatment with lasers

Minimizing skin necrosis
- Inject with low pressure
- Stop immediately if you see blanching or bleb

CEAP classification for venous disease

Clinical (C)		Etiology (E)	Anatomy (A)	Pathophysiology (P)
C0-	No visible sign	Ec- Congenital	As- Superficial	Pr- Reflux
C1-	Telangiectasia < 3 mm	Ep- Primary	Ap- Perforator	Po- Obstruction
		Es- Secondary (Post thrombotic)	Ad- Deep	Pr,o- Both
C2-	Varicose veins > 3 mm			
C3-	Edema			
C4-	a. Pigment/Eczema			
	b. LDS/ Atrophie Blanche			
C5-	Healed ulcer			
C6-	Active ulcer			

Venous clinical severity score

Attribute	Absent (0)	Mild (1)	Moderate (2)	Severe (3)
Pain	None	Occasional	Daily	Daily limiting w/meds
Varicose veins	None	Few	Confined to calf or thigh	Involves both calf and thigh
Edema	None	Limited to foot/ankle	Extends above ankle	To knee and above
Pigmentation	None	Limited to perimalleolar	Diffuse lower 1/3 calf	Above lower 1/3 calf
Inflammation	None	Limited to perimalleolar	Diffuse lower 1/3 calf	Above lower 1/3 calf
Induration	None	Limited to perimalleolar	Diffuse lower 1/3 calf	Above lower 1/3 calf
No active ulcer	None	1	2	>2
Active ulcer size (largest)	None	<2 cm diameter	2–6 cm	>6 cm
Ulcer duration (longest active)	None	<3 mo	3 mo–1 yr	>1 yr
Compression therapy	None	Intermittent	Most days	Fully compliant

Part 3
Drugs and Therapies

DRUGS AND THERAPIES

Handbook of Dermatology: A Practical Manual, Second Edition.
Margaret W. Mann and Daniel L. Popkin.
© 2020 John Wiley & Sons Ltd. Published 2020 by John Wiley & Sons Ltd.

Medication Quick Reference

Topical steroids

CLASS 1 – SUPERPOTENT

Betamethasone dipropionate*	Diprolene	O/G	0.05%	15, 50 g
Clobetasol propionate*	Clobex	L/Sp/Sh	0.05%	2, 4 oz
	Cormax	S	0.05%	25, 50 ml
	Temovate	O/Cr	0.05%	15, 30, 45 g
	Temovate	S	0.05%	25, 50 ml
	Olux	F	0.05%	100 g
	Olux E	F	0.05%	100 g
Desoximetasone	Topicort	Sp	0.25%	100 g
Diflorasone diacetate	Psorcon	O	0.05%	15, 30, 60 g
	Psorcon E	O	0.05%	15, 30, 60 g
Fluocinonide	Vanos	Cr	0.05%	30, 60, 120 g
Flurandrenolide	Cordran	Tape	0.05%	Small, large
Halobetasol propionate*	Ultravate	O/Cr	0.05%	15, 50 g

CLASS 2 – POTENT

Amcinonide*	Cyclocort	O	0.1%	30, 60 g
Betamethasone dipropionate	Diprolene AF	Cr, L	0.05%	15, 50 g
Desoximetasone*	Topicort	O/Cr	0.25%	15, 60 g
	Topicort	G	0.05%	15, 60 g
Diflorasone diacetate*	Florone	G	0.05%	15, 60 g
	Psorcon	Cr	0.05%	15 g
Fluocinonide *	Lidex	O/Cr	0.05%	15, 30, 60,
		G		120 g
Halcinonide	Halog	O/Cr	0.1%	15, 30, 60,
				240 g
Triamcinolone acetonide*	Kenalog	O	0.5%	15 g

CLASS 3 – UPPER MID-STRENGTH

Amcinonide*	Cyclocort	Cr, L	0.1%	30, 60 g
Betamethasone dipropionate	Diprosone	Cr	0.05%	15, 50 g
Betamethasone valerate	Luxiq	F	0.12%	100 g
Diflorasone diacetate	Florone, Maxiflor	Cr	0.05%	15 g
Fluticasone propionate	Cutivate	O	0.005%	15, 30, 60 g
Mometasone furoate	Elocon	O	0.1%	15, 45 g
Triamcinolone acetonide*	Kenalog	Cr	0.5%	15 g

continued p.296

---

* Available in generic.

CLASS 4 – MID-STRENGTH

Desoximetasone	Topicort LP	Cr, O	0.05%	15, 60 g
Fluocinolone acetonide	Synalar-HP	Cr	0.2%	15, 60 g
	Synalar	O	0.025%	60 g
Flurandrenolide	Cordran	O	0.05%	15, 30, 60 g
Mometasone furoate	Elocon	Cr	0.1%	15, 45 g
Triamcinolone acetonide	Kenalog	O	0.1%	15, 60, 240 g, 1 lb

CLASS 5 – LOWER MID-STRENGTH

Betamethasone dipropionate	Diprosone	L	0.05%	20, 60 g
Betamethasone valerate	Valisone	Cr/L	0.1%	15, 45 g
Clocortolone	Cloderm	Cr	0.1%	15, 45, 90 g
Fluocinolone acetonide	Capex	Sh	0.01%	120 ml
	Synalar	Cr	0.03%	15, 60 g
	Dermasmooth/FS	Oil	0.01%	4 oz
Flurandrenolide	Cordran	Cr, L	0.05%	15, 30, 60 g
Fluticasone propionate	Cutivate	Cr, L	0.05%	15, 30, 60 g
Hydrocortisone butyrate	Locoid	Cr	0.1%	15, 45 g
Hydrocortisone valerate	Westcort	Cr	0.2%	15, 45, 60 g
Prednicarbate	Dermatop	Cr	0.1%	15, 60 g
Triamcinolone acetonide	Kenalog	Cr/L	0.25%	15, 60, 80 g

CLASS 6 – LOW

Alclometasone dipropionate	Aclovate	O/Cr	0.05%	15, 45, 60 g
Betamethasone valerate	Valisone	L	0.1%	60 g
Desonide	DesOwen	Cr	0.05%	15, 60, 90 g
	Tridesilon	Cr	0.05%	5, 15, 60 g
	Desonate	G	0.05%	60 g
	Verdeso	F	0.05%	50, 100 g
Fluocinolone acetonide	Synalar	Cr/S	0.01%	15, 60 g
Triamcinolone acetonide	Aristocort	Cr/L	0.1%	15, 60, 240 g

CLASS 7 – LEAST POTENT

Topicals with hydrocortisone 0.5, 1.0, and 2.5% (Cortisporin, Hytone, U-cort, and Vytone), dexamethasone, flumethasone, methylprednisolone, and prednisolone

Cr: Cream; F: Foam; G: Gel; L: Lotion; O: Ointment; S: Solution; Sp: Spray; Sh: Shampoo.

Nonsteroidals

Crisaborole	Eucrisa	O	2%	60, 100 g
Tacrolimus	Protopic	O	0.03, 0.1%	30, 60 g
Pimecrolimus	Elidel	Cr	0.1%	15, 30, 100 g

Commonly used drugs in dermatology
Acne Vulgaris
Isotretinoin 0.5–1 mg/kg/d divided qd-bid (Goal = 120–150 mg/kg) 10, 20, 30, and 40 mg.
Acanya (BP 2.5%/Clindamycin 1.2%) G – 50 g
Akne-mycin (Erythromycin) 2% O – 25 g
Azelex 20% Cr – 30, 50 g
Benzaclin (BP 5%/Clindamycin 1%) G – 25, 50 g
Benzamycin (BP 5%/Erythromycin 3%) G – 46 g
BP 5%/Erythromycin 3% Generic G – 23, 46 g;
Cleocin T 1% S, L – 60 ml, 1% G – 30, 60 g, 1% pledgets – 60/box;
Differin/Adapelene 0.1% Cr, G – 15, 45 g; 0.3% G – 45 g; 0.1% L – 2 oz
Duac (BP 5%/Clindamyin1.2%) G – 45 g
Erythromycin 2% O – 25 g; 2% G – 27, 50 g
Epiduo 0, 1% G – 45 g
Evoclin 1% F – 50,100 g
Finacea 15% G – 30 g
Klaron (Sodium sulfacetamide 10%)L – 59 ml
Retin-A Micro 0.04%, 0.1% G – 20, 45 g; Generic 0.025%, 0.05%, 0.1% Cr – 20, 45 g; Generic 0.025%, 0.1% G – 15, 45 g
Sulfa 5%/Sodium sulfacetamide 10% L – 25 ml; Gel 15, 45 g; cream 30, 60 g;
Tazorac 0.05%, 0.1% Cr – 15, 30, 60 g
Vanoxide (BP 5%/hydrocortisone 0.05%) L – 25 g

Antibiotics – topical
Mupirocin/Bactroban/Centany bid/tid 2% Cr, O – 15, 30 g
Polysporin – (bacitracin + polymyxin) – OTC
Silvadene 1% Cr – 20, 50, 400, 1000 g

Antibiotics – systemic
Bactrim DS bid
Keflex 500 mg bid–qid; 250, 500 mg tab
Tetracycline 500 mg bid; 250, 500 mg tab
Doxycycline 100 mg bid; 50, 100 mg tab
Minocycline 100 mg bid; 50, 100 mg tab

Antibiotic preoperative prophylaxis

One hour prior to surgery
Cephalexin: 2 g × 1; 500 mg tab
Dicloxacillin: 2 g × 1; 500 mg tab

If allergic to penicillin
Azithromycin: 500 mg × 1; 500 mg tab
Clarithromycin: 500 mg × 1; 500 mg tab
Clindamycin: 600 mg × 1; 300 mg tab

If oral site
Amoxicillin 2 g × 1; 500 mg tab

If lower extremity/groin
Cephalexin 2 g × 1; 500 mg tab
Bactrim DS × 1; 1 tab
Levofloxacin 500 mg × 1; 500 mg tab

Antifungal

Ciclopirox (Penlac) 8% nail S – 6.6 ml
Diflucan/Fluconazole 150–300 mg Qwk 150 mg
Efinaconazole (Jublia) 10% nail qd × 48 wk – 4, 8 ml
Griseofulvin 20 mg/kg/d; 250, 500 mg, 125 mg/5 ml
Lamisil/Terbinafine 250 mg po qd, 250 tab; OTC 1% C, S, spray
Loprox/Ciclopirox 1% Cr, L – 15, 30, 90 g
Luliconazole (Luzu) 1% cr – 60 g
Mentax/Butenafine1% Cr – 15, 30 g
Micatin/Miconazole 2% Cr – 15, 30, 90 g
Nizoral/Ketoconazole 2% Cr – 15, 30, 60 g; 2% wash – 120 ml
Sertazconazole (Ertazco) 2% Cr – 30, 60 g
Specatazole/Econazole 1% Cr – 15, 30, 85 g
Sporanox/Itraconazole 200 mg qd or pulse dose 200 mg bid × 7 days q
    month
Tavaborole (Kerydin) 5% nail qd × 48 wk – 4, 10 ml
Thymol 4% in alcohol: 30 cc dispense with dropper.
Naftin 1% G, Cr – 15, 30, 60 g
Zeasorb – AF powder/miconazole 2%

Antiparasitics

Elimite/Permethrin – Cr 5% – 60 g
Ivermectin 0.2 mg/kg × 1; 6 mg tab

Antivirals

Abreva/Docosanol 5×/day for 5-10d OTC Cr 10% – 2 g
Acyclovir 400 mg tid × 19 days; 400 mg tab

Aldara/Imiquimod 3×/week qhs; Cr 5% – 1 box = 12 pks
Denavir/Penciclovir Q2 h × 4 days; Cr 1% – 2 g
Valtrex 2 g bid × 1 day; 500,1000 mg tab
Veregen/Sinecatechins TID × 16 weeks; O 15% – 15, 30 g
Zovirax/Acyclovir Q3 h × 5–7 days; O 5% 5×/d for 5 d – 2,10 g

Antipruritic
Capsagel, Salonpas, Zostrix/Capsaicin 0.025% Cr
Elavil/Amitriptyline 10–25mg qd for anxiety, neuropathic pain; 10, 25, 50 mg tab
Naltrexone 25–50mg qd; 25, 50 mg tab
Neurotin/Gabapentin 300mg qd, titrate up to 1200 mg tid; 10, 25, 50 mg tab
Pramosone/Pramoxine L 60, 120 ml; Cr – 30, 60g; O – 30g
Phenergan/Promethazine 12.5 mg qid or 25 mg qhs; 12.5, 25 mg tab
Sarna Lotion OTC
Sinequan/Doxepin 10–75mg qhs; 10, 25, 50 mg tab
Zofran/Ondansetron 8 mg bid; 4, 8, 24 mg tab
Zonalon/Doxepin 5% Cr – 30, 45 g

Anxiolytics/Sedation
Valium/Diazepam 2 – 10mg po, onset 15 min, long duration; 2, 5, 10 mg tab
Versed/Midazolam 0.25 – 0.5 mg/kg po, onset 10 min, short duration; 2mg/ml syrup
    IM 0.07 mg/kg, ~ 5 mg for adult, quick onset, short duration
Xanax/Alprazolam 0.5 - 4mg po, onset 30 min; 0.25, 0.5, 1 mg tab

Antihistamines
Allegra/Fexofenadine 60 mg bid or 180 mg qd; 60, 180 mg tab
Atarax/Hydroxyzine 10–50 mg q4–6 h; 10, 25 mg, 10 mg/5 ml
Clarinex/Desloratadine 5 mg qd; 5 mg tab
Claritin/Loratadine 10 mg qd; OTC 10, 5/5 ml
Doxepin 10–75 qhs; 10, 25, 50 mg tab
Perlactin/Cyproheptadine 4 mg tid; 4 mg tab
Phenergan/Promethazine 12.5 mg qid or 25 mg qhs; 12.5, 25 mg tab
Zyrtec/Cetirizine 5–10 mg; 5, 10, 5/5 ml

Bleaching agents
Azelex 20% Cr – 30, 50 g
Hydroquinone (EpiQuin Micro, Lustra, Triluma, others) bid. 4% Cr – 30, 60 g

Chemotherapy
Aldara/Imiquimod. For AK, BCC qhs × 8–12 weeks. Cr 5% – 1 box = 12 single-use 250 mg packets
Efudex/Fluorouracil. For AK qd–bid × 2–6 weeks. 5% Cr – 25 g; 2%, 5% S – 10 ml
Picato/Ingenol mebutate. For face/scalp qd x 3 d; 0.015% G. For trunk/ext qd x 2 d; 0.05% G
Solaraze/diclofenac bid × 3 months; Cr 5% – 30, 45 g

Sonidegib/Odomzo. For advanced BCC. 200 mg qd; 200 mg tab
Vismodegib/Erivedge. For advanced BCC. 150mg qd; 150 mg tab

CTCL
Bexarotene tabs 200–300 mg/m2 qd; 75 tab
Nitrogen mustard bid.10 mg% in Aquaphor 2 lb
Targretin/Bexarotene Gel qd–bid. 1% G – 60 g

Hair
Bimatoprost/Latisse 0.03% qhs – 3ml
Minoxidil/Rogaine 2%, 5% bid to scalp – 60 ml
Propecia/Finesteride 1 mg qd; 1 mg tab
Spironolactone 25–200 mg qd, start 25–50mg; 25, 50, 100 mg
Vaniqa/Eflornithine bid. Cr 13.9% – 30 g

Hyperhidrosis
Clonidine start 5 mg, titrate to effect; 5, 10, 15 mg
Ditropan/Oxybutynin start 5mg, titrate to effect; 5, 10, 15 mg
Drysol 20%/CertainDry 12.5%/Xerac-AC 6.25% qhs until effective then
    spaced out; S – 35, 37.5, 60 ml
Robinul/Glycopyrrolate start 1mg, titate to effect; 1 mg

Psoriasis
Dovonex/Calcipotriene bid. 0.005% O, Cr – 30, 60, 100 g; scalp S – 60 ml
Dermazinc with clobetasol spray. Write Dermazinc 4 oz. compound with 50
    mcg micronized clobetasol, disp. 4 oz.
Liquor Carbonis Detergens (LCD): must be compounded: TMC 0.1% oint
    compounded with 10% LCD, disp.1 lb.
Oxsoralen ultra 0.4–0.6 mg/kg 1–2 h prior to PUVA. 10 mg tab
Tazorac/Tazorotene qd. Cr 0.05%, 0.1% – 15, 30, 60 g, G 0.05%,
    0.1% – 30, 100 g

Rosacea
Azelex 20% Cr – 30, 50 g
Finacea 15% G – 30 g
Klaron (Sodium sulfacetamide 10%)L – 59 ml
Metronidazole 1% Cr – 30 g; 0.75% Cr – 30,45 g; 0.75% G – 29 g;
    0.75% L – 59 ml
Mirvaso/Brimonidine 0.33% G - 30,45 g
Rhofade/Oxymetazoline 1% Cr - 30, 60 g
Soolantra/Ivermectin 1% Cr - 30,45, 60g
Sulfa 5%/Sodium sulfacetamide 10% L – 25ml; Gel 15, 45g; cream 30, 60g;

Miscellaneous

Biotin 2.5 mg qd

Colchicine 0.3 mg, titrate to diarrhea; 0.6 mg tab

Elidel/Pimecrolimus bid; Cr 1% – 15, 30, 100 g

Folic acid 1 mg qd; 1 mg tab

Lac-hydrin (lactic acid) bid; Cr 12% – 140, 385 g; L 12% – 150, 360 ml

Niacinamide 500 mg Tid; 500 mg tab

Protopic/Tacrolimus bid; Cr 0.03, 0.1% – 30 g

Trental 400 mg Tid; 400 mg tab

Systemic Medications

Antimalarials

Drug (Brand name) Trade size	Dose	Labs to follow	Mechanism	Adverse events	Interactions	♀
Diaminodiphenyl sulfone (Dapsone) 25, 100 mg	50 mg/d then increase to 100–200 mg/d (take with food)	Baseline: CBC, **G6PD**, CMP, UA, neuro exam (check reflex) F/U: CBC qwk × 4, qmo × 6, then q6 mo; CMP, neuro exam q3–4 mo	*Antimicrobial* (antagonist of dihydropteroate synthetase → prevents formation of folic acid) and *anti-inflamm* (inhibits PMN chemotaxis, Ig binding; inhibits myeloperoxidase)	**Hemolysis** (dose-related), **methemoglobinemia** (dose- related; decreased incidence with cimetidine), **agranulocytosis** (idiosyncratic), hypersensitivity syndrome – mono-like, **neuropathy** (motor), hepatitis	Rifampin, antimalarials, sulfonamides, probenecid, folate antagonists, and TMP	C
Hydroxychloroquine (Plaquenil) 200 mg	200–400 mg/d (6.5 mg/kg/d)	Baseline: eye exam, **G6PD**, CBC; F/U: **eye exam**: q1–5 yr; CBC qmo (→ q6mos)	ALL antimalarials: Intercalate In to DNA preventing transcription; disrupt UV O2 radical formation; inhibit IL-2 synthesis; inhibit chemotaxis; reduce platelet aggregation; Inhibit endosome acidification	Blue pigment, GI upset (brand name medication with decreased GI upset), corneal deposition, hemolysis, **retinopathy (peripheral fields)**, psoriasis/ PCT flares, cardiac toxicity with overdose (2–6 g), CNS stimulant	Cimetidine, digoxin, kaolin, magnesium trisilicate; Avoid combination of chloroquine/ hydroxychloroquine	C
Chloroquine (Aralen) 250, 500 mg	250 mg/d (4.0 mg/kg/d)	Same as Plaquenil		SAME as Plaquenil PLUS bleaches hair, increased ocular risk	Smoking decreases effectiveness and worsens underlying lupus	C
Quinacrine (Atabrine) 100 mg	100 mg/d	Same as Plaquenil EXCEPT no eye exam, no G6PD		SIMILAR to Plaquenil BUT **no ocular toxicity, yellow hyperpigment,** no hemolysis	SAME as above BUT safe to use with chloroquine or hydroxychloroquine	C

Immunosuppressive agents

Drug	Dose	Labs to follow	Mechanism	Adverse events	Interactions	♀
Prednisone (1, 2.5, 5, 10, 20, 50 mg)	Variable	If long-term therapy (>3 mo of >20 mg/d):BP, PPD, DEXA-scan; supplement Ca++ (1000 mg)/ Vit D (1000 IU) and bisphosphonate	Decreases AP-1 cyclooxygenase, NF-kB. Decreases proinflammatory cytokines (esp. IL-2)	Hyperglycemia, insomnia, HTN, infection, osteoporosis, avascular necrosis, poor wound healing, peptic ulcer, water retention, adrenal insufficiency, cushingoid, glaucoma, myopathy, electrolyte imbalance (hypoK, hyperNa)	Metabolized by CYP3A4	C
Methotrexate (Rheumatrex) 2.5 mg	Begin at 5 mg up to 25 mg qwk PO/IM **dose with folate** 1 mg qd	Baseline CBC, CMP, Hep panel F/U: CBC/LFTs qwk x 4 → q3 mo; **LIVER BX**: q1–1.5 g; Grade I/ II = continue; IIIA (mild fibrosis) = continue, rebx in 6 mo; IIIB (severe)/IV (cirrhosis) = stop	Inhibits **dihydrofolate reductase;** Cell-cycle specific (**S phase**); inhibits thymidylate synthetase, methionine synthetase, and AICAR; increases local adenosine (anti-inflammatory effects related to adenosine)	**Hepatotoxic,** cancer, **BM depression,** HA, pulm fibrosis/pneumonitis, alopecia, photosensitivity, UV burn recall, GI; increases homocysteine (↑ CV risk), anaphylactoid rxn reported (test dose at 5 mg); Leucovorin rescue	EtOH, NSAIDs, TCNs, retinoids, TMP/SMX, dapsone cyclosporin, probenecid, phenytoin, dipyridamole, chloramphenicol, phenothiazines	X
Azathioprine (Imuran) 50 mg	1–3 mg/kg/d, increase by 0.5 mg/kg/d q4 wk	Baseline: CBC, LFT, **TPMT;** F/U: CBC, LFT qmo x 3 → q2 mo Consider PPD	6-Thioguanine (active metabolite via HGPRT) incorporates into DNA; inhibits de novo purine synthesis (lymphocytes)	N/V, **BM suppression,** oral ulcers, **hepatotoxicity, cancer** (lymphoma, SCC), infxn, curly hair, hypersensitivity syndrome at 14 d (fever/shock)	Allopurinol (↓ dose by 75%) warfarin, ACE-I, TMP/SMX, sulfasalazine, IUDs	D

continued p.304

DRUGS AND THERAPIES

Drug	Dose	Labs to follow	Mechanism	Adverse events	Interactions	♀
Mycophenolate mofetil (Cellcept 500 mg; Myfortic 180, 360 mg)	0.5–2 g bid (cellcept 1000 = myfortic 720)	Baseline: CBC, LFTs; F/U: CBC: qwk × 4 → qmo, LFTs qmo	Inhibits **inosine monophosphate dehydrogenase → de novo** purine biosynthesis (lymphs)	GI symptoms (Myfortic = enteric coated, less GI effects), BM depression, hepatotoxicity	Cholestyramine, iron, magnesium/ aluminum hydroxide, acyclovir	D
Tofacitinib (Xeljanz) 5, 10mg tab; 11mg XR tab	Tablets 5 mg bid; extended release 11 mg qd	Baseline: CBC; lipid panel	JAK inhibitor	URI, headache, diarrhea, and nasopharyngitis	Inhibitor of CYP3A4 and CYP inducers	C
Thalidomide (Thalidomid) 50 mg	50–300 mg qh	Baseline: hCG, neuro exam, **SNAP**; F/U: hCG qwk× 4 then q2–4 wk; neuro q3 mo; SNAP prn	Decreases TNF-α; inhibits angiogenesis; inhibits PMN phagocytosis; inhibits monocyte chemotaxis	Birth defects, sedation, constipation, peripheral **neuropathy** (sensory), and leukopenia	Sedatives, histamine, serotonin, prostaglandin	X
Cyclosporine (Neoral) 25, 100 mg	Start at 2.5 mg/ kg/d max 5 mg/kg/d (without food)	Baseline, q2 wk (→ qmo): CBC, BMP, LFTs, FLP, Mg, Uric Acid, and BP; F/U: **Creatinine Cl** q6 mo; Trough levels if >5 mg/kg/d	Binds cyclophilin → inhibits calcineurin activation of NF-AT; Inhibits IL-2, IFN-γ synthesis	**Nephrotoxic, HTN** (use CCB, no ACE/ diuretic), hyperlipidemia, infxn, cancer, HA, acne, hyperK/uricemia, hirsutism, hypoMg, paresthesias, and gingival hyperplasia	Metabolized by CYP3A4 (liver), P-gp (intestine) – Azoles, Macrole, CCB, **grapefruit juice**, MTX, SSRI, ticlopidine; additive toxicity with nephrotoxic drugs	C

Cyclophosphamide (Cytoxan) 25, 50 mg	1–3 mg/kg/d or IV pulse 1 g/m2 qmo; increase fluid intake (>3 l/day)	Baseline: CBC, CMP, and UA; F/U: CBC qwk × 8 then qmo; CMP qmo; **UA** qwk × 12 then q2–4 wk **forever**; cystoscopy: yearly or if microscopic hematuria; **urine cytology** at >50 g	**Cell cycle-independent;** Covalent DNA binding; B-cell suppression	**BM depression, hemorrhagic cystitis** (acrolein metabolite), **carcinogenesis** (esp. TCC of bladder), hepatotoxicity, reproductive toxicity, anagen effluvium, mucositis, SIADH, pneumonitis/fibrosis, infections, nail ridging, pigmented bands on teeth, and diffuse hyperpigmentation	Allopurinol, chloramphenicol, succinylcholine, digoxin, doxorubicin, barbiturates, cimetidine, halothane, and nitrous oxide	D
Apremilast* (Otezla) 10, 20, 30 mg	Titration schedule per instructions: Day 1: 10 mg qam to Day 6 and thereafter: 30 mg BID	No monitoring	PDE4 inhibitor "selective immunosuppressant"	Depression and suicidal thoughts, weight decrease	Metabolized by strong P450 inducers	C

* Available in generic.

DRUGS AND THERAPIES

305

Systemic retinoids

Drug	Dose	Labs to follow	Mechanism	Adverse events	Interactions	♀
Isotretinoin (Accutane) 10, 20, 30, 40 mg	0.5–1 mg/kg/d with food. Total dose based on body weight = 120–150 mg/kg	Baseline: hCG, LFT, and FLP; F/U: hCG, LFT, FLP q3 mo. Half Life: 10–20 h pregnancy Avoidance = 30 d	*All retinoids:* Affect cell growth/ differentiation, morphogenesis, inhibit malignant cell growth, alter cellular cohesiveness, inhibit AP-1, NF-kB, ornithine decarboxylase, TLR-2; Increase dermal collagen ↓, hyaluronic acid, elastic fibers, fibronectin, transglutaminase, and Th1 skewing	**Dryness,** myalgia/arthralgia, tendinitis, hyperostosis (long term), HA, depression, transaminase elevation, alopecia (telogen effluvium), decreased night vision, PGs, photosensitivity, staph infxns, and IBD association	Tetracyclines (risk of pseudotumor cerebri), MTX (hepatotoxicity), Vitamin A, macrolides, azoles, rifampicin, alcohol, phenytoin, mini-pill contraceptive, photosensitizers, and carbamazepine	X
Acitretin (Soriatane) 10, 25 mg	25–50 mg/d with food	Baseline: CBC, LFT, FLP, hCG, and BUN/Cr; F/U: hCG, CBC qmo; LFT, FLP q2 wk → qmo → q3 mo Half-life: 50 h pregnancy Avoidance = 3 yr	*Isotretinoin:* no specific receptor; *Acitretin:* all RAR receptor subtypes *Bexarotene:* all RXR receptor subtypes	SAME as Accutane but difference is duration of tx; **longer pregnancy avoidance** (3 yr), more alopecia, more hyperostosis. Alcohol can convert acitretin to etretinate (accumulates in fat)		X
Bexarotene (Targretin) 10, 75 mg	300 mg/m2/day with food (fatty foods improve bioavailability for retinoids)	Baseline: FLP, CBC, LFT, **TSH/T4,** and hCG; F/U: FLP qwk until stable then q1–2 mo; CBC, LFT, hCG qmo × 3–6 mo; TSH/T4 q8 wk Half-life: 7 h pregnancy Avoidance = 30 d		SAME as other retinoids PLUS more marked **hypertriglyceridemia, central hypothyroidism, leukopenia,** cataracts, and hypoglycemia	Same as above; gemfibrozil	X

Biologics

Drug	Dose	Labs to follow	Mechanism	Adverse events	Interactions	♀
Adalimumab (Humira) 40 mg/0.8 ml autoinjector pen or prefilled syringe	80 mg, then 40 mg SQ qow staring 1 wk later	Baseline: PPD and/or CXR, Tb testing f/u annually. Consider CBC, CMP, HepB, HepC, and HIV	IgG1 to TNF-α; binds **soluble and transmembrane TNF-α**	SAME as Enbrel	None	B
Anakinra (Kineret) 100 mg	RA dosing: 100 mg SQ daily Indicated for Periodic fever syndromes	Baseline: PPD and/or CXR, Tb testing f/u annually. Consider CBC, CMP, HepB, HepC, and HIV.	IL-1 receptor antagonist	SAME as Enbrel	None	B
Brodalumab (Siliq) 210 mg prefilled syringe	210 mg SQ at weeks 0, 1, 2, and q2w thereafter	Baseline: PPD and/or CXR, Tb testing f/u annually. Consider CBC, CMP, HepB, HepC, and HIV. Must enroll in SILIQ REMS Program to monitor suicidal thoughts and behavior	IgG2 selectively binds to receptor blocking IL-17A, C, E, and F	SAME as secukinumab, and counsel for suicidality	None	N/A
Dupilumab (Dupixent 300 mg prefilled syringe)	600 mg SQ followed by 300 mg qow	Consider CBC	IgG1 selectively binds to IL-4a receptor blocking IL-4 and IL-13	Injection site rxn, potential increased risk for infections, **increased conjunctivitis and keratitis**	None	N/A

continued p.308

DRUGS AND THERAPIES

307

Drug	Dose	Labs to follow	Mechanism	Adverse events	Interactions	♀
Etanercept (Enbrel) 25, 50 mg	25–50 mg SQ 2× per wk × 3 mo then 50 mg qw	Baseline: PPD and/or CXR, Tb testing f/u annually. Consider CBC, CMP, HepB, HepC, and HIV	Recombinant fusion protein Fc IgG1 to TNF receptor; binds **soluble TNF-α**	Injection site rxn, infection (**TB** reactivation), cancer, CHF, **demyelinating disease**, lupus-like syndrome, paradoxical pustular psoriasis	None	B
Guselkumab (Tremfya) 100 mg prefilled syringe	100 mg SQ at weeks 0, 4, and q8w thereafter	Baseline: PPD and/or CXR, Tb testing f/u annually. Consider CBC, CMP, HepB, HepC, and HIV	IgG1 selectively binds to IL-23 subunit (p19)	Injection site rxn, increased risk for infections, potential increased risk for cancer	None	N/A
Infliximab (Remicade)	3–10 mg/kg IV; Week 0, 2, 6 then q8 wk	Baseline: PPD and/or CXR, Tb testing f/u annually. Consider CBC, CMP, HepB, HepC, and HIV	Murine chimeric monoclonal IgG1 antibody to TNF-α; binds **soluble and transmembrane TNF-α**	SAME as Enbrel but slightly increased risk; infusion reactions	None	B
IVIg	2 g/kg over 2–5 d. Also see TEN protocol	Baseline: IgA levels (use Gammagard in IgA deficiency), BMP, and evaluate for heart failure	Immunomodulatory	Fluid overload, anaphylactic shock (in IgA deficiency), rare reports of hemolytic anemia, ARF, and aseptic meningitis	None	C
Ixekizumab (Taltz) 80 mg autoinjector or prefilled syringe	160 mg SQ at week 0; 80 mg at weeks 2, 4, 6, 8, 10, 12; 80 mg q4 wk	Baseline: PPD and/or CXR, Tb testing f/u annually.	IgG4 neutralizing IL-17A	SAME as secukinumab	CYP450 drugs and live vaccinations	N/A

Drug	Dosing	Monitoring	Mechanism	Side effects	♀
Omalizumab (Xolair) 75 mg/0.5 ml, 150 mg/ml prefilled syringe	150 or 300 mg SC q4w. Dosing in CIU is not dependent on serum IgE level or body weight	None for CIU	IgG1 to free IgE	**Anaphylaxis,** hypersensitivity reactions	None	B
Rituximab (Rituxan)	Chemo: 375 mg/m² × 4, q week. RA: 1 g × 2, qow	Baseline: CBC Follow CD19 q6–12 mo	Murine chimeric IgG1 to CD20	Infusion rxn (worst with first infusion), JC virus infx resulting in PML, severe mucocutaneous reactions	None	C
Secukinumab (Cosentyx) 150 mg autoinjector or prefilled syringe	300 mg SQ at weeks 0, 1, 2, 3, and 4, q4w thereafter	Baseline: PPD and/or CXR, Tb testing f/u annually. Consider CBC, CMP, HepB, HepC, and HIV	IgG1 selectively binds to IL-17A	Injection site rxn, increased risk for infections, potential increased risk for cancer, **caution in UC and Crohn's Dx**	None	B
Ustekinumab (Stelara) 45, 90 mg prefilled syringe	45 mg for <=100 kg, 90 mg for >100 kg SQ at weeks 0, 4, and q12w thereafter	Baseline: PPD and/or CXR, Tb testing f/u annually. Consider CBC, CMP, HepB, HepC, and HIV	IgG1κ to p40 common subunit of IL-12 and IL-23	Injection site rxn, increased risk for infections, especially fungal; potential increased risk for cancer	None	B

Nomenclature of biologics: mab (monoclonal antibody); ximab (chimeric); zumab (humanized); umab (human); cept (receptor–antibody fusion protein).

♀: Pregnancy category.

DRUGS AND THERAPIES

General Reference

Metric measurements
15 ml = 15 cc = 1 tablespoon
5 ml = 5 cc = 1 teaspoon
250 ml = 8 oz
454 g = 16 oz
30 g = 1 oz

Dose calculations
1% = 1 g/100 ml = 10 mg/cc
0.1% = 0.1 g/100 ml = 1 mg/cc

Topical medication dispensing and absorption
1 g Cream (or ~0.95 g Ointment) → covers 100 cm^2
1 Fingertip Unit (FTU) = 2 cm of cream on fingertip = 0.5 g

	1 Application (G)	bid × 1 week(G)
Adult full body	10–30	170
Head and neck	2	10
Hands and feet	2	10
Single arm	3	15
Single leg	4–6	30
Trunk	7–8	60

Percutaneous absorption by anatomic site: scrotum > cheeks > abdomen and chest > scalp and axillae > back > forearms > palms > ankles > soles.

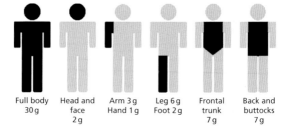

| Full body 30 g | Head and face 2 g | Arm 3 g Hand 1 g | Leg 6 g Foot 2 g | Frontal trunk 7 g | Back and buttocks 7 g |

Age	Number of FTU				
3–6 mo	1	1	1.5	1	1.5
1–2 yr	1.5	1.5	2	2	3
3–5 yr	1.5	2	2	3	3.5
6–10 yr	2	2.5	4.5	3.5	5
Adult	4	8	16	14	14

Corticosteroid Dosage Equivalence

	Equivalent dose (mg)	Glucocorticoid potency	Mineralo-corticoid potency	Duration (h) (half life)
Hydrocortisone	4	1	1	8–12
Cortisone acetate	5	0.8	0.8	8–12
Prednisone	1	3.5–5	0.8	18–36
Prednisolone	1	4	0.8	18–36
Triamcinolone	0.8	5	0	18–36
Methylprednisolone	0.8	5–7.5	0.5	18–36
Dexamethasone	0.15	25–80	0	36–54
Betamethasone	0.12–0.15	25–30	0	36–54

Acne – Topical

Antibiotics/antimicrobial

Drug name (Trade Name)* –Formulation, dosage	Trade size	♀
Benzoyl peroxide/clindamycin*		
Acanya gel (2.5% BP, 1.2% C)	50 g pump	C
Benzaclin gel (5% BP, 1% C)	25, 50 g	C
Duac gel (5% BP, 1.2% C)	45 g	C
Benzoyl peroxide 5%/erythromycin 3%*		
Generic gel	23, 46 g	C
Benzamycin	46 g, 60/box	C
Benzoyl peroxide 5%/hydrocortisone 0.05%		
Vanoxide HC Lotion	25 g	C
Clindamycin*		
Cleocin T 1% solution, lotion	60 ml	B
1% gel	30, 60 g	B
1% swabs	60/box	B
Clindagel 1% gel	7.3, 40, and 75 ml	B
ClindaReach (1% solution with applicator arm)	1 kit	B
Clindacin PAC (1% pledget and cleanser)	1 kit	B
Evoclin 1% foam	50, 100 g	B

continued p.312

*Available in generic.   ♀: Pregnancy category.

Drug name (Trade Name)* –Formulation, dosage	Trade size	♀
Erythromycin*		
Akne-Mycin 2% ointment	25 g	B
Emgel 2% gel	27, 50 g	B
Sodium sulfacetamide 10%		
Klaron lotion	59 ml	C
Sulfa 5%/sodium sulfacetamide* 10%		
Generic lotion	25 ml	C
Avar Gel; Avar Green gel	45 g	C
Clarifoam EF	60, 100 g	C
Clenia emollient cream	1 oz	C
Novacet lotion	30, 60 ml	C
Plexion TS cream	30, 90 g	C
Rosula gel	45 ml	C
Rosanil	6 oz	I
Sulfacet R lotion	25 ml	C
Sumadan (sulfur 4.5/ SS 9%)	16 oz	I
Sumaxin pads (sulfur 4%/ SS 10%)	60 pads	I
Sumaxin wash (sulfur 4%/ SS 9%)	16 oz	I
Sumaxin TS (sulfur 4%/ SS 8%)	16 oz	I

Keratolytics

Azelaic acid		
Azelex 20% cream	30, 50 g	B
Finacea 15% gel	30 g	B

Benzoyl peroxide* (BP) – Antibacterial/keratolytic for comedonal acne; may bleach clothing

Rx	Benzac AC 2.5%, 5%, 10% emollient gel	60, 90 g	C
	Benzac gel 5%, 10% gel	45 g	C
	Benzac W 5%, 10% wash	8 oz	C
	BenzaShave 5%, 10% shaving cream	4 oz	C
	BenzFoam 5.3% foam	60, 100 g	C
	Brevoxyl 4%, 8% gel, lotion/cleanser	42.5, 90 g	C
	Generic BP 2.5%, 5%, 10% gel, wash		C
	Inova Easy Pad 4%, 8%		C
	Triaz 3%, 6%, 10% gel	42.5 g	C

*Available in generic.   ♀: Pregnancy category.

OTC	Clearasil 10% cream, lotion		C
	Oxy balance 10% gel		C
	OC8 7% gel	45 g	C
	Panoxyl Bar 5%, 10% bar soap		C

Resorcinol – antimicrobial/keratolytic

OTC	Acnomel 2% Resorcinol/ 8% sulfur	28 g	

Retinoids

Adapalene* *(specific for RAR-beta and gamma)*

Differin 0.1%, 0.3% gel	45 g	C
Differin 0.1% cream	45 g	C
Differin 0.1% lotion	2 oz	C
Epiduo 0.1% (+benzoyl peroxide 2.5%) gel	45 g	C

Tretinoin* *(binds all RAR, no RXR)*

Retin-A Micro 0.04% (gray tube), 0.1% gel (purple tube)	20, 45 g	C
Generic 0.025% (gray), 0.05% (blue), 0.1% (red) cream	20, 45 g	C
Generic 0.01% (green), 0.025% (orange) gel	15, 45 g	C
Atralin 0.05% gel	45 g	C
Avita 0.025% cream, gel	20, 45 g	C
Refissa 0.05% cream	40, 60 g	C
Renova 0.02% cream	40, 60 g	C
Tretin-X 0.0375% cream, 0.01%, 0.025% gel	35 g	C
Veltin 0.025% (+ clindamycin 1.2%) gel	30, 60 g	C
Ziana 0.025% (+ clindamycin 1.2%) gel	30, 60 g	C

Tazarotene *(specific for RAR-beta and gamma)*

Avage 0.1% cream	15, 30 g	X
Fabior 1% foam	50, 100 g	X
Tazorac 0.05%, 0.1% cream	15, 30, 60 g	X
Tazorac 0.05%, 0.1% gel	30, 100 g	X

Others

Dapsone

Aczone 5% gel	30, 60 g	C
7.5% gel	30, 60, 90 g	

Spironolactone 5% Compounding pharmacy – compound with niacinamide or benzoyl peroxide

*Available in generic.

Acne – Oral

Antibiotics

Tetracycline* (Sumycin)	250, 500 mg	D
Dose: 250–500 mg po bid-qid	Susp 125/5 ml	
Do not use in age < 8 years		
Doxycycline* 50–100 mg	50, 100 mg	D
Dose: 50–100 mg po qd-bid		
Adoxa (doxycycline monohyclate)	150 mg	
Doryx (doxycycline hyclate)	75, 100 mg ER	
Monodox (doyxcycline monohyclate)	50, 75, and 100 mg	
Vibramycin (doxycycline hyclate)	100 mg	
Periostat po bid	20 mg	
Oracea po qd	40 mg	
SE: photosensitivity, dizziness, esophagitis: take w/8 oz water. Do not take w. calcium. Not for age <8 years		
Minocycline* (Dynacin, Minocin)	50, 75, 100 mg	D
Dose: 50–100 mg po qd-bid	50 mg/5 ml	
Solodyn brand qd	55, 65, 80, 105, and 115 mg ER	
Generic (Ximino) qd	45, 90, and 135 mg ER	

Dosing table

45–59 kg: 45 mg qd

60–90 kg: 90 mg qd

91–136 kg: 135 mg qd

SE: gray discoloration of skin/teeth, lupus-like syndrome, pseudotumor cerebri. Not for age <8 years

Erythromycin* (E-mycin, Erytab)	250, 333, and 500 mg	B
Dose: 250–500 mg po qid or 333 mg po tid, or 500 mg po bid	Susp 200/5, 400/5 l	
PEDs: 50 mg/kg/d divided qid		
SE: nausea, diarrhea		

*Available in generic.

Retinoids

Isotretinoin* (13-cis retinoic acid)		
Amnesteem, Sotret, and Claravis	10, 20, and 40 mg	X
Absorica (more bioavailable, can be taken without food)	10, 20, 30, and 40 mg	X

0.5–1 mg/kg/d divided qd–bid; may need 2 mg/kg/d for severe acne

✓ LABS: Baseline – 2 neg βhcg, lipids, LFTs, +/– CBC, glucose.
  Monthly – βhcg, lipids, and LFTs.

SE: dryness, teratogen, HA, arthralgias/myalgias, ↓ night vision, depression, lipid and LFT abnormalities, pseudotumor cerebri.

Elevated triglycerides- dosage related and reversible; if 300–500: low-fat diet, no alcohol; lower dose; if > 500: stop medication to prevent pancreatitis if persistent

Contraindication/Interactions: pt cannot donate blood while on treatment and for 1 mo afterwards; Tetracycline with increased risk of psuedotumor cerebri

Others

Spironolactone* (Aldactone)	25, 50, and 100 mg	X

25–200 mg qd, start 25–50 mg

Weakly antiandrogenic effects for PCOS patients

SE: hyperkalemia, gynecomastia, and hypotension. Careful with ACE inhibitors, digoxin.

Analgesics

Acetaminophen and nonsteroidal anti-inflammatory drugs are very effective and should be first-line drugs for postoperative pain (may alternate every three hours). Opioids only in rare circumstances.

Acetaminophen	500 mg po q4–6 h	500 mg	B
	Inhibits prostaglandin synthesis, COX-3 pathway		
Ibuprofen	200–800 mg po q4–6 h	200 mg	B**
	Reduce inflammation through COX-2 inhibition		

**ibuprofen is pregnancy category D in third trimester.

Opioids Dose: 1–2 tabs po q4–6 h PRN pain (in increasing strength)

Tylenol #3*	Codeine + Acetaminophen	15/300 mg (#2)	C
	Can cause constipation-Rx with Colace 100 bid	30/300 mg (#3)	
		60/300 mg (#4)	
Vicodin*	Hydrocodone + Acetaminophen	5/500 mg	C
		7.5/500 mg	
Percocet*	Oxycodone + Acetaminophen	2.5/325 mg	C
	Strong, rarely prescribed in Dermatology. Use 5/325 mg for major abd surgeries, etc.	5/325 mg	
		7.5/325 mg	

*Available in generic.

Anesthetics – topical

				B
EMLA Lidocaine 2.5% + prilocaine 2.5%			5, 30 g	

May cause prilocaine-induced methemoglobinemia in children, at large doses.

Age area	Weight (kg)	Max dose (g)	Max area (cm^2)
1–3 mo	<5	1	10
4–12 mo	5–10	2	20
1–6 yr	10–20	10	100
7–12 yr	>20	20	200

LMX 4 Lidocaine 4% cream	15,30 g	B
LMX 5 Lidocaine 5% cream	15, 30 g	B
Lida-Mantle Lidocaine 3% cream	28, 85 g	B
Lida-Mantle HC Lidocaine 3% + 0.5% HC	28, 85 g	C
Lidoderm Lidocaine 5% patch (10 × 14 cm)	Box of 6	B
Pramosone Pramoxine + 1% or 2.5% HC	60, 120 ml solution	C
– topical for itching	30, 60 g cream	
	30 g ointment	
Synera Lidocaine 3% + tetracaine 0.5% patch	10 patch/box	B
Topicaine Lidocaine 4%, 5% gel	10, 30, 113 g	B

Anesthetics – topical compounded

BLT benzocaine 20%, lidocaine 6%, tetracaine 4%
TAC tetracaine 0.5%, epinephrine 1:2000, cocaine 11.8%
LET lidocaine 4%, epinephrine 1:2000, tetracaine 0.5%
Lasergel lidocaine 10%, tetracaine 10%
23/7 lidocaine 23%, tetracaine 7%

Antibiotics

Topical/antiseptic

Mupirocin*		B
2% cream (Bactroban)	15, 30 g	
2% ointment (Bactroban)	1, 22 g	
2% ointment (Centany)	30 g	
apply bid–tid for impetigo, wound infections; for nasal MRSA eradication, use 0.5 g in each nostril bid × 5 days		

*Available in generic.

Bacitracin – Polymyxin* (Polysporin)	OTC	C
Silver sulfadiazine* (Silvadene) 1% cream	20, 50, 400, and 1000 g	B
Retapamulin (Altabax) 1% ointment bid×5 days for methicillin sensitive s. aureus or s. pyogenes	5, 10, and 15 g	B
Chlorhexidine* (Hibiclens 4% cleanser) Good antimicrobial agent for bacteria, fungus, and yeast. For MRSA eradication	120, 240, 480, 960, and 3840 ml	B
Gentamicin* (Garamycin cream/ointment 0.1%) For pseudomonas coverage (i.e. nails, wound)	15 g	D
Ciprofloxacin otic drops For pseudomonas nails, drop to nails daily	10 g	C

For pseudomonas nails (green nails)

1. Vinegar soaks – 50:50 with water
2. Clorox bleach soaks (1 tbsp in cup of water)
3. Vinegar: isoprophyl alcohol mix (50:50) drops under nail and let dry
4. Ciprofloxacin otic drops to nails
5. Oral agents

Systemic

Amoxicillin* (Amoxil) aminopenicillin 250–500 mg po tid Child: 20–40 mg/kg/d po divided tid	250, 500 mg Susp 125 mg/5 ml 250 mg/5 ml	B
Augmentin* (Amoxicillin + Clavulanic acid) 500–875 mg po bid/250–500 mg po tid Peds: 20–40 mg/kg/d divided bid/tid	250, 500, and 875 mg Susp 200 mg/5 ml 400 mg/5 ml	B
Azithromycin* (Zithromax) macrolide. B 500 mg po × 1; then 250 mg qd 5 d 500 mg po qd for 3 d	Zpak: 250 mg TriPak: 500 mg	
Cefaclor* (Ceclor) second gen. cephalosporin. 250–500 mg po tid. 250 mg/5 ml Susp 125/5, Peds: 20–40 mg/kg/d po divided tid	250, 500 mg 250 mg/5 ml	B
Cefadroxil* (Duricef) first gen cephalosporin. 1 g po qd or 500 mg po bid. Susp 250/5, Peds: 30 mg/kg/d po divided bid	500 mg, 1 g 500 mg/5 ml	B

continued p.318

*Available in generic.

Cephalexin* (Keflex) first gen cephalosporin 250–500 mg po qid Peds: 40 mg/kg/d po divided bid	250, 500 mg Susp 250 mg/5 ml	B
Ciprofloxacin* (Cipro) second gen. quinolone. 250–750 mg po bid Interactions: antacids, sucralfate, Fe, Zn, theophylline, warfarin, and cyclosporine. Prolong QT interval. Risk of tendiopathy/ tendon rupture esp in > 60 yo and concomitant corticosteroid use	250, 500, and 750 mg	C
Clarithromycin* (Biaxin) macrolide 250–500 mg po bid Peds: 7.5 mg/kg po bid	250, 500 mg Susp 125 mg/5 ml, 250 mg/5 ml	C
Clindamycin* (Cleocin) lincosamide 150–450 mg po qid Peds: 8–25 mg/kg/d divided tid–qid May cause C. difficile colitis	75, 150, and 300 mg Susp 75 mg/5 ml	B
Doxycycline* (Adoxa, Doryx, and Vibramycin) 50–100 mg po qd–bid SE: photosensitivity, dizziness, and esophagitis: take w/8 oz water. Do not take with calcium. Not for age <8 years	50, 100 mg	D
Erythromycin*– macrolide E-mycin, Erytab 250–500 mg po qid or 333 mg po tid, or 500 mg po bid Erythromycin ethyl succinate – EES,Eryped 400 mg po qid Peds: 50 mg/kg/d divided qid SE: nausea, diarrhea	 250, 333, and 500 mg 400 mg 200 mg/5 ml 400 mg/5 ml	B B B B
Levofloxacin* (Levaquin) quinolone. 500 mg po qd (need to adjust dose in renal impairment) Interactions: antacids, sucralfate, Fe, and warfarin. Prolong QT interval. Risk of tendiopathy/tendon rupture esp. in > 60yo and concomitant corticosteroid use	250, 500, and 750 mg 25 mg/ml	C
Minocycline* (Dynacin, Minocin) 50–100 mg po qd–bid. SE: blue-gray discoloration of skin/teeth, lupus-like syndrome, pseudotumor cerebri. Not for age <8 years	50 mg/5 ml 50, 75, 100 mg	D

*Available in generic.

Rifampin* 10–20 mg/kg/d, max 600 mg qd   150, 300 mg   C
   P450 drug interactions: antacids, calcium
      channel blockers, steroids, cyclosporine,
      digoxin, dapsone, quinolones, warfarin,
      and L-thyroxine.

Tetracycline* (Sumycin)   250, 500 mg   D
   250–500 mg bid–qid
   Not for age < 8 years

Trimethoprim-sulfamethoxazole* (Septra,   Sulfa (mg)/TMP (mg)   C
Bactrim)   400/80
   1 tab (double-strength) po bid   800/160 (DS)
   Peds: 0.5 mg/kg po bid;   Sus 200/40 per 5 ml
      10 kg – 1 tsp bid
      20 kg – 2 tsp bid
      30 kg – 3 tsp bid
      >40 kg – 4 tsp bid or 1 DS tab bid
   Avoid in G6PD deficiency. May interfere with
      warfarin

Antibiotic preoperative prophylaxis
See p. 135–6 for use of antibiotic prophylaxis for endocarditis indicated for
surgical procedure on infected tissue in patients with high-risk cardiac lesion.

Antibiotic postoperative skin infection
Perform wound culture and adjust antibiotics accordingly. Treat for 7–14 days.

	Medication	Spectrum of coverage
First line	Cephalexin 500 mg TID–QID	Great: gram+ (MSSA, Strep)
	or Cefadroxil 500 mg BID	+/–: gram– (E. coli, Kleb)
	(same sensitivity as cefazolin)	No: anaerobic
PCN allergic	Azithromycin 500 ×1, then 250 mg QD	Good: gram+ (MSSA, strep), anaerobic
		Limited: gram–

continued p.320

*Available in generic.

	Medication	Spectrum of coverage	
MRSA	Bactrim DS BID	First line for CA-MRSA, broad spectrum	Avoid in G6PD deficiency and coumadin
	Tetracycline 500 BID DCN or MCN 100 BID	Great: CA-MRSA, atypicals	May increase INR with coumadin
	Linezolid 600 mg BID		Reserve for highly resistant MRSA
			Very expensive
Oral	Clindamycin 300 mg QID	Great: gram+, anaerobic	Increase risk of *C. diff*
		No: gram-	
		+/−: MRSA, some resistance	
	Amoxicillin/ clavulanate 875mg BID–TID	Good: anaerobic, gram+ (MSSA, strep), gram− (*E. coli*)	
	Amoxicillin 500 BID	Great: strep, *E. coli*	
		No: *S. aureus*	
Pseudomonas/ ear	Ciprofloxacin 500mg BID	Great: gram−, Pseudomonas	Avoid with coumadin
		+/−: gram +	
		No: anaerobic	
	Levofloxacin 500mg QD	Great: gram-	Avoid with coumadin
		Good: gram+, *S. aureus*	
		+/− Pseudomonas	

Antibiotic sensitivity

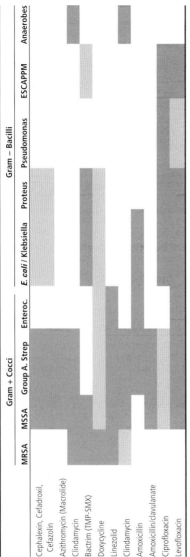

ESCAPPM = Enterobacter, Serratia, Citrobacter, Aeromonas, Proteus, Providencia, Morganella
Dark grey=strong coverage; light grey= moderate coverage; no shading = no coverage.

Antibiotic regimens

	First line	Second line
Acne, perioral dermatitis	MCN 50–100 mg qd–bid DCN 50–100 mg qd–bid TCN 500 mg bid	Erythromycin TMP-SMZ
Anthrax	Cipro 500 mg bid × 60 d Peds: 20–30 mg/kg/d divided q12 × 60 d	DCN 100 mg bid × 60 d Peds > 8 yr 2.2 mg/kg bid × 60 d
Bacillary angiomatosis	Clarithro 500 mg bid Azithromycin 250 mg qd Cipro 500–750 mg bid	Erythromycin 500 mg Qid DCN 100 mg bid
Bite: Cat *Pasteurella multocida*	Augmentin 875/125 mg bid Or 500/125 mg tid	Cefuroxime 0.5 g q12 h DCN 100 mg bid
Bite: Dog *Pasteurella multocida*	Augmentin 875/125 mg bid Or 500/125 mg tid	Clinda 300 Qid +TMP-SMX Cinda + Floroquinone
Bite: Human	Augmentin 875/125 mg bid × 5 d	If infxn: Clinda + Cipro
Bite: Spider – (Brown Recluse)	Dapsone 50 mg qd may help	
Borrelia recurrentis	Doxycycline	Erythromycin
Campylobacter jejuni	Floroquinone	Erythromycin
Cellulitis (extremity)	Nafcillin 2 g Q4 h IV Dicloxacillin 500 Q6 h Cefazolin 1 g Q8 h IV	Erythromycin, Z-Pak Augmentin 875/125 mg bid
Cellulitis (Face)	Vancomycin 1 g IV Q12h	Amoxicillin/Penicillin
Clostridium perfringens	Clindamycin + PCN G	Doxycyline
Erythrasma (*Corynebact. minutissimum*)	Erythro 250 mg Qid × 14 d	Topical agents
Kawasaki syndrome	IVIG 2 g/kg over 12 h + ASA 80–100 mg/kg/d divided in four doses then 3–5 mg/ kg/d qd × 6–8 wk	
Impetigo	Dicloxacillin 125–500 mg Qid Bactroban topically	Azithromycin, Clarithromycin Erythromycin

	First line	Second line
Lyme disease (*Borrelia burgdorferi*)	Exposure: DCN 200 mg ×1 Tx: for 14–21 d DCN 100 bid Amoxicillin 500 Tid Cefuroxime 500 bid	Erythromycin 250 Qid
Meningococcus (*N. meningitides*)	PCN G	Cefuroxime
Mycoplasma	Azithromycin Clarithromycin Erythromycin Fluoroquinone	Doxycyline
Pseudomonas aeruginosa	Cipro 500–750 mg bid	Third-generation Cephalo Imipenem, Aztreonam
Rickettsia: RMSF	DCN 100 mg bid × 7 d	Chloramphenicol 500 mg Qid × 7 d
Staphylococcus	Clindamycin TMP-SMX	Erythromycin
Staph scalded skin divided Q6 h	Nafcillin or Oxacillin 2 g IV Q4 h × 5–7 d Ped: 150 mg/kg	
Streptococcus	PCN G	Erythromycin Azithromycin Clarithromycin

Bites: need tetanus prophylaxis.
Modified from the Sanford Guide 2006.

STDs

Disease	Symptoms	First-line therapy	Second-line therapy
Gonorrhea (and treat for Chlamydia)	Male: urethritis with discharge	Cefixime 400 mg	Gatifloxacin 400 mg
	Female: endocervicits with discharge	Cipro 500 mg Ofloxacin 400 mg and Azithromycin 1 g DCN100 mg bid × 7 d	Enoxacin 400 mg Lomefloxacin 400 mg and Azithromycin 1 g DCN 100 mg bid × 7 d
Chancroid (*Haemophilus ducreyi*)	Deep ulcer, pain, 50% adenopathy	Azithromycin 1 g × 1 Ceftriazone 250 mg IM ×1	Erythromycin 500 mg Qid × 7 d Cipro 500 mg bid × 3 d
Lymphogranuloma Venereum (*Chlamydia trachomatis*)	Herpetiform vesicle, NO PAIN, +LAD/ Groove sign	DCN 100 mg bid × 21 d	Erythromycin 500 mg Qid × 21 d

continued p.324

Disease	Symptoms	First-line therapy	Second-line therapy
Granuloma Inguinale (*Klebsiella granulomatis*, formerly *Calymmatobacterium granulomatis*)	Ulcer with beefy granulation tissue, NO PAIN, NO LAD + Donovan bodies	DCN 100 mg bid × 21 d TMP-SMX DS bid × 21 d	Erythromycin Cipro
Syphilis (*Treponema pallidum*)	Indurated chancre, NO PAIN, +LAD	Benzathine PCN G** 2.4 million units IM × 1, repeat in 1 wk	DCN 100 mg bid × 14 d TCN 500 mg Qid × 14 d

**Pregnant mothers who are PCN allergic should get desensitization, then treat with PCN.

Antifungals

Topical

Classes: polyenes bind ergosterol; azoles inhibit 14-alpha demethylase; allylamines inhibit squalene epoxidase. Topical oxaborole — inhibit fungal protein synthesis by inhibiting tRNA synthetase.

Rx			
Butenafine* (Mentax) 1% cream	15, 30 g	B
Ciclopirox (Loprox) 1% cream, lotion	15, 30, 90 g	B
Ciclopirox (Loprox) 0.77% gel	30, 45, 100 g	B
Ciclopirox* (Penlac) 8% nail solution	6.6 ml	B
Econazole* (Spectazole) 1% cream	15, 30, 85 g	C
Econazole (Ecoza) 1% foam	70 g	C
Efinaconazole (Jublia) 10% solution	4 ml	C
Genadur hydrosoluble nail lacquaer	12 ml	
Iodoquinol (Alcortin A) 1% cream + 1% hydrocortinsone	48 g	C
Iodoquinol (Aloquin) 1% gel	60 g	C
Ketoconazole* (Nizoral) 2% cream	15, 30, and 60 g	C
Ketoconazole (Extina) 2% foam	50, 100 g	C
Ketoconazole* (Nizoral) 2% shampoo	120 ml	C
Ketoconazole (Xolegel) 2% gel	45 g	C
Ketoconazole (Extina) 2% foam	50, 100 g	C
Luliconazole (Luzu) 1% cream	60g	C
Miconazole* (Micatin) 2% cream, powder, spray	15, 30, and 90 g	C
Miconazole 0.25%, zinc oxide, petrolatum (Vusion)	50 g	C
Naftifine* (Naftin) 1% gel, cream	15, 30, and 60 g	B

*Available in generic.

Naftifine (Naftin) 2%	15, 30, and 60 g	B
Oxiconazole (Oxistat) 1% cream, lotion	15, 30, and 60 g	B
Selenium suilfide (TersiFoam) 2.25% foam	70 g	C
Sertazconazole (Ertazco) 2% cream	30, 60 g	C
Tavaborole (Kerydin) 5% topical solution	4, 10 ml	C
Thymol 4% in alcohol	30 ml with dropper	

OTC	**Clotrimazole** (Lotrimin, Mycelex) 1%cream, solution, and lotion	10, 15, 30, 60 g	B
	Ketoconazole (Nizoral) 1% cream, shampoo	125, 200, 251 mL	C
	Miconazole (Desenex, Lotrimin AF, Micatin, Zeasorb-AF) 2% powder	71, 100 g	C
	Miconazole (Monistat) 2% cream	100, 200 g	C
	Tolnaftate (Tinactin) cream, powder, spray	15, 30, 60 g	
	Terbinafine (Lamisil) 1% cream, solution, spray	15, 30 g	B
	Selenium sulfide (Selsun, Head and Shoulder)1%, 2.5% shampoo	100, 118, 135 g	C

Oral

Amphotericin B (Amphocin)   B
For systemic fungal infection, the dose varies
0.3–1 mg/kg/d IV, start 0.25 mg/kg/d and increase by
5–10 mg/d. Max 1.5 mg/kg/d
✓ Check renal function, Mg, K+, LFT, CBC.
Mechanism: associates with ergosterol to produce pores

Griseofulvin*   C

(Grifulvin, Grisactin, and Fulvicin U/F) *Microsize:* 500–1000 mg po qd.	250, 500 mg
(Gris-PEG, Fulvicin P/G) *Ultra micro*: 375–750 mg po qd *Peds:* 20–25 mg/kg/d divided bid, max 1 g/d x 6–8 weeks ✓ Consider check CBC every 2 wk × 1 mo, then q3 mo	125, 250 mg 125 mg/5 ml

Take with food (fatty meals increase absorption)
Do not take if pregnant, h/o hepatic failure, porphyria, lupus
May cause agranulocytosis, OCP failure, lupus,
 photosensitivity, disulfiram-like reaction
CYP3A4 inducer: decreases levels of warfarin, CSA, OCPs;
 increase effect of alcohol
Mechanism: inhibits microtubules

continued p.326

---

*Available in generic.

DRUGS AND THERAPIES

Fluconazole* (Diflucan)　50, 100, 150,　C

Onychomycosis: 150–300 mg　and 200 mg

1 dose q wk, for 3–12 mo　10 or 40

Peds: 3–6 mg/kg/d　mg/ml

Do not take: cisapride – fatal arrhythmia

Increases effects of: warfarin, CSA, phenytoin, zidovudine,
theophylline, and terfenadine
(CYP2C9 and 3A4 inhibitor)

Rifampin decreases Fluconazole levels and HCTZ increases
Fluconazole levels

Mechanism: inhibits lanosterol 14-α demethylase

Itraconazole* (Sporanox)　100 mg　c

Onychomycosis: 200 mg qd or pulse dose 200 mg bid ×　10 mg/ml
1 wk/mo

Peds: pulse dose 1 wk/mo (10–20 kg = 50 mg qd; 20–30
mg = 100 mg qd; 30–40 mg = 100/200 alternate; 40–50
kg=200 mg qd; >50 kg = 200 mg bid)

✓ Check LFTs after 4 wk.

Treat 6 wk-fingernails, 12 wk-toenails

Tinea versicolor: 200 mg × 1, repeat in 1 wk

Tinea capitis: 3–5 mg/kg/d divided qd–bid
for 1 mo

Take with orange juice/carbonated beverage

Do not take: cisapride (arrhythmia)

Contraindication ventricular dysfunction

CYP3A4 inhibitor: increases effects of: felodipine, CSA,
digoxin, warfarin, statins, and oral hypoglycemics

Mechanism: inhibits lanosterol 14-α demethylase

Ketoconazole* (Nizoral) 200 mg po qd　200 mg　C

Not usually recommended due to potential hepatotoxicity

✓ Check LFTs if long-term use, Q2 wk × 2 mo

Take with orange juice/carbonated beverage

CYP3A4 inhibitor

Do not take: cisapride, pimozide, and quinidine (arrhythmia)

Increases effects of: warfarin, CSA, phenytoin, and
theophylline

Rifampin, PPI decrease Ketoconazole levels

Mechanism: inhibits lanosterol 14-α demethylase

Nystatin* Swish and swallow 4–6 ml Qid　100 000　C

For oral candidiasis　units/ml

Mechanism: associates with ergosterol to produce pore

*Available in generic.

Terbinafine* (Lamisil)   250 mg   B

Onychomycosis: 250 mg po qd × 12 wk, or pulse dose 250
   mg bid for 1 wk/mo × 3 mo
Tinea capitis: Peds 3–6 mg/kg/d for 1 mo.
<20 kg – ¼ tab po qd; 20–40 kg – ½ tab po qd;
>40 kg – 1 tab po qd.
✓ Check LFTs baseline and q6wks.
May cause SCLE, taste or visual disturbance, headache,
   and diarrhea. Major side effects: hepatotoxicity, severe
   neutropenia, pancytopenia, and agranulocytosis.
Lowers CSA level. CYP2D6 inhibitor: increases theophylline,
   TCA, narc levels. Rifampin decreases and cimetidine/
   terfinadine increases terbinafine levels. Caution with
   hepatic or renal insufficiency.
Mechanism: inhibits squalene epoxidase

Antifungal regimens
Candidal infection
Perleche: Ketoconazole cream, Miconazole cream bid until resolve
Intertrigo: Clotrimazole cream, Miconazole cream bid until resolve then
   use Miconazole or Zeasorb AF powder to keep area dry
Oral candidiasis/Thrush: Nystatin swish and swallow qid
   Clotriamazole troche 5×/day
Chronic paronychia: Thymol solution bid
Potency against candida: ciclopirox > ketoconazole/ miconazole/
   clotrimazole/ econazole ≫ butenafine > terbenafine/naftifine

Pityrosporum folliculitis: (*P. ovale* or *P. orbiculare*)
Topical: Loprox cream, lotion; Nizoral cream, shampoo; Selenium sulfide
Oral: Nizoral 200–400 mg qd

Onychomycosis
Also need to use topical antifungal cream bid indefinitely

Topical	**Ciclopirox* (Penlac)**: Apply lacquer to affected nails qd; apply new coats on top of previous coats.	6.6 ml	B
	Thymol 4% in alcohol Drip onto and around affected nails bid	30 ml with dropper	
	Efinaconazole 10% (Jublia) apply to nail qd × 48 wk	4, 8 ml	C
	Tavaborole 5% (Kerydin) Mechanism of action: Topical oxaborole – inhibit fungal protein synthesis by inhibiting tRNA synthetase apply to nail qd × 48 wk	4, 10 ml	C

continued p.328

*Available in generic.

Oral	Treat fingernails for 6 wk, toenails for 12 wk.		
	Terbinafine (Lamisil) 250 mg po qd	250 mg	B
	✓ Labs: LFTs baseline, Q6 wk		
	On label use: QD × 6 wk for fingernails, ×12 wk for toenails		
	Off label: 250 mg QD × 1 wk for every other or third month until nail clears		
	Itraconazole (Sporanox) 200 mg po qd	100 mg	C
	Use when resistant or nonresponsive to terbinafine		
	On label: 200 mg po qd		
	Off label: pulse dose 200 mg po qd for 7 d/mo (off 21 d) for 3 mo		

Tinea versicolor (*Malassezia*)

Mild: Topical treatments
Ketoconazole (Nizoral) shampoo/ cream, Tersi Foam QD or BID × 2 wk
Clotrimazole, Econazole, etc. are also effective
Severe: Oral agents

Fluconazole (Diflucan) [150 mg]
    300 mg weekly dose for two weeks

Itraconazole (Sporanox) [100 mg]
    200 mg po qd × 5–7 days

Ketoconazole (Nizoral) [200 mg] – *no longer recommended due to potential hepatotoxic side effects*
    200 mg po qd × 5 days
Or 400 mg po × 1, 1–2 h before exercise. Let sweat dry, leave on as long as possible. Repeat in one week

Maintenance treatment with Ketoconazole (Nizoral) shampoo/ cream

Tinea capitis (almost exclusively in children)

Griseofulvin: 20 mg/kg/d divided bid × 6–8 weeks (250, 500 mg, or 125/5 ml)
Itraconazole (Sporanox): 3–5 mg/kg/d × 4–6 weeks (100 mg or 10 mg/ml)
Concomitent use of topical antifungal treatment first two weeks to decrease transmission (e.g. ketoconazole shampoo, terbinafine cream)

Tinea corporis

Rx: Spectazole, Naftin 1% bid; Naftin 2% qd; Oxistat qd; Luliconazole (Luzu) qd (one week treatment) to area until resolve
OTC: Lamisil, Lotrimin bid to area until resolve

Potency against dermatophytes: butenafine/terbenafine > ciclopriox/naftifine > clotrimazole/econazole/oxistat > ketoconazole, miconazole

Tinea pedis

Potency against *T. rubrum, T. mentagrophytes, E. Floccosum*:
Luliconazole > butenafine/terbinafine > ciclopriox/naftifine > clotrimazole/econazole/oxistat > ketoconazole, miconazole

Topical agents – usually apply for four to six weeks until resolve.

- Use weekly antifungal spray/powder in footwear (Tinactin, Micatin, and Zeasorb AF powder)
- Avoid occlusive footwear and wear cotton/wool socks to reduce moisture
- For moccasin distribution: apply to bottom and sides of feet; may need concomitant use of urea/keratolytic
- For interdigital: apply to interdigital area and soles; sometimes dermatophytes and *Candida*
- For vesiculation/maceration: antifungal + domeboro soaks

Topical	In order of potency		
	Luliconazole (Luzu)	qd × 1–2 wk	Rx
	Terbinafine (Lamisil)	bid × 4 wk	OTC
	Ciclopirox 1% cream (Loprox)	bid × 4 wk	Rx
	Naftifine (Naftin) 1%	bid × 4 wk	Rx
	Naftifine (Naftin) 2%	qd × 4 wk	Rx
	Clotrimazole 1%	bid × 2–6 wk	OTC
	Ketoconazole (Nizoral)	bid × 4 wk	OTC
	Econazole (Ecoza)	bid x 4–6 wk	Rx
	Oxiconazole (Oxistat)	qd × 4 wk	Rx
	Sertaconazole (Ertaczo)	bid × 4 wk	Rx
Oral	**Terbinafine** (Lamisil)	250 mg po qd	B
		×1 wk for interdigital	
		× 2 wk for moccasin	
	Itraconazole (Sporanox)	100–200 mg po qd	C
		×2–4 wk	

Antiparasitics

For Scabies:

Permethrin* (Elimite, Acticin) FDA approved > 2 mo   5% cream   B
    Apply from neck to soles of feet, leave on overnight   60 g
    for 8–12 h, wash off in am; repeat in 1 wk

Ivermectin (Stromectol) – not FDA approved for scabies   3 mg   C
Single dose of 0.2 mg/kg with empty stomach. In some cases, 2 doses seven days apart may be necessary.

Weight:(kg)	Dose
15–24	½ tab (3 mg)
25–35	1 tab (6 mg)
36–50	1½ tab (9 mg)
51–65	2 tab (12 mg)
66–79	2½ tab (15 mg)
≥80	0.2 mg/kg

Mechanism: blocks invertebrate glutamate-gated Cl channels, leading to paralysis and death

Precipitated sulfur   6% in petrolatum   C
    Apply to entire body below head on three successive
    nights; bathe 24 h after each application

Crotamiton (Eurax) FDA approved in adults   10% in cream/lotion   C
    Apply to entire body below head, leave on for 24 h,   60 g
    bathe, and repeat next day.

Lindane (Kwell) For scabies   1% lotion or cream   C
    Adults: apply thin layer from chin to toes; use on dry skin and shower off 10 h later;
    repeat in 1 wk
    *Second-line secondary to neurotoxicity (not for use in neonates or infants. Avoid in
    disrupted skin)*

For lice

Malathion* (Ovide) FDA approved > 6 yr   0.5% lotion   B
Apply to clean dry hair/scalp. Wash out after 8–12 h. Repeat   59 cc
in 1 wk. Use nit comb. Stinks! *(Best efficacy among
chemical pediculicides – kills lice, some nits)*

Permethrin* (Nix) FDA approved >2 mo   1% lotion   B
Apply to clean dry hair/scalp, leave on 10 min, then rinse.   60 ml
Repeat in 1 wk. Use nit comb. Do not use if allergic to
ragweed or chrysanthemum

*Available in generic.

Pyrethrin* (RID, Pronto, Butoxide, A-200) FDA approved > 2 mo		1% lotion	B
Apply to clean dry hair/scalp, leave on 10 min, then rinse. Repeat in 1 wk. Use nit comb. Do not use if allergic to ragweed or chrysanthemum		60 ml	
Benyzl alcohol (Ulesfia) FDA approved > 6 yo		5% lotion	B
Apply to clean dry hair/scalp, leave on 10 min, then rinse. Repeat in 1 wk. Use nit comb		227 g	
Ivermectin (Sklice) FDA approved > 6 mo		0.05% lotion	C
Apply to clean dry hair/scalp, leave on 10 min, then rinse.		117 g	
Spinosad (Natroba) FDA approved > 6 yo		0.09% suspension	B
Apply to clean dry hair/scalp, leave on 10 min, then rinse. Repeat in 1 wk. Use nit comb		120 cc	

Antivirals

For HSV labialis – topical agents

Acyclovir (Zovirax)	Apply ointment 5×/d for 5 d	5% cream 2, 10 g 5% ointment, 30 g	B
Acyclovir 5% + HC 1% (Xerese)	Apply cream 5×/d for 5 d	2, 5 g	B
Docosanol (Abreva)	Apply cream 5×/d for 5–10 d (efficacy same as placebo)	OTC 2 g	B
Penciclovir (Denavir)	Apply cream to lesions q2 while awake × 4 d	1% cream 1.5, 5 g	B

*Available in generic.

For HSV 1 or 2 – oral agents

	Primary	Recurrent	Suppression	Dosage	
Valacyclovir (Valtrex)	Labialis: 2 g q12 h × 1 d, OR 500 mg bid × 5 d	500 mg bid × 5 d		500 mg, 1 g	B
	Genital: 1 g bid × 10 d		<10×/yr: 500 mg qd >10×/yr: 1 g qd		
Famciclovir (Famvir)	Labialis: 500 mg tid × 5 days	125 mg bid × 5 d	250–500 mg bid	120, 250, 500 mg	B
	Genital: 250 mg tid × 7–10 d				
Acyclovir* (Zovirax)	400 mg tid × 10 d, OR 200 mg 5 ×/d ×10 d, OR 5 mg/kg/d IV q8 h	400 mg tid × 5 d, OR 800 mg bid × 5 d	400 mg bid	200, 400, and 800 mg 200 mg/5 ml 250, 500 mg IV	B
(Sitavig)	Labialis:	Apply 1 tab to canine fossa within 1 h onset of prodrome × 1 dose		50 mg Bucca tablet	B

*Available in generic.

For HSV disseminated disease

Acyclovir* (Zovirax)	5–10 mg/kg IV q8 h for 7 d if > 12 yr	200, 400, and 800 mg	B
	Neonatal: 400 mg tid during third trimester	250, 500 mg IV	

For herpes zoster/VZV

Valacyclovir (Valtrex)	1 g po tid × 7 d	500 mg, 1 g	B
Famciclovir (Famvir)	500 mg po qid × 7 d	125, 250, and 500 mg	B
Acyclovir* (Zovirax)	800 mg 5×/d × 7–10 d	200, 400, and 800 mg	B

Mechanism: These nucleoside analogs are phosphorylated by viral thymidine kinase to form a nucleoside triphosphate which then inhibits HSV DNA polymerase action.

For genital warts

Tips on counseling:

- Genital HPV is common (90% sexually active men and 80% sexually active women have at least 1 type of HPV infection). Most are asymptomatic. Very difficult to know WHEN or HOW a person becomes infected with HPV.
- Diagnosis of HPV is not indicative of sexual infidelity in the other partner.
- Women should get regular pap test.
- Pt with active genital wart should avoid sexual activity until warts are gone.
- Consider vaccine – 90% effective if given as indicated. Best if given before sexual activity.
  - Cervarix: HPV 16/18 – most common cervical cancer
  - Gardasil: HPV 16/18 and 6/11 (anogenital warts)
  - Gardasil 9: HPV 16/18; 6/11, and 31, 33,45,52,58
- Recurrence after treatment is common, especially in first 3 months

Imiquimod (Aldara)	Apply to genital warts 3× weekly at night for up to 16 wk. Wash off in 6–10 h.	5% cream 1 box = 12 or 24 pks of 250 mg each	C
Podofilox (Condylox)	Apply to genital warts bid 3 d/ wk consecutively then 4 d no treatment for 4-wk cycle	0.5% gel, 3.5 g; 0.5% soln, 3.5 ml	C
Podophyllin/ Benzoin (Podocon-25)	MD applies. Allow to air-dry before contact with clothes. Leave pt leave on for 1–6 h then wash off	25% powder, 15 ml	X
Veregen (sinecatechins)	Apply to genital warts TID for up to 16 wk (Extract from green tea leaves)	15% ointment, 15, 30 g	C

*Available in generic.

For verruca vulgaris

Compound W pad	40% Salicylic acid	OTC	/
Compound W gel	17% SA with colloidion		
Canthacur-PS	30% SA, 5% podophyllin, 1% cantharidin	MD applies	
Cidofovir	3% topical ointment bid until resolve	Compound by pharm	C
Bleomycin	Place 0.5–1 mg/ml solution onto wart, then prick it into wart with needle		
Candida antigen	Inject intradermally into wart by MD. Dilute 1:1 with 1% Lidocaine. Inject 0.1–0.2 cc per wart. Limit total to 0.3–0.5 cc. Repeat q 3 wk x 3 visit to see if respond.		
Cimetidine	30–40 mg/kg/d divided BID–TID upto 800 mg BID	300,400, and 800 mg	B
Ranitidine	150 mg BID	150, 300 mg	B
DPCP sensitization	Apply 2% DPCP to 3 warts to sensitize, then 0.01% DPCP once weekly for 2–3 wks, increase to twice weekly as tolerated		
WartPeel	Fluorouracil 2% and Salicylic acid 17%. Apply qhs, small amount to wart under occlusion.		

For molluscum

Canthacur	0.7% cantharidin. Apply by MD with toothpick
Currettage	Currette lesions in office
Cryotherapy	Brief freeze with cotton tip every 2–3 wk
TCA 70%	Drip onto molluscum lesions and let dry
Tazorac gel	Apply to areas qhs.
Veregen	Sinecatechin, off-label use for molluscum, variable efficacy
Imiquimod (Aldara)	Variable efficacy

Antihistamines

	Antihistamine effect	Anticholinergic effect	Sedative effect
Cetirizine (Zyrtec)	Strong	Weak	Some
Cyproheptadine (Periactin)	Moderate	Moderate	Mild
Desloratadine (Clarinex)	Strong	Weak	Rare
Diphenhydramine (Benadryl)	Mild	Strong	Strong
Fexofenadine (Allegra)	Strong	Weak	Rare
Hydroxyzine (Atarax, Vistaril)	Strong	Moderate	Strong

	Antihistamine effect	Anticholinergic effect	Sedative effect
Loratadine (Claritin)	Strong	Weak	Rare
Promethazine (Phenergan)	Very strong	Strong	Strong

Sedating (usually use at night)

Cyproheptadine* (Periactin)	4 mg tid; max 32 mg/d Peds (2–5 yr): 2 mg bid–tid Peds (6–12 yr): 4 mg bid–tid	4 mg Susp 2 mg/5 ml	B
Diphenhydramine* (Benadryl)	25–50 mg q6–8 h. Peds: 5 mg/kg/d divided q4–6 h	OTC 25, 50 mg 12.5 mg/5 ml	B
Hydroxyzine* (Atarax, Vistaril)	10–50 mg po q4–6 h. Peds (<6 yr): 2 mg/kg/d divided q6 h	10, 25, and 50 mg Susp 10 mg/5 ml	C
Promethazine* (Phenergan)	12.5 mg QID or 25 mg qhs	12.5, 25, and 50 mg	C

Nonsedating

Loratadine* (Claritin, Alavert)	10 mg po qd Peds (2–5 yr): 5 mg qd	OTC 10 mg Susp 5 mg/5 ml	B
Desloratadine* (Clarinex)	5 mg po qd	5 mg	C
Fexofenadine* (Allegra)	60 mg po bid or 180 mg po qd Peds (6–12 yr): 30 mg bid	30, 60, 180 mg	C
Cetirizine* (Zyrtec)	5–10 mg qh Peds (2–6 yr): 2.5 mg qh max 5 mg qd. *(may be sedating)*	5, 10 mg Susp 5 mg/5 ml	B

H2-blockers for angioedema, systemic mastocystosis

Famotidine (Pepcid)	20 mg qd–bid	20, 40 mg 40 mg/5 ml	B
Cimetidine (Tagamet)	400 mg qd–qid	300, 400, and 800 mg	B
Ranitidine (Zantac)	150 mg qd–bid	150, 300 mg 15 mg/ml	B

*Available in generic.

Antipruritic

Topical

Pramoxine (Pramosone) – topical anesthetic + 1 or 2.5% hydrocortisone	30 g O 30, 60 g C 60, 120 ml L	C
Doxepin (Zonalon) 5% Cream – Apply q 3–4 h × 1 wk max; may cause systemic effect if applied to >10% BSA	30, 45 g C	B
Capsaicin (Capsagel, Salonpas-Hot, Zostrix) 0.025% cream	OTC	/
Sarna lotion (Menthol 0.5%, Camphor 0.5%)	OTC	/
Aveeno anti-itch cream (calamine 3%, Camphor 0.47%, Pramoxine 1%)	OTC OTC	/
Calamine lotion	OTC	
Gold bond cream (Menthol 1%, Pramoxine 1%)	OTC	/
Amitriptyline 2%/ Ketamine 1%/Lidocaine 2% cream	Compounded by pharmacy Compounded by pharmacy	
(may be helpful in neurodermatitis)	Compounded by pharmacy	
Amitriptyline 2%/ Ketamine 1% in lipoderm cream	Compounded by pharmacy	
(may be helpful in neurodermatitis)		
Amitriptyline 1%/ Ketamine 0.5% cream		
(may be helpful in neurodermatitis)		
Doxepin 6-10%/ Hydrocortisone 2.5% cream		
(may be helpful in neurodermatitis)		

Oral

Doxepin (Sinequan)	10–75 mg qh Tricyclic antidepressant with high affinity for H1 receptor. Do NOT use with MAOI	10, 25, 50 mg	B
Promethazine hydrochloride (Phenergan)	12.5 mg Qid, 25 mg qh CNS depressant, antiemetic, anticholinergic, sedative antihistamine (H1)	12.5, 25, and 50 mg	C
Amitriptyline (Elavil)	10–25 mg to 150 mg qd for anxiety, neuropathic pain. TCA	10, 25, and 50 mg	D
Gabapentin (Neurotin)	Start at 300mg qd, titrate up to 1200 mg TID as tolerated. Do not discontinue abruptly but taper off gradually. For neurogenic, uremic, hematologic, and idiopathic pruritis SE:sedation, pancytopenia, cholestasis, hypersensitivity syndrome, and dyskinesia.	10, 25, and 50 mg	D

Naltrexone (RevVia, Depade)	25–50 mg qd Opioid antagonist	25, 50 mg	C
Ondansetron (Zofran)	8 mg bid Blocks serotonin 5HT3 and opioid receptors	4, 8, and 24 mg	B
Cholestyramine (Questran)	4–16 mg qd For cholestastic pruritus. Bile acid resin. Do not take other meds for 4 h	4, 378 g	B
Rifampin	300–600 mg qd (10 mg/kg/d) For pruritus from primary bilary cirrhosis. Increases metabolism/ excretion of bile acid	150, 300 mg	C
Pimozide (Orap)	Start 1 mg qd to 0.2 mg/kg/d For delusions of parasitosis Increases toxicity of MAOI, CNS depressant May cause extrapyramidal effects ✓ Check ECG – may cause long QT	1, 2 mg	C

Anxiolytics/Sedation

Always make sure patient has a designated driver and consent is obtained prior to administration.

Benzodiazepines can be used as perioperative anxiolytic and amnestic effects.

	Dosage	Onset	Duration	how supplied	Indications
Clonazepam (Klonopin)	<10 yr: 0.125–0.5 mg >10 yr: 0.25–2 mg	30–60 min	6–8 h ½ life (20–80 h)	0.5, 1 mg tab	For kids
Xanax (Alprazolam)	0.5–4 mg po	30 min, Peak 30–60 min	3–4 h ½ life (11–16 h)	0.125, 0.25, 0.5, and 1 mg oral dissolving tab 0.25, 0.5, and 1 mg	Moderate procedure
Diazepam (Valium)	2–10 mg po 2–10 mg IM	15 min, Peak 1–2 h	4–6 h ½life (>100 h)	2, 5, and 10 mg	Long procedure
	Very long duration of effect. Caution: neonates, elderly, and pts with severe hepatic dysfunction may experience ≫ duration of 50–100 h. Metabolized by P450 3A4. Contraindicated: myasthenia gravis, severe respiratory insufficiency, severe hepatic insufficiency, sleep apnea syndrome, or acute narrow- angle glaucoma				
Lorazepam (Ativan)	0.5–4 mg po 0.05 mg/kg IM (max 4 mg)	30–60 min 20–30min IM Peak 1–2 hrs	4–6 h ½life (10–20)	0.5, 1, and 2 mg 2 mg/ml	Moderate procedure

Good for longer appointments (>3 h). Contraindicated: acute narrow-angle glaucoma or severe respiratory insufficiency. No active metabolites, so less affected by age, hepatic dysfunction, or drug–drug interaction compared to diazepam.

Midazolam (Versed)	0.25–0.5 mg/kg po for kids	10–20 min		2 mg/ml	Short procedure
	0.07 mg/kg IM	<5 min IM			
		Peak 20–50 min			
	Caution: reduce dose in elderly, COPD, concomitant narcotic, or other CNS depressants; congestive heart failure or renal failure; contraindicated: narrow-angle glaucoma				
Triazolam (Halcion)	0.125–0.5 mg po	15–30 min	1.5–5 h	0.125, 0.25 mg	Short procedure
	Best for short to moderate appointments (2–4 h)				
	Caution: neonates, elderly, and pts with severe hepatic dysfunction may experience >> duration of 50–100 h. Metabolized by P450 3A4.				

Antihistamines

can be used as perioperative anxiolytic due to its sedative/ hypnotics effects.

	Dosage	Onset	Half-life	How supplied
Diphenhydramine (Benadryl)	25–50 mg po	15–60 min	2–9 h	25, 50 mg
Hydroxyzine (Atarax, Vistaril)	50–100 mg po	15–60 min	14 h	10, 25, 50, and 100 mg
Promethazine (Phenergan)	25–50 mg po	15–60 min	7–15 h	12.5, 25, 50, and 100 mg

Bleaching Agents/Depigmenting Agents

All contain hydroquinone which inhibits enzymatic oxidation of tyrosine to 3-(3,4-dihydroxyphenyl-alanine [dopa]). Some agents also contain topical steroids, retinoids, sunscreen (SS), and glycolic acid (G).

Hydroquinone* 4% cream		$30, 60	30, 60 g	C
Aclaro 4% emulsion	SS	$190	1.5 oz	C
Aclaro PD 4% bioadhesive emulsion	SS	$140	1.5 oz	C
EpiQuin Micro/Hydroquinone time release*		$40	30 g	C
Lustra 4% cream	0.3% Tretinoin	$120	56.8 g	C
Lustra AF 4% cream/ Alphaquin HP*	G, SS	$20, 40	28.4, 56.8 g	C
Melpaque HP	SS	$40	28.4 g	C
Melquin 3% topical solution		$20	30 ml	C
Melquin 4% HP cream		$30	28.4 g	C
Nuquin 4% HP gel	SS	$30	28.4 g	C
Triluma 4% cream	0.01% Fluocinolone	$190	30 g	C

Compounded HQ (adapted from Dr. Alison Tam)

Compounded HQ/Kojic acid with variable of these ingredients:

- Hydroquinone 6–12% (Fitz II: 6; Fitz III: HQ 8; Fitz IV: HQ 10; Fitz V: HQ 12)
- Kojic acid 1–6% (do NOT use if PCN/mushroom allergy)
- Vitamin C (can help for stability of compound)
- Fluocinolone 0.01% or hydrocortisone 2.5% – if PIH component
- Tretinoin 0.025–0.05%
- Glycolic acid 2–3%
- Niacinamide 5%

*Available in generic.

Bleaching cream – others

Azelex cream 20%	Bid to affected area	30, 50 g	B
Finacea gel 15%	Bid to affected area	30 g	B

Depigmenting agent

Benoquin 20% cream – final depigmentation for vitiligo	Monobenzone 20% Apply bid until effect (2–4 mo)	$50–70	35.4 g	C

Oral agent

Tranexamic Acid (Lysteda)	Half tab po BID × 3 mo, then QD × 3 mo	$50–70	650 mg	B
Off label for Melasma	May compound as 250 mg tab po BID			

Hair

Alopecia – androgenic

Finasteride (Propecia)	1 mg	X
Androgenetic alopecia in men: 1 mg po qd		
Inhibitor of type II 5a-reductase		
Minoxidil* (Rogaine)	2% women; 5% men	C
For men or women: usually use 5% solution.	60 ml	
1 ml bid to dry scalp		
Spironolactone* (Aldactone)	25, 50, and 100 mg	X
25–200 mg qd, start 25–50 mg		
Weakly antiandrogenic effects for PCOS patients		
SE: hyperkalemia, gynecomastia, and hypotension. Careful with ACE inhibitors, digoxin.		

Alopecia – areata

Anthralin ointment or cream	2% women; 5% men	C
Apply to area for 5–10 min, then wash off. Increase time to 60 min as tolerated		

continued p.342

*Available in generic.

DPCP or Squaric acid sensitization (see pg 9 gen derm)

For alopecia areata. 2 g DPCP in 100mL acetone for 2%.

Sensitize with 2%, then start treatment with 0.001% every 1–3 weekly, increase
to 0.01%, then 0.1, 0.5, 1, and 2% until irritated

Minoxidil* (Rogaine)		2% women; 5% men	C
For men or women: usually use 5% solution. 60 ml	60 ml		
1 ml bid to dry scalp			

Hypertrichosis

Eflornithine 13.9% (Vaniqa)	Apply to affected area bid	30 g	C

Hypotrichosis – eyelash

Bimatoprost 0.03% (Latisse)	Apply to upper eyelid qhs	3 ml	C

Hyperhidrosis

Aluminum Cl (Drysol 20% CertainDry 12.5% Xerac-AC 6.25%)	Apply to underarms every night was off in the AM until desired effects, then space out. If too sensitive, start off every other night. Mechanism: combines with intraductal keratin to produce a functional closure.	35, 37.5, and 60 ml	/
Glycopyrrolate (Robinul)	Start 1 mg, titrate to effect (usually 1–2 mg BID)	1 mg	B
	Antimuscarinic anticholinergic – inhibits ACh at parasympathetic sites (smooth muscle, CNS, and secretory glands). SE: anhidrosis/hyperthermia, dry mouth, blurred vision, urinary retention, constipation, and tachycardia		
Oxybutynin (Ditropan)	Start 5 mg, titrate to effect (5–7.5 mg BID)	5, 10, and 15 mg	B
	Antimuscarinic anticholinergic – see glycopyrrolate		
Clonidine	Start 5 mg, titrate to effect (5–7.5 mg BID)	5, 10, and 15 mg	B
	Antimuscarinic anticholinergic – see glycopyrrolate		
Botulinum Toxin A (Botox, Dysport, Xeomin)	25–50 units per palm, axilla, or sole q4–6 mo		C
	Blocks release of ACh via inhibiting SNAP-2		

Other treatment modalities include iontophoresis, sympathectomy, Miradry, and liposuction.

*Available in generic.

Psoriasis

Topical agents (see also topical steroids)

Dermazinc with Clobetasol spray	DermaZinc 4 oz compound with 50 mcg micronized clobetasol	4 oz	C
Clobetasol spray (Clobex)	0.05% Solution	2, 4.25 oz	C
Calcipotriene (Dovonex)	0.005% Ointment	30, 60, and 100 g	C
	0.005% Cream	30, 60, and 100 g	
	Scalp solution	60 ml	
Calcitrol (Vectical)	Ointment (3 mcg/g)	100 g	C
Tazorotene (Tazorac)	0.05%, 0.1% Cream	15, 30, and 60 g	X
	0.05%, 0.1% Gel	30, 100 g	
Betamethasone/ calcipotriene (Taclonex) (Taclonex scalp)	0.064%/0.005% ointment	60, 100 g	C
	Topical suspension	60 g	

Tar (apply in direction of hair growth)

Crude coal tar (CCT)	1–10% Compound in petrolatum base		C
Tar gel (Estar 5%, Psorigel 7.5%)	Cover with vaseline to prevent drying	90, 120 ml	C
Liquor carbonis detergens (LCD)	Triamcinolone 0.1% ointment compound with 10% LCD	1 lb	C
Tar shampoo Neutrogena T-Gel	Apply to scalp, leave for 5–10 min then rinse	OTC	C

Anthralin/dithranol (stains normal skin and clothes)

Micanol 1%	Apply to affected area, leave for 10–30 min then rinse	C
Dithro-crème 1%, 50g		
Zithranol		

Systemic agents

Methoxypsoralen (Oxsoralen Ultra)	0.4–0.6 mg/kg po 1–2 h prior to PUVA		10 mg	C
	Weight (kg)	Dose (mg)		
	<30	10		
	30–65	20		
	65–90	30		
	>90	40		

See toxic drug chart pg. 302.

Retinoids: **acitretin** (Soriatane); Biologics: **Adalimumab** (Humira), **Brodalumab** (Siliq), **etanercept** (Enbrel), **Guselkumab** (Tremfya), **infliximab** (Remicade), **Ixekizumab** (Taltz), **Secukinumab** (Cosentyx), **Ustekinumab** (Stelara).

Rosacea

Antibiotics/antimicrobial – topical

Metronidazole		
Noritate 1% cream	30 g	B
MetroCream 0.75%	30, 45 g	B
MetroGel 0.75% gel	29 g	B
MetroLotion 0.75% lotion	59 ml	B
Sodium sulfacetamide 10%		
Klaron lotion	59 ml	C
Sulfa 5%/sodium sulfacetamide* 10%		
Generic lotion	25 ml	C
Avar Gel; Avar Green gel	45 g	C
Clarifoam EF	60, 100 g	C
Clenia emollient cream	1 oz	C

Keratolytics
Azelaic acid

Azelex 20% cream	30, 50 g	B
Finacea 15% gel	30 g	B

Vasoconstrictor

Brimonidine 0.33% gel (Mirvaso)	30, 45 g	B
Alpha adrenergic agonist		
Oxymetazoline 1% cream (Rhofade)	30, 60 g	
Alpha1A adrenoceptor agonist		

Other

Ivermectin 1% cream (Soolantra)	30, 45, and 60 g	C

Antibiotics – systemic

Tetracycline* (Sumycin)	250, 500 mg	D
250–500 mg bid–qid	Susp 125/5 ml	
Do not use in age < 8 yr		
Doxycycline* 50–100 mg	50, 100 mg	D

*Available in generic.

50–100 mg qd–bid			
Adoxa (doxycycline monohyclate)	150 mg		
Doryx (doxycycline hyclate)	75, 100 mg ER		
Monodox (doyxcycline monohyclate)	50, 75, and 100 mg		
Vibramycin (doxycycline hyclate)	100 mg		
Periostat po bid	20 mg		
Oracea po qd	40 mg		

SE: photosensitivity, dizziness, and esophagitis:
take w/8 oz water. Do not take w. calcium. Not
for age <8 yr

Seborrheic Dermatitis

(see Topical Steroids, Keratolytics)

Carmol scalp treatment	Sodium sulfacetamide 10% lotion	90 ml Lotion	B
Derma-Smoothe/FS	Fluocinolone acetonide 0.1%, peanut oil, mineral oil	120 ml Oil	C
Ovace	Sodium sulfacetamide 10% wash	180, 360 ml wash	B
Nizoral	Ketoconazole 2% cream	15,30, and 60 g	C
	Ketoconazole 2% shampoo	120 ml	C
	Ketoconazole 1% shampoo	OTC	C
Selsun, Head and Shoulders	Selenium sulfide 1%, 2.5% shampoo	OTC	C

Skin Cancer – Topical and Oral Chemotherapy

Actinic keratoses (AK)

5-Fluorouracil (Efudex)	Apply qd–bid × 2–6 wk or until irritated	5% Cream 40 g	X
		2% solution 10, 25 ml	
		5% solution 10, 25 ml	
(Fluoroplex)	Apply qd–bid × 2–6 wk or until irritated	1% cream 30 g	X
(Carac)	Apply qd–bid × 2–6 wk or until irritated	0.5% cream 30 g	X
Diclofenac (Solaraze)	Apply bid × 8–12 wk	3% gel	B
	NSAID	100 g	
Ingenol mebutate (Picato)	Face and scalp: QD × 3 d	0.015% gel	C
	Trunk and extremities: QD × 2 d	0.05% gel	C
Imiquimod (Aldara)	Apply qh × 8–12 wk	5% cream	C
		1 box = 12 pks of 250 mg each	
(Zyclara)	Apply qhs × 2 wk, off 2 wk, then qhs × 2 wk	3.75% cream	

Aminolevulinic acid/ ALA – office use (see PDT protocol pg. 165)

Levulan® Kerastick® topical solution 20% – use with Blue light (Blu-U)

Ameluz®

78 mg/g nanoemulsion gel 10% – use with Red Light (BF-RhodoLED)

Basal cell carcinoma (BCC)
Topical agents – *for superficial BCC*

Imiquimod (Aldara)	Apply qh × 8–12 wk	5% Cream 1 Box = 12 pks of 250 mg each	C

Oral agent – for advanced BCC

Vismodegib (Erivedge)	1 tab po QD with or without food	150 mg	X

Hedgehog pathway inhibitor – Treatment of metastatic or locally advanced BCC

Side effects: Muscle spasm (72%); Alopecia (64%); Dysgeusia (55%); weight loss (45%); fatigue (40%); amenorrhea (30%)

Sonidegib (Odomzo)	1 tab po QD on empty stomach	200 mg	X

Monitoring: obtain creatine kinase (CK) level and real function test prior to initiation. Interrupt medication if CK > 2.5–10×, resume when CK normal. If recurrent CK >2.5× and worsening renal function, stop permanently

Hedgehog pathway inhibitor – treatment of locally advanced BCC

Side effects: Muscle spasm (54%); Alopecia (53%); Dysgeusia (46%); fatigue (41%); nauseal (39%); weight loss (30%)

CTCL
Topical agents (see also Class I topical steroids and CTCL in General Dermatology section for systemic treatments)

Bexarotene (Targretin Gel)	Apply to area qd–bid as tolerated	1% gel 60 g tube	X
Nitrogen mustard Mechlorethamine (Mustargen)	Apply to plaques of CTCL bid	10 mg% in Aquaphor. 2 lb	D

Oral agent

Bexarotene (Targretin)	200–300 mg/m2 qd with meal	75 mg	X

Other agent

Interferon α 2a (Roferon A)	6–9 million IU SC 3Xper/wk Use in combination with PUVA	3, 6, an d9 million IU prefilled syringes	C

Melanoma
Oral agent

Dabrafenib (Tafinlar) Use in combination with PUVA		50, 75 mg	D
Trametinib (Mekinist) Use in combination with PUVA		50, 75 mg	D

Vasoactive/Antiplatelet Agents

Ca+ Channel Blockers:

Nifedipine	30–180 mg qd. Start with lowest dose titrate as tolerated	10 mg	C
	biotin deficiency		
Amlodipine	5–20 mg qd. Start with lowest dose, titrate as tolerated	2.5, 5, and 10 mg	C
Pentoxifiline (Trental)	400 mg po TID (up to 800 mg TID)	400 mg	C
	Increase RBC/WBC deformability, inhibits neutrophil adhesion, reduces platelet agreegation.		
	For treatment of peripheral vascular disease, painful diabetic neuropathy, and venous ulcer		
	✓ Check serum creatinine/BUN baseline		
Stanozolol (Winstrol)	2 mg po BID–TID (up to 10 mg QD)	2 mg	x
	Anabolic steroid with fibrinolytic properties		
	For treatment of hereditary angioedema, urticarial, Raynaud's, cryofibrinogenemia, and lipodermatosclerosis		
	✓ Check BP, lipids, LFT, PSA, CBC, and creatinine		
Topical nitroglycerin	Apply 0.5 in. locally for Raynaud's. Can be titrated to 2 in. every 4–6 h with 12 h nitrate-free period	1–2%	C
	SE: headache, dizziness		

Vitamins/Nutritional Supplements

Biotin (Appearex 2.5 mg)	1 tab qd – for nails/biotin deficiency Note: biotin supplementation may interfere with certain immunoassays such as thyroid hormones tests (falsely elevated T4, T3, and cortisol).	30 tabs	/
Folic acid (Vitamin B9)	1 mg qd for MTX toxicity prophylaxis	100 tabs	A
Niacinamide (Nicotinamide) (water-soluble form of Vitamin B3; NOT niacin, no flushing)	500 mg tid in Bullous pemphigoid in combination with tetracycline 500 mg bid - May reduce in AKs and NMSC, antiaging effects	500 mg	C
Nicomide (NOT niacin)	Contains nicotinamide 750 mg + copper 1.5 mg, folic acid 0.5 mg, zinc 25 mg for acne rosacea	60 tabs	A

Wound Care

Acetic acid		35, 37.5, and 6 ml	C
Burow's solution/Domeboro Aluminum acetate	Dissolve one pack into 1 pint of water	12, 100, and 1000 tabs/box	/
Dakin's solution	0.25% Solution	480, 3840 ml	C
Sodium hypochlorite	0.5% Solution	480 ml	

Miscellaneous Meds

Colchicine	Start 0.3 mg qd – titrate to diarrhea 0.6 mg po bid–tid Prevents assembly of microtubules ✓ Check CBC, U/A, BMP q3 mo	0.6 mg	C
SSKI/Potassium **iodide** 1 drop = 47 mg KI	5–15 drops Tid Alters host immune/nonimmune response, for use in EM, E. nodosum, Sporothrichosis ✓ Check TSH, T4. Monitor for Wolff–Chaikoff effect – excess iodide can inhibit binding of iodine in the thyroid gland resulting in cessation of thyroid hormone synthesis	30, 240 ml	D

Cytochrome P-450 interactions

CYP2D6	Substrates	Amiodarone, Antipsychotics, Beta blockers, Antidepressants (TCA's, SSRIs, and Venlafaxine) Narcotics (Codeine, Tramadol)
	Inducers	**Rifampin, Dexamethasone**
	Inhibitors	Potent: Amiodarone, SSRIs, Ritonavir, antipsychotics, and Celecoxib
		H1-Antagonists: Cimetidine, Hydroxyzine
CYP3A4	Substrates	Antiarrhythmic (Amiodarone, Digoxin, and Quinidine), Anticonvulsant (Carbamazepine, Verapamil), Antidepressant (Amitriptyline, SSRI), Immunosuppressive (Steroids, Dapsone, Tacrolimus, Cyclophosphamide, and Cyclosporine) Others: Antihistamines, Benzodiazepine, CCBs, Estrogens, Erythromycin, Omeprazole, Statins, Protease inhibitors, and Theophylline
	Inducers	**Anticonvulsants (Phenobarbital, Phenytoin, and Carbamazepine)** **Anti-TB (INH, Rifampin), Glucocorticoids, St. John's Wort, Efavirenz, Nevirapine, Glitazones, and Griseofulvin**
	Inhibitors	Antibiotics (Erythromycin, Clarithromycin, and Fluoroquinolone) Azoles, CCBs, Cimetidine, Protease Inhibitors, SSRI,Grapefruit Juice
CYP1A2	Substrates	TCA's, Theophylline, Haloperidol, Propranolol, Verapamil, R-Warfarin Estradiol, Tacrine, Clozapine, Naproxen, Zileuton, and Zolmitriptan
	Inducers	**Omeprazole, Rifampin, Ritonavir** **Nafcillin, Phenobarbital, Phenytoin** **Smoking, Charbroiled meats** **Broccoli, Brussel Sprouts, and Cabbage**
	Inhibitors	Fluoroquinolones, Fluvoxamine, Paroxetine, Amiodarone, Cimetidine, Ticlopidine Grapefruit Juice
CYP2C9	Substrates	Phenytoin, S-Warfarin, NSAIDs, Sartans (Losartan), Sulfonylureas, Tricyclic antidepressants, and Valproic acid
	Inducers	**Rifampin, Secobarbital, Ethanol**
	Inhibitors	Azoles, Ritonavir, INH, TMP-SMX Statins, Fluvoxamine, Zafirlukast, and Amiodarone

Pregnancy Categories of Commonly Used Dermatologic Agents

Class B	Class C
Acyclovir	Adapalene (Differin)
Alefacept (Amevive)	Bacitracin preps (Polysporin)
Amoxicillin	Benzaclin and Benzamycin
Amphotericin topical	Benzoyl peroxide
Augmentin	Calcipotriene (Dovonex)
Azithromycin (Zithromax)	Carmol
Azelaic acid (Azelex, Finevin)	Ciprofloxacin
Butenafine (Mentax)	Clarithromycin
Cephalexin (Keflex)	Cyclosporine
Cetirizine (Zyrtec)	Desloratadine (Clarinex)
Chlorhexidine (Hibiclens)	Econazole (Spectazole)
Ciclopirox (Loprox, Penlac)	Eflornithine (Vaniqa)
Clindamycin	Fexofenadine (Allegra)
Clotrimazole topical	Fluconazole (Diflucan)
Cimetidine	Griseofulvin – po
Cyproheptadine	Hydroquinones – topical
Diclofenac (Solaraze)	Hydroxychloroquine (Plaquenil)
Diphenhydramine	Hydroxyzine
Docosanol (Abreva)	Imiquimod
Doxepin	Itraconazole (Sporanox)
Erythromycin po/ topical	Ivermectin
Etanercept (Enbrel)	Ketoconazole (Nizoral)
Famciclovir	Levofloxin
Famotidine (Pepcid)	Methoxypsoralen
Glycopyrrolate (Robinul)	Miconazole (Micatin, Zeasorb)
Imiquimod	Minoxidil
Infliximab (Remicade)	Neomycin preps (Neosporin)
Lidocaine cream (LMX)	Nystatin
Loratadine (Claritin)	Pimecrolimus
Metronidazole topical	Rifampin
Mupirocin (Bactroban)	Sertaconazole (Ertaczo)
Naftifine (Naftin)	Sirolimus (Rapamune)
Oxiconazole (Oxistat)	Sodium sulfacet/sulfur (Avar, Plexion, and Rosula)
Penciclovir topical	Sodium sulfacetamide (Klaron)
Penicillin	Steroids – systemic and topical
Permethrin (Elimite, Nix)	Sulfonamides
Silvadene	Tacrolimus – systemic and topical

Class B	Class C
Solaraze	Tretinoin (Renova)
Terbinafine – po and topical	Trimethoprim-sulfamethoxazole
Valacyclovir	
Zithromax	

Class D	Class X
Azathioprine (Imuran)	Acitretin
Doxycycline	Finasteride (Propecia), Gentamicin
Topical	Fluorouracil (Efudex, Carac)
Minocycline	Isotretinoin (Accutane, Amnesteem)
Mycophenolate mofetil (Cellcept)	Methotrexate
Nitrogen mustard	Tazarotene (Tazorac)
Tetracycline	Thalidomide

B: Generally considered safe to use. C: No evidence of harm to fetus.

D: Some significant risks. Use only if benefits outweigh risks.

X: Evidence of fetal abnormalities. Should not be used in pregnancy.

Common Dermatologic Drugs and Teratogenic Effects

	Medication	Teratogenic effects
Analgesics	Acetaminophen	Analgesic of choice, low dose not linked with identifiable risk throughout pregnancy
	NSAIDs	Caution in final trimester: fetal/neonatal hemorrhage and premature closure of ductus arteriosus
	Opioids	Respiratory depression and withdrawal symptoms
Antimicrobial	Tetracyclines	Dental staining and enamel hypoplasia (limited data for minocycline and doxycycline)
	Voriconazole	Known teratogen
	Lindane, malathion, permethrin	Although FDA category B, low risk and historically, well tolerated, precipitated sulfur is often preferred given theoretical toxicity
Miscellaneous	Prednisone	Small risk of orofacial clefts
	Lidocaine with epinephrine	No appreciable risk for small excisional biopsies

From Leachman and Reed. The use of dermatologic drugs in pregnancy and lactation. *Dermatol Clin.* 2006 24: 167–197.

DRUGS AND THERAPIES

Dermatologic Drugs Reportedly Associated with Contraceptive Failure

Medication	Contraceptive agent	Proposed mechanism
Azathioprine	Intrauterine devices	Unknown
NSAIDs	Intrauterine devices	Unknown
Griseofulvin	Oral contraceptives	Increased estrogen metabolism by hepatic microsomal enzyme induction
Rifampin	Oral contraceptives	Increased estrogen metabolism by hepatic microsomal enzyme induction or reduced enterohepatic circulation of estrogens
Tetracycline	Oral contraceptives (unlikely to play causal role in contraceptive failure)	Reduced enterohepatic circulation of estrogens
Sulfonamides	Oral contraceptives (unlikely to play causal role in contraceptive failure)	Reduced enterohepatic circulation of estrogens

Drug Eruptions

Common medications that can cause cutaneous eruptions. When these diseases start abruptly, flare, or are not controlled by conventional therapies, reevaluate diagnosis and consider complicating factors such as medication list.

Disease	Medications
Acne	Corticosteroids, oral contraceptives, androgens, ACTH, lithiu, phenytoin, halogens, isoniazid, haloperidol, radiation, and sirolimus
AGEP	Beta-lactam antibiotics (most common), macrolides, mercury (association with loxocelism), diltiazem, hydroxychloroquine, terbinafine, and imatinib
Alopecia	ACE inhibitors, allopurinol, anticoagulants, antidepressants, antiepileptics, azathioprine, bromocriptine, beta-blockers, cyclophosphamide, didanosine, ECMO, hormones, indinavir, interferons, NSAIDs, oral contraceptives, methotrexate, retinoids, and tacrolimus
Beau lines/ onychomadesis	Carbamazepine, cefaloridine, chemotherapy (taxanes), cloxacillin, dapsone, fluorine, itraconazole, lithium, metoprolol, phenophtaleine, psoralens, retinoids, radiation, sulfonamides, and tetracyclines

Disease	Medications
Bullous pemphigoid	Ampicillin, captopril, chloroquine, ciprofloxacin, enalapril, furosemide, neuroleptics, penicillamine, penicillins, phenacetin, PUVA, salicylazosulfapyridine, sulfasalazine, and terbinafine
Dermatomyositis-like	Dermatomyositis-like Hydroxyurea (most common), lovastatin, simvastatin, omeprazole, BCG vaccine, penicillamine, tegafur, and tamoxifen
Hypersensitivity/DRESS	Phenobarbital, phenytoin, carbamazepine, minocycline, sulfonamides, dapsone, allopurinol, gold, nevirapine, abacavir, and lamotrigine
Erythema nodosum	Oral contraceptives (most common), echinacea, halogens, penicillin, sulfonamides, and tetracycline
Fixed drug eruptions	Trimethoprim-sulfamethoxazole, phenolphthalein, NSAIDs, anticonvulsants, and tetracyclines
GA-like	Gold therapy, diclofenac, allopurinol, quinidine, intranasal calcitonin, and amlodipine
Hair curling/kinking	Retinoids, indinavir, antineoplastics, valproate, and azathioprine
Hair straightening	Interferon, lithium
Hypertrichosis	Acetazolamide, cyclosporin, minoxidil, phenytoin, psoralens, steroids, streptomycin, and zidovudine
Interstitial granulomatous drug reaction	Anti-hypertensives (ACE inhibitors, calcium channel blockers, and beta-blockers), antidepressants, anticonvulsants, antihistamines, and lipid-lowering agents
Leukocytoclastic vasculitis	Allopurinol, penicillins, sulfonamides, anti-TNF agents, quinolones, hydantoins, insulin, tamoxifen, OCP, phenothiazines, thiazides, retinoids, anti-influenza vaccines, interferons, and sympatomimetic illicit drugs (ANCA+ vasculitis: hydralazine, propylthiouracil, MCN, leukotriene inhibitors; Necrotizing – bortezomib)
Linear IgA dermatosis	Vancomycin, atorvastatin, captopril, carbamazepine, diclofenac, glibenclamide, lithium, phenytoin, amoidarone, and piroxicam
Lupus erythematosus, definite association	Minocycline, methyldopa, chlorpromazine, procainamide, hydralazine, quinidine, and isoniazide
Lupus erythematosus, possible association	Beta-blockers, methimazole, captopril, nitrofurantoin, carbamazepine, penicillamine, cimetidine, phenytoin, ethosuximide, propylthiouracil, sulfasalazine, levodopa, sulfonamides, lithium, and trimethadione
Lupus erythematosus, unlikely association	Allopurinol, penicillin, chlorthalidone, phenylbutazone, gold, salts, reserpine, griseofulvin, streptomycin, methysergide, and oral contraceptives
Lupus erythematosus, subacute cutaneous	Thiazides>terbinafine, verapamil, diltiazem, buproprion, enalapril, nifedipine, infliximab, etanercept, statins, interferon-alfa, leflunomide, and acebutolol

continued p.354

Disease	Medications
Melanonychia	Chemotherapy, hydroxyurea, psoralens, and zidovudine
Nail brittleness	Antiretrovirals, chemotherapy, and retinoids
Nail, decreased growth	Cyclosporin, heparin, lithium, methotrexate, and zidovudine
Nail, increased growth	Azoles, levodopa, and oral contraceptives
Nail pigmentation	Antimalarials (blue-brown), anthraline (brown-black), clofazamine (dark brown), gold (yellow), minocycline (blue-gray), tar (brown-black), and tetracyclines (yellow)
Paronychia	Antiretrovirals, cyclophosphamide, EGF receptor antagonists, fluorouracil, methotrexate, and retinoids
Pemphigus	*Thiols*: ACE inhibitors, penicillamine, gold sodium thiomalate, mercaptopropionylglycine, pyritinol, thiamazole, and thiopronine
	Nonthiols: aminophenazone, aminopyrine, azapropazone, cephalosporins, heroin, hydantoin, imiquimod, indapamide, levodopa, lysine acetylsalicylate, montelukast, oxyphenbutazone, penicillins, phenobarbital, phenylbutazone, piroxicam, progesterone, propranolol, and rifampicin
Photoonycholysis	Quinolones, tetracyclines, psoralens, quinine, captopril, chlorpromazine, thiazides, and taxanes
Photosensitivity	ACE inhibitors, amiodarone, amlodipine, celecoxib, chlorpromazine, diltiazem, furosemide, griseofulvin, lovastatin, nifedipine, phenothiazine, piroxicam, quinolones, sulfonamides, tetracycline, and thiazides
Pseudolymphoma	Phenytoin, ACE inhibitors, and penicillamine
Pseudoporphyria	Amiodarone, bumetanide, chlorthalidone, cyclosporine, dapsone, etretinate, fluorouracil, flutamide, furosemide, hydrochlorothiazide/triamterene, isotretinoin, NSAIDs, oral contraceptives, and tetracycline
Pseudotumor cerebri	Minocycline, tetracycline, doxycycline (most frequently reported tetracyclines in descending order), vitamin A analogs, corticosteroids (especially in withdrawal), nalidixic acid, sulfonamides, lithium, thyroxine, growth hormone, amiodarone, and tamoxifen
Psoriasis	Antimalarials, beta-blockers, NSAIDs, penicillin, tetracycline, ACE inhibitors, G-CSF, interferons, lithium, corticosteroid withdrawal, and anti-TNF agents
Pyogenic granulomas	Cyclosporin, EGF receptor antagonists, indinavir, and retinoid
Raynaud phenomenon	Ergot compounds (methysergide), OCPs containing estrogen and progesterone, nonselective beta-blockers (propranolol), chemotherapy, and polyvinyl chloride
Serum sickness	Antithymocyte globulin, penicillin, and vaccines (pneumococcal, rabies, and horse serum derivatives)

Disease	Medications
Serum sickness-like	Cefaclor (most common), other beta-lactams, minocycline, propranolol, streptokinase, sulfonamides, NSAIDs, rituximab, buproprion, and infliximab
SJS/TEN	Sulfonamides, antiepileptics, allopurinol, NSAIDs, and antiretrovirals
Sweet syndrome	All-*trans*-retinoic acid, celecoxib, GCSF, nitrofurantoin, oral contraceptives, tetracyclines, and trimethoprim-sulfamethoxazole
Thrombotic microangiopathy	CSA, mitomycin C, and tacrolimus
Urticaria	Opiates, ibuprofen, aspirin, polymyxin B, tartrazine, beta-lactams (immunologic), and dextran

Medications that rarely (less than 3 per 1000) cause cutaneous eruptions.
Antacids, antihistamines (oral), atropine, benzodiazepines, corticosteroids, digoxin, ferrous sulphate, insulin, laxatives, local anesthesics (other than topical), muscle relaxants, nitrates, nystatin, propranolol, spironolactone, theophylline, thyroid hormones, and vitamins.

Adapted from Knowles and Shear. Recognition and management of severe cutaneous drug reactions. *Dermatol Clin.* 2007; 25:245–253; Callen JP. Newly recognized cutaneous drug eruptions. *Dermatol Clin.* 2007; 25:255–261; Piraccini and Iorizzo, Drug reactions affecting the nail unit: diagnosis and management. *Dermatol Clin.* 2007; 25:215–221; Bolognia, Jorizzo and Rapini. *Dermatology.* St. Louis: Mosby, 2003.

Chemotherapeutic Agents and Skin Changes

Cutaneous manifestation	Chemotherapeutics
Alopecia (most common reaction to chemotherapy, usually anagen effluvium)	
Irreversible alopecia	Cyclophosphamide, busulfan
Hair texture change upon regrowth *(dry and dull)*	Doxorubicin
Hyperpigmentation	
Serpentine supravenous hyperpigmentation	Fluorouracil, fotemustine, vinorelbine, docetaxel, sometimes with combination chemotherapy
Hair color change from light to black	Cyclophosphamide

continued p.356

Cutaneous manifestation	Chemotherapeutics
Flag sign	Methotrexate
Flagellate streaks with pruritus	Bleomycin
Dusky pigmentation, similar to Addison's except no mucous membrane involvement	Busulfan – "busulfan tan"
Areas of pressure	Cisplatin
Acral	Tegafur
Occluded areas	Thiotepa, BCNU
Banded hyperpigmentation of nails	Bleomycin, cyclophosphamide, daunorubicin, doxorubicin, fluorouracil, melphalan, and vincristine
Oral hyperpigmentation: mucous membrane	Doxorubicin, fluorouracil
Oral hyperpigmentation: gingival	Cisplatin (transient lead line)
Oral hyperpigmentation: teeth	Cyclophosphamide
Yellowish discoloration	Sunitinib
Interaction with ultraviolet light	
Most phototoxic	Fluorouracil, dacarbazine, and methotrexate
Photoallergy	Flutamide, tegafur
Photo-onycholysis	Mercaptopurine, taxanes
Ultraviolet recall	Methotrexate, suranim
Reverse UV recall (reactivation of healed extravasation ulcer)	Mitomycin
Squamous cell carcinoma	Fludarabine
Inflammation of keratoses	
Actinic keratosis	Fluorouracil, doxorubicin, sorafenib, and capecitabine
Seborrheic keratosis	Cytarabine
Hypersensitivity reactions	
Type I hypersensitivity (i.e. urticaria, anaphylaxis) most common	L-asparaginase, paclitaxel, docetaxel, and mitomycin-C
Type I hypersensitivity (i.e. urticaria, anaphylaxis) severe	Methotrexate
Type IV hypersensitivity (i.e. contact dermatitis)	Mitomycin-C (groin), mechlorethamine, and carmustine
Fixed drug in patients with SLE on cyclophosphamide	Mesna
Flushing (results in skin thickening and hyperpigmentation, stop treatment)	Mithramycin, mitomycin, and plicamycin

Cutaneous manifestation	Chemotherapeutics
Nail dystrophies	
Subungal abscess	Docetaxel (subungual hemorrhage – docetaxel, sunitinib)
Nail bed changes	EGFR inhibitors (splinter hemorrhages – sunitinib, sorafenib)
Onycholysis	Bleomycin, cyclophosphamide, fluorouracil, methotrexate, mitoxantrone, doxorubicin, and paclitaxel
Leukonychia	Anthracyclines, cisplatinum, cyclophosphamide, and vincristine
Miscellaneous	
Raynaud's phenomenon (vasoconstriction)	Bleomycin, vinblastine, cisplatin, gemcitabine, and rituximab
Flushing (vasodilation)	Anthracyclines, asparaginase, bleomycin, cisplatin, dacarbazine, and taxanes
Capillary leak syndrome – edema (skin and lungs), erythema, pruritus, and vascular collapse	Taxanes, gemcitabine, IL-2, sirolimus, docetaxel, and G-CSF
Scleroderma-like reaction	Bleomycin, docetaxel, paclitaxel, melphalan, and gemcitabine
Ulcers	Hydroxyurea (leg), methotrexate, interferon, and bleomycin
Acanthosis nigricans	Diethylstilbestrol
Furunculosis	Fluoxymesterone, methotrexate
Pustular psoriasis	Aminoglutethimide
Sticky skin (acquired cutaneous adherence)	Doxorubicin, ketoconazole
Acute intermittent porphyria	Chlorambucil, cyclophosphamide
Dermatomyositis-like reaction	Hydroxyurea, tamoxifen, and tegafur
Discoid lupus	Fluorouracil, tegafur (SCLE-taxanes)
Bullous pemphigoid	Dactinomycin, methotrexate
Exacerbation of psoriasis and autoimmune disorders (also injection site reactions)	Interferons, IL-2
Sweet's syndrome	GCSF erythema
Nodosum	Azathioprine Increased
skin neoplasms	Hydroxyurea, suranim
Folliculitis	Dactinomycin
Lichen planus	Hydroxyurea, tegafur

continued p.358

Cutaneous manifestation	Chemotherapeutics
Leukoderma	Topical thiotepa
Acneiform follicular eruption	EGF receptor inhibitors (i.e. cetuximab), actinomycin D, and docetaxel
Edema (>eyes and ankles), pigmentation changes	Imatinib (edema is through PDGFR)
Conjunctivitis	Cytarabine
Excessive lacrimation	Docetaxel
Blue sclera	Mitoxantrone
Pseudolymphoma	Gemcitabine (also erysipelas-like reaction)
Baboon syndrome	Hydroxyurea (also amoxicillin, ampicillin, nickel, heparin, and mercury)
Neutrophilic eccrine hidradenitis	Cytarabine, bleomycin, GCSF
Acral erythema = hand–foot; Syndrome = Burgdorf's; Syndrome = "Palmar-plantar erythrodysesthesia"	Cytarabine, doxorubicin, fluorouracil, and sorafenib (bullous variant: cytarabine, methotrexate, tegafur [PPK])
Radiation recall	Dactinomycin, doxorubicin, docetaxel, etoposide gemcitabine, and methotrexate
Radiation enhancement	Doxorubicin, dactinomycin, and 5-bromodeoxyuridine
Extravasation	
Necrosis (vesicant)	
Rx: aspiration, cold packs, except vinca alkaloids require heat. Otherwise, specific antidotes as below	Doxorubicin, daunorubicin (large ulcerations), bleomycin, doxorubicin, vinblastine, and vincristine

Antidote to extravasation of chemotherapeutic agents

Antidote	Specific drug
Sodium thiosulfate (neutralizes vesicant)	Mechlorethamine cisplatin
Dimethlysulfoxide (free radical scavenger), dexrazoxane	Anthracyclines, mitomycin C
Vinca alkaloids	Hyaluronidase

Source: Adapted from Sanborn and Sauer. Cutaneous reaction to chemotherapy: commonly seen, less described, little understood. *Dermatol Clin.* 2008; 26:103–119; Guillot et al. Mucocutaneous adverse events of antineoplastic therapy. *Expert Opin Drug Saf.* 2004; 579–587; Bolognia, Jorizzo, and Rapini. *Dermatology.* St. Louis: 2003.

DRUGS AND THERAPIES

UV Light Treatment

UVA/UVB dosing

Skin type		UVA			UVB	
		Initial dose (J/cm²)	Increment (J/cm²)	Max	Initial dose (mJ/cm²)	Increment (mJ/cm²)
I		0.5	0.5	5	20	5
II		1.0	0.5	8	25	10
III	2.0	0.5–1.0	12	30	15	
IV	3.0	0.5–1.0	14	40	20	
V	4.0	1.0–1.5	16	50	25	
VI	5.0	1.0–1.5	20	60	30	

Classify patient with erythroderma as Type I skin.

NBUVB dosing

Skin type	Initial dose (mJ)	Increase (mJ)	Estimated goal ~4× initial dose
I	130	15	520
II	220	25	880
III	260	40	1040
IV	330	45	1320
V	350	60	1400
VI	400	65	1600
Vitiligo	170	30	Unknown

PUVA

- *Absolute contraindication*: Photosensitivity (lupus, albinism, and XP), porphyria, pregnancy, and lactation.
- *Relative contraindication*: Melanoma or family history of melanoma, personal history of non-melanoma skin cancer, prior radiation, arsenic, photosensitizing meds (simply note use then "start slow and go slow"), severe cardiac/liver/renal disease, pemphigus/pemphigoid, immunosuppression, inability to understand details of tx.
- *Photosensitizing meds*: Griseofulvin, phenothiazine, nalidixic acid, salicylanilides, sulfonamides, TCN, thiazides, MTX, and retinoids.

Choosing appropriate patients

- Usually reserved for severe disease or patients unresponsive to UVB.
- Good choice for patients whose disease will likely require maintenance (i.e. long history of severe psoriasis or CTCL).

DRUGS AND THERAPIES

- Good choice for thicker plaques, palmar/plantar disease, or erythematous/pustular disease due to deeper penetration.
- Better in darker skin (Type III or above).

General precautions
- *Eye protection*: It is absolutely necessary on day of treatment.
- *General sun protection*: Patients need to be more cautious with sun exposure to avoid risk of burning, worsening photoaging, and "hardening" their skin with natural sunlight which makes them less responsive to phototherapy.
- *Genital coverage for men*: Wear athletic support or sock over genitals. No full coverage underwear as most psoriasis and CTCL patients have involvement of their buttocks

8-METHOXYPSORALEN = Oxsoralen Ultra 10 mg caps
Dose 0.6 mg/kg
   Take 1.5–2 hours before treatment with food/milk.

Adverse events: Nausea, anorexia, dizziness, HA, malaise, and phototoxic reaction
   Nausea: decrease dose by 10 mg, take with food, rarely antiemetics.
   Treatment for nausea: Divide dose, take with food.
   PUVA burns: UVB burns present within 12–24 hours, PUVA burns are delayed 48 hours but can be as late as 96 hours. Prevent repeat burns by careful questioning of patients by phototherapy nurses, patient education, and always skipping a day between tx (i.e. MWF) to give a burn time to present itself.
   PUVA itch: It can be intractable and can last for weeks. Make sure patient's skin is hydrated and then back off on light as soon as patients complain (see below). This itch usually does NOT respond to antipruritic agents.

Long-term adverse events: Photoaging, non-melanoma skin cancer, potential for increased melanoma risk, cataracts (prevent with eye protection), and genital cancer (shield).

Clearing schedule
- Usually takes 10 treatments to tell if responsive
- If no response, increase additional 0.5 J/tx
- If after 15 treatments and no response, increase dose by 10 mg
- Correctable causes for non-response: missed tx, inadequate oxsoralen concentration in the skin (patient not pigmenting), patient not taking med, or taking medication which increases liver enzyme (i.e. carbamazepine, phenytoin)
- Takes 25–30 treatments to achieve control (three months)

Maintenance schedule

- Once clearance is achieved, maintain dose but space out visits (i.e. qwk ×4, then qow ×4, then q mo).

Missed treatment

Missed 1 tx	Hold dose as previous
Missed >1 tx	Decrease by 0.5 J for each tx missed
Missed >3 tx	May need to return to starting dose

Pruritus protocol (i.e. PUVA itch)

Mild	Use moisturizer, increase UVA by 0.5 J
Severe	Stop UVA for a few days to see if light induced. (If yes, then decrease by 2–3 J)
Intractable	Localized: shield area, keep UVA constant
	Generalized: Stop tx until clear, then resume 2–3 J below pruritic dose

Erythema protocol

None	Increase per skin type
Minimal	(Erythema occurs but resolves by next appointment)
	Hold UVA dose content, do not increase until resolve
Marked	(Erythema occurs and does not resolve by next appointment)
	Stop tx until erythema resolve
Edema	Do not treat

Toxic Epidermal Necrolysis (TEN) Protocol

Based on current published data and reviews on the treatment of TEN. 1st edition – Courtesy of Dr. Amy Cheng and Dr. Grace Bandow – Washington University Dermatology Protocol 2008

Diagnosis of TEN

History

- Prodrome of fever, cough, sore throat, and constitutional sxs may occur one to three days prior to rash.
- Burning eyes, photophobia, and burning/painful skin starts on torso/face.
- Drug exposure one to three weeks prior.

Physical exam
- Initial lesions are poorly defined macules with dusky centers/bullae with surrounding erythema, that is, two zones of color, not a classic target with three zones.
- Full-thickness necrosis leads to Nikolsky sign (lateral shearing) and wrinkled paper skin. Detachment occurs in areas of pressure (palms/soles). Denuded areas are oozing dark red.
- Mucosal involvement: urethra, GI, vulva, anus, eyes, mouth, and tracheobronchial tree.

SJS and TEN – Continuum of disease affected by epidermolysis

SJS	< 10% TBSA
SJS/TEN	10–30% TBSA
TEN	>30% TBSA

Common culprits: Sulfa, PCN, quinolones, cephalosporins, carbamazepine, phenobarbital, phenytoin, valproic acid, NSAIDs, allopurinol, lamotrigine, and HAART. Can also occur following *mycoplasma pneumonia* infection.

Genetic association
- Carbamazepine and HLA-B 15:02 in Han Chinese (FDA recommend screening)
- Carbamazepine and HLA-A 31:01 in European and Japanese
- Allopurinol and HLA-B 58:01 in Asian and European

Workup for suspected TEN
- CBC, CMP, LFTs, albumin, lytes, and baseline CXR.
- Skin biopsy from skin adjacent to blister for frozen section and H&E for full-thickness epidermal necrosis
- Skin biopsy from periblister skin for DIF – IgA to rule out drug-induced IgA bullous dermatosis.
- Do not need to culture the skin unless you think they are septic.

Triage algorithm for TEN patients

1. What is the total body surface area affected?
   - **A.** <10% TBSA (including areas of erythema) →Continue to Step 2
   - **B.** >10% TBSA →Continue to Step 4
2. Is the patient:
   - **A.** <10 year old or >50 year old →Continue to Step 4
   - **B.** Between 11 and 49 year old →Continue to Step 3

3. Does the patient have underlying medical problems?
   A. Yes (CHF, renal, pulm, diabetes, others) →Continue to Step 4
   B. No → OK To: Manage on the floor with wound care consult
   Reevaluate daily: If progresses or needs more extensive wound care, then transfer to ICU for care. Wound care alone justifies ICU transfer.
4. ICU care: (If no Burn Unit is readily available) Transfer to Unit based on underlying concerns.
   A. Significant medical comorbidities:
   - MICU
   - Wound care consult
   B. No significant medical comorbidities:
   - SICU
   - Wound care consult

Treatment for all TEN patients

1. Identify culprit drug and STOP ALL non-vital medications.
2. Transfer to specialized burn unit or ICU.
3. Consider additional dialysis if needed for patients with ESRD.
4. Consultations:
   a. Ophthalmology. 40% of TEN survivors have disabling ocular symptoms including scarring and blindness.
   b. Nutrition. Massive protein loss may require enteral or parenteral feeding.
   c. Consult additional services (pulmonary, GI, urology, and OB-GYN for mucosal involvement) prn system involvement.
5. Evaluate percentage of TBSA affected daily.
6. Evaluate mucosal involvement daily: eyes, GU, and pulmonary.
7. Wound care:
   a. Swab mouth, nose, involved orifices with saline daily. Apply mupirocin ointment. Non-sulfa antibiotic ointments and eye drops are usually recommended by ophtholmology. They should follow daily to break up synechiae.
   b. Vaseline with vaseline gauze to denuded skin (alternatives: Exudry, Telfa, or Acticoat dressings, kept wet with sterile saline). Vaseline on intact blisters. Leave necrotic intact epidermis in place. Leave normal skin alone. Do not use Silvadene! (It has a sulfa moiety.)
8. Monitor electrolytes, albumin, fluids, and replace accordingly – patients lose a lot transdermally but can get overloaded with high volume of IVIg if CHF or renal failure.
9. Warming to combat massive heat loss.
10. Avoid taping, debridement, or skin trauma.

DRUGS AND THERAPIES

11. Prophylactic antibiotics are not recommended: may cause worsening drug reactions and increase resistance.
12. Systemic treatment of TEN is controversial
    a. IVIG – Use high-dose IVIG early in the disease process in the absence of alternative evidence-based alternatives. Benefits outweight risks. Though efficacy is questionable with recent study by Lee 2013 and Firoz 2012 have not shown mortality benefits from predicted SCROTEN outcomes. (see Appendix III for IVIG dosing.)
    b. Cyclosporine – may have greater improvement in mortality compared to IVIG. Usual dose: 3 mg/kg over seven days, then taper.
    c. Prednisone- High-dose Prednisone is controversial. Questionable benefit of short course in early TEN. Most do not recommend because of increased infections and mortality in septic patients.
    d. TNF-α anatgonists – infliximab and etanercept show promising results in reducing mortality, while thalidomide is detrimental.
13. Output follow up: ophtho, GI, GYN, urology, etc. based on involvement for evaluation and tx of strictures, phimosis, synechiae, etc.

Appendix I: American Burn Assocation Burn Center Referral Criteria

1. Second- or third-degree burns >10% body surface area in patients <10 year old or >50 year old.
2. Second- and third-degree burns >20% TBSA any age group.
3. Significant burns of face, hands, feet, and genitalia.
4. Full-thickness burns that involve more than 5% of TBSA in other age groups.
5. Significant electric injury, including lightning injury.
6. Significant chemical injury.
7. Lesser burn injuries w/ associated inhalation injury, concomitant mechanical trauma or significant preexisting medical disorders.
8. Burn injury in patients who will require special social, emotional, or long-term rehab support.

Appendix II   SCORTEN Score

(Risk factors for death in both SJS and TEN)
One point for each factor:

Age > 40
Malignancy
Heart rate > 120
BUN > 10 mmol/l
Serum glucose > 250 mg/dl
Bicarb < 20 mEq/l
Initial BSA involved with epidermal detachment > 10%

Mortality rates are as follows:

SCORTEN 0–1	= 3.2%
SCORTEN 2	= 12.1%
SCORTEN 3	= 35.3%
SCORTEN 4	= 58.3%
SCORTEN >5	= 90%

Appendix III   IVIg

Avoid in patients with known IgA deficiency and anaphylaxis to previous IVIg infusions.

Need monitored bed for administration (especially if IgA levels not available, frequently test not available over the weekend at many hospitals).

Gammagard is the IgA-deficient brand that needs to be specially ordered for IgA deficient or unknown status patients.

Dose 3 g/kg/total over three to four days as tolerated (slow infusion rate if necessary for ESRD or CHF patients; some cases demonstrated benefit w/2 g or 1.5 g)

Write orders to dose the infusion rate at

> 30 cc per hour × 1 h
> 60 cc per hour × 2 h
> 120 cc per hour after that
> For example 70 kg patient would get 70 g/d × 3 d
> 70 g is about 1600 cc of Gammar P. This would take ~12.5 h to infuse.

Appendix IV   Further Reading for TEN/SJS

1. Magina, S., Lisboa, C., Leal, V. et al. (2003). Dermatological and ophthalmological sequels in toxic epidermal necrolysis. *Dermatology* 207: 33–36.
2. Freedberg IM, Eisen A *et al. Fitzpatrick's Dermatology in General Medicine.* 2003.
3. Bologna, J.L. (2003). Jorizzo JL *et al.* In: *Dermatology.*
4. Townsend C, Evers MB. *Sabiston Textbook of Surgery.* 2004.
5. Lissia, M., Figus, A., and Rubino, C. (2005). Intravenous immunoglobulins and plasmapheresis combined treatment in patients with severe toxic epidermal necrolysis: preliminary report. *Br J Plast Surg.* 58: 504–510.
6. Tan, A.W., Thong, B.Y. et al. (2005). High-dose immunoglobulins in the treatment to toxic epidermal necrolysis: an Asian series. *J Dermatol.* 32: 1–6.
7. Nassif, A., Moslehi, H. et al. (2004). Evaluation of the potential role of cytokines in toxic epidermal necrolysis. *J Invest Dermatol.* 123: 850–855.
8. Chave, T.A., Mortimer, M.J., Sladden, M.J. et al. (2005). Toxic epidermal necrolysis: current evidence, practical management and future directions. *Brit J Dermatol.* 153: 241–245.
9. Huang, Y.C., Li, Y.C., and Chen, T.J. (2012). The efficacy of intravenous immunoglobulin for the treatment of toxic epidermal necrolysis: a systematic review and meta-anlaysis. *Br. J. Dermatol.* 167: 424–432.
10. Firoz, B.F., Henning, J.S., Zarzabal, L.A., and Pollock, B.H. (2012). Toxic epidermal necrolysis: five years of treatment experience from a burn unit. *J Am Acad Dermatol.* 67: 630–635.
11. Lee, H.Y., Lim, Y.L., Thirumoorthy, T., and Pang, S.M. (2013). The role of intravenous immunoglobulin in toxic epidermal necrolysis: A retrospective analysis of 64 patients managed in a specialised centre. *Br J Dermatol.* 169: 1304–1309.
12. Enk, A.H., Hadaschik, E.N., and Eming, R. (2016). European Guidelines (S1) on the use of high-dose intravenous immunoglobulin in dermatology. *JEAVD* 30: 1657–1669.
13. Kirchhof, M., Miliszewski, M., Sikora, S. et al. (2014). Retrospective review of Stevens–Johnson syndrome/toxic epidermal necrolysis treatment comparing intravenous immunoglobulin with cyclosporine. *J Am Acad Dermatol.* 71: 941–947.
14. Valeyrie-Allanore, L., Wolkenstein, P., Brochard, L. et al. (2012). Open trial of ciclosporin treatment for Stevens Johnson syndrome and toxic epidermal necrolysis. *Br J Dermatol.* 163: 847–853.

DRUGS AND THERAPIES

Index

Handbook of Dermatology: A Practical Manual, Second Edition.
Margaret W. Mann and Daniel L. Popkin.
© 2020 John Wiley & Sons Ltd. Published 2020 by John Wiley & Sons Ltd.